BIOIDENTICAL HORMONES 101,

MADE EXCEEDINGLY SIMPLE BY JEFFREY DACH MD

www.bioidenticalhormones101.com

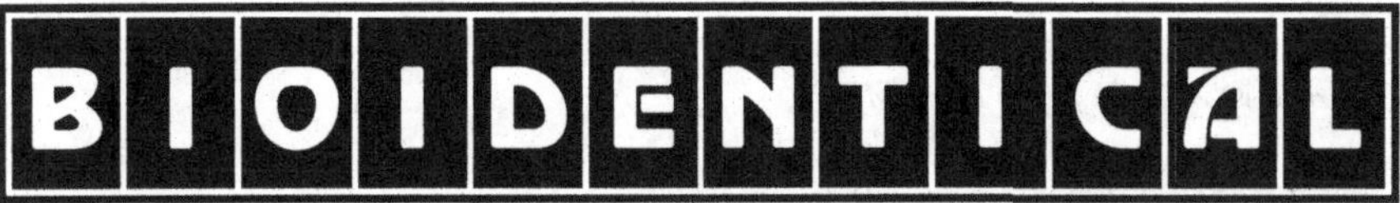

HORMONES 101

MADE EXCEEDINGLY SIMPLE BY
JEFFREY DACH MD

Bioidentical Hormones, Natural Thyroid, and Natural Medicine

www.bioidenticalhormones101.com

iUniverse, Inc.
Bloomington

BIOIDENTICAL HORMONES 101
BIOIDENTICAL HORMONES, NATURAL THYROID, AND NATURAL MEDICINE

www.bioidenticalhormones101.com

The information, ideas, and suggestions in this book are not intended as a substitute for professional medical advice. Before following any suggestions contained in this book, you should consult your personal physician. Neither the author nor the publisher shall be liable or responsible for any loss or damage allegedly arising as a consequence of your use or application of any information or suggestions in this book.

iUniverse books may be ordered through booksellers or by contacting:

iUniverse
1663 Liberty Drive
Bloomington, IN 47403
www.iuniverse.com
1-800-Authors (1-800-288-4677)

ISBN: 978-1-4620-3499-4 (sc)
ISBN: 978-1-4620-3655-4 (hc)
ISBN: 978-1-4620-3654-7 (ebk)

Printed in the United States of America

iUniverse rev. date: 08/18/2011

TABLE OF CONTENTS

Section Five:
Screening Mammography, and Breast Cancer

Section Six:
Low Testosterone Diagnosis and Treatment

Section Seven:
Testosterone and PSA Screening for Prostate Cancer

Section Eight: Selenium, Why We Need It.

Section Nine: Your Drug May Be The Problem. Are You Taking A Bad Drug?

Section Ten: Preventing and Reversing Heart Disease

Section Eleven: Vitamins B5, B6, E and Wheatgrass

Section Twelve:
Is Your Food Making You Sick?

Section Thirteen:
Mind Body Connection and Spirituality

Section Fourteen:
The Future of Medicine

ACKNOWLEDGEMENTS

First of all, I wish to thank my wife, Judith, who is the light of my life, and whose help this book would not have been possible. This book is dedicated to my children, Ari, Benjamin and Karina who are all grown up and no longer children, so they know how much work goes into this.

I wish to thank all the people who have influenced the book, my friends, colleagues, mentors:

Burton Berkson MD, Kenton Bruice MD, John Crisler, DO, David Brownstein MD, Mayer Eisenstein MD, George Flechas MD, Larry Frieders, Nicholas Gonzalez MD, Kent Holtorf MD, Ron Hoffman MD, Steven Hotze MD, Russell Jaffe MD, Joel Kauffman PhD, Bruice Kenton MD, Joseph McWherter MD, Sangeeta Pati MD, David Perlmutter MD, C.W. Randolph MD, Uzzi Reiss MD, James C Roberts MD, Ron Rothenberg MD, Erika Schwartz MD, Steven Sinatra MD, Michael Schachter MD, Frank Shallenberger MD, Eugene Shipman MD, Jacob Teitelbaum MD, Sherry TenPenny MD, Julian Whitaker MD, and Jonathan Wright MD.

Special recognition and acknowledgement goes to Jonathan Wright MD, who deserves credit as the inventor and first pioneer of bioidentical hormones, also known as Bi-Est and Tri-Est. Dr Wright's monthly newsletter is strongly recommended to the reader as a source of invaluable information, much of it original, about natural medicine and bioidentical hormones.

Additional acknowledgement goes to Suzanne Somers and Oprah Winfrey for their insight and courage to step forward into the public spotlight with the bioidentical hormone story.

Also, this book is dedicated to the memories of these great medical pioneers: Broda Barnes MD, Bernard Bihari MD, Robert Crayhon, Abram Hoffer MD, John R Lee MD, Sheri Lieberman, William McK Jefferies MD, and Linus Pauling PhD.

Also thanks and acknowledgement goes to the many people on the internet on blogs, message boards, groups, and with emails that have interacted, communicated, shared knowledge and influenced this book. Medical education is an ongoing process that starts with medical school and never stops. My second medical education began with installation of high speed internet, a key learning tool in the medicine of the future.

Finally I must acknowledge that this book is merely a milestone along a long road that leads from the early days when Rembrandt painted the Anatomy Lesson of Doctor Nicoleas Tulp (1632), to today's state of the art. The history of medicine will march forward into the future, as we marvel at how much has been accomplished in a few hundred years.

Disclaimer

This book is not intended as medical advice nor should it be regarded as such. It is important to discuss any treatment plan with your personal physician. Do not start or stop a treatment, drug, supplement or lifestyle change based on information from this book. Even if a drug is on a ligation, recall or black box list, any decision to start or stop a drug should be made in consultation with your own doctor, who should help you weigh the comparative risks and benefits to arrive at an informed decision.

The information contained in this book is NOT intended to diagnose or treat any existing disease or ailment, or to replace in any way the patient /physician relationship with your own personal physician.

Regarding the nutritional supplements which may be mentioned: These have not been evaluated by the FDA and are not intended to treat disease. Any comments made about nutritional supplements are of a general nature and not intended to provide personal advice. The reader should seek the advice of a trusted health care professional regarding the use, risks, benefits, indications, and contra-indications of the various nutritional supplements which may be mentioned.

Regarding FDA approved pharmaceutical drugs mentioned: Any comments made about drugs are of a general nature and not intended to provide personal advice. The reader should seek the advice of a trusted health care professional regarding the use, risks, benefits, indications, and contra-indications of drugs.

The reader is advised to discuss the comments on these pages with his/her personal physicians and to only act upon the advice of his/her personal physician

Some treatment options do not require a prescription and can be obtained over the counter. Even so, it is recommended that one should always work closely with a knowledgeable physician, found by consulting one of the following organizations:

http://www.worldhealth.net/
American Academy of Anti-Aging Medicine (Chicago Office)
1510 W. Montana Street
Chicago, IL 60614 USA
Directory of members, to find a doctor: Telephone is 800-558-1267

http://www.acamnet.org/
ACAM—American College for the Advancement of Medicine
24411 Ridge Route Ste 115Laguna Hills, CA 92653
ACAM doctor's directory to find a physician: Toll free telephone: 800-532-3688

http://icimed.com/
International College of Integrative Medicine
122 Thurman St. Box 271, Bluffton, OH 45817, Telephone: (866) 464-5226, (419) 358-0273, ICIM doctor's directory

http://www.holisticmedicine.org/
American Holistic Medical Association
One Eagle Valley Court, Suite 201, Broadview Heights, Ohio 44147
Phone: (440) 838-1010

Introduction by David Brownstein MD

Once in a while, a book comes out questioning the prevailing medical dogma, the things we are all used to hearing. Such a book makes you step back, ask a few questions, and do some critical thinking about the information handed down by the powers-that-be. " Bioidentical Hormones 101" by Jeffrey Dach MD is one of those books.

The book covers a wide range of topics. The first chapter sets the tone for the book and is titled, "Less is More, Mainstream Goes Alternative." This chapter describes medical studies which show that more health care is not necessarily better health care, and actually results in worse health outcomes. One example is the use of synthetic hormones which causes heart disease and cancer. Other examples include arthroscopic surgery for osteoarthritis and SSRI antidepressant medications for treating mild to moderate depression, both of which have been shown to be no better than placebo therapy. Dr. Dach provides ongoing commentary with these studies which provide the reader with a clear path: stay away from many commonly used conventional therapies, in preference to safe and effective natural alternatives.

Dr. Dach points out the conventional approach to diagnosing and treating thyroid disorders leaves much to be desired. He describes the limitations of relying on TSH levels to treat and diagnose hypothyroidism. He feels it is best to check all of the thyroid function tests, the TSH and the free T3 test. Many people who have the signs and symptoms to make the diagnosis of hypothyroidism are being denied the therapy they need because doctors are solely relying on TSH levels instead of doing more comprehensive testing. I could not agree more with the analysis in this book.

The bioidentical hormone controversy is covered in great detail. Reviewing the medical journals compromised by use of ghost writers, Dr. Dach presents a scary picture with mainstream medicine nonchalantly handing out synthetic hormones while there is clear evidence for the safety and efficacy of bioidentical hormones. There are 15 chapters dedicated to reviewing the literature on synthetic and bioidentical hormones. At the end of reading these chapters, it becomes blatantly obvious that the use of bioidentical hormones is indicated in a number of medical conditions and that synthetic hormones have no place in medicine.

There are many other topics covered in this book including questioning the usefulness of mammograms, acid blocking drugs, osteoporosis drugs and antidepressant drugs. Reading this manuscript should empower the reader to embrace a more holistic approach to one's health care.

I have been practicing holistic medicine for nearly 20 years. I have seen the failure of conventional medicine at treating many chronic illnesses. Furthermore, the use of most commonly prescribed drugs leads to further health problems in the vast majority of individuals. This book provides the reader with the information necessary to make better health care choices. It challenges the conventional wisdom about mammograms, hormone therapies, depression medications and many other conditions. I found the information in this book to be extremely worthwhile. I would recommend this book for both doctors and patients alike who are willing to question the conventional dogma and search for safe and effective natural therapies.

David Brownstein MD, The Center for Holistic Medicine
www.drbrownstein.com
5821 W. Maple Rd., Ste. 192, West Bloomfield, MI 48322, Tel: (248) 851-1600

Introduction by Mary Shomon

You can't open a newspaper or women's magazine, or turn on the health segment of the morning television shows or an afternoon talk shows without hearing about hormones. Whether it's Oprah, Suzanne Somers, your coworker, brother, mother, or your best friend, it seems that after the age of 40, many of us start to pay closer attention to what's happening to us hormonally, and the impact hormones have on our health and happiness.

Unfortunately, hormones are a complicated topic. Endocrinologists study them from a technical standpoint, but don't often understand their workings and interactions physiologically. Some gynecologists or urologists look at them more as the product of the organs and glands they treat, rather than as system unto itself. And women and men, well, we understand that hormones are at the core of almost every process in the body — from thinking, to energy, to digestion . . . but how they all work together? Often, a mystery!

Unraveling this mystery is what Dr. Jeffrey Dach does in this terrific book. Dr. Dach offers a comprehensive, understandable, and eye-opening look at debilitating hormonal issues, including thyroid disorders, adrenal fatigue, and low testosterone, as well as an unbiased, step-by-step look at the timely topic of bioidentical hormones.

I also appreciate Dr. Jeffrey Dach's decades-long commitment to researching and communicating information about hormonal and natural health — especially in an environment where physicians are routinely looked down upon for bringing sound judgment, new ideas, clinical experience, and common sense into their medical practice. More patients in the United States now visit integrative, functional, holistic, complementary and alternative practitioners than conventional physicians in the United States, and there is a reason: patients are looking for solutions, and conventional medicine falls short in many areas where complementary medicine shines.

Nowhere is that more evident than in hormonal medicine. We don't have a specialty called "hormonologist," but we in fact need one. In the meantime, doctors from a variety of disciplines — family practice, gynecology, anti-aging medicine, integrative and functional medicine and more — are increasingly becoming experts in the art and science of diagnosing and treating hormone imbalances. They are discovering that they spend an increasing amount of their time with patients being a hormone detective. These hormone detectives — with doctors like Dr. Dach on the front lines — are breaking new ground, looking at the role of the thyroid, the adrenal glands, the reproductive organs, and the body's management of insulin and glucose, as key components of our health, and as smoking guns responsible for many of today's worst health challenges, like heart disease, inflammation, and obesity.

As a thyroid patient advocate, I wouldn't be honest if I didn't say that I'm pleased to see that Dr. Dach's first key hormone section in the book focuses on the thyroid. The thyroid rarely enjoys top billing — it's usually overlooked, misdiagnosed, denigrated, stigmatized, and otherwise ignored by the medical establishment. So Dr. Dach's upfront, accurate and knowledgeable discussion of thyroid issues is a welcome change. Dr. Dach also delves into one of today's hot button's — adrenal issues — so often the topic of debate between conventional doctors , and the more cutting-edge integrative physicians. He also clearly explains the controversy, including pros and cons, of bioidentical hormones. There are patients, and many doctors, who will find this information enlightening and life-changing. To that end, I have to say that the book is a must-read for anyone who wants unbiased information on hormones.

Dr. Dach also discusses some of the politics of medicine — the role pharmaceutical companies in the health care and medications you receive (or don't receive) — as well as natural treatments you may not hear about, due to the oppressive control that conventional medicine has when it comes to innovative ideas. This is the type of information you rarely hear from an MD — most of them are too busy accepting their honoraria from drug companies and lunching with lobbyists to realize how influenced they are by the business of medicine. Dr. Dach is not afraid to tell the truth.

Overall, there is so much information packed into this book that an introduction can't really do it justice. My best advice is to read, highlight, make notes in the margin, add some sticky notes, go back to it again, and keep it handy, because it will become a resource you return to regularly to make smart decisions that will help improve your health and your life.

Live well,
Mary Shomon, Thyroid Patient Advocate and author of 11 books on thyroid disease and health. The Guide to Thyroid Disease at About.com, a New York Times Co., since 1997.
http://www.thyroid-info.com
http://thyroid.about.com
http://www.facebook.com/thyroidsupport
http://www.twitter.com/thyroidmary
PO Box 565, Kensington MD 20895 / Phone: 888-810-9471

Introduction by Jeffrey Dach MD

The introduction to this book is actually my previous book, Natural Medicine 101, available on Amazon or on the internet as a free e-book at http://naturalmedicine101.com. I would encourage you to read my earlier work, Natural Medicine 101 which introduces many topics covered in more depth here. I apologize in advance for redundancy in a few of the chapters, especially those dealing with bioidentical hormones. However, repetition may be a good thing. Also, I would encourage you to visit the web site where you will find this entire book and references hyperlinked at: http://www.bioidenticalhormones101.com.

Reaching a New Extreme

As I write this introduction, corporate control of the media and government has reached a new extreme, bringing us the Gulf Oil Spill disaster, the Subprime Mortgage Debacle, the Genetically Modified (GMO) Food Scandal, and of course, a dysfunctional medical system. Large health care corporations have created the "for-profit medical system" which places financial gain before any consideration for individual health. Even our access to information about health, drugs and food is meticulously controlled by the Health Care Lobby. In this confusing information war, where can we find the truth about drugs, healthcare and medicine?

Why Write This Book?

This book was written to provide the missing information your doctor will not tell you, and may not be available in the mass media. Considering the misinformation in the news media, there has never been a better time to write this book. This book chronicles my learning and discovery process as each topic was researched and meticulously referenced as a blog entry at http://www.jeffreydach.com. Unlike the old days when books first appeared in print, this book was originally written on my blog with references hyperlinked. The advantage for the reader is the ability to use the hyperlinked references, allowing the reader instant access to the reference article. Therefore you may find it advantageous to use the internet version of this book at http://www.bioidenticalhormones101.com for the convenience of the hyperlinked references. While you are there, I would also encourage you to sign up for the free monthly newsletter email where you can observe the creative process for the next book as it is written.

The Great Achievements of Modern Medicine

Among the great achievements of modern medicine is the invention of antibiotics and the conquest of infectious disease. Perhaps this would not have been possible without the drug patent system which provides financial incentive for new drugs. The patent drug system has also created the most profitable industry in the world, the pharmaceutical industry, which controls and dominates the practice of medicine. This highly profitable drug industry liberally funds medical research, advertising, marketing, education, and of course, "sales reps" to present "educational" literature in doctor's offices. Major corporations such as the drug industry and the health insurance industry influence government legislative bodies and regulatory agencies such as the FDA and USDA, and determine how NIH research grants are allocated.

The Patented Drug Paradigm

For centuries, our medicines came from the plant and natural world. Only recently in the 19th century, everything changed with the creation of patent law system, granting economic protection and profitablitity to the patent holder of a chemical formula or new invention. Patented drugs are chemically altered versions of natural substances not found in nature or in the human body, and are actually foreign to the human body. This patent protection eliminates the competition and insures massive profit at inflated prices for the newly patented drug. Thus, the patent system has created the pharmaceutical industry, the most profitable business on the planet.

Another feature of patent law is that the natural world has been excluded, and cannot be patented, so there is little financial incentive for drug companies to invest in natural substances. For example, both Vitamin C and bio-identical hormones are natural substances, and therefore their chemical structures cannot be patented.

Drug patents have a limited life time, with eventual expiration, so the Drug Company must have a steady stream of new drugs in the pipeline. In order to bring these new drugs to market, clinical trials must be submitted for FDA approval showing benefit greater than placebo. Once approved, the next step is a massive advertising campaign to convince both the public and the medical professionals they need the drug.

Somewhere along the way things went wrong, and we find the clinical trials are manipulated to show benefit for drugs which are marginal, ineffective or actually harmful. We find the drug marketing advertising to be deceitful and misleading. We also find that drug companies behave like any other self interested corporation. They lobby the government and peddle influence to gain favor for their products, while using their clout to change the rules and suppress competition in natural medicine.

Medical Ghostwriting

Medical ghostwriting is the insidious practice of paying an "opinion leader" academic physician to lend their name to an article in the medical literature. Unknown to the reader, the article is actually written by paid-for-hire writers to promote the synthetic hormone drug agenda, by downplaying adverse effects, hyping the benefits, and casting doubts about bioidentical hormones.

FDA "GAG" Rule

An FDA "gag rule" makes it unlawful for vitamin companies to give information to the public about their products. This FDA rule makes it illegal for a vitamin manufacturer to inform customers about the benefits of vitamins, supplements and natural medicines. Obviously, this rule is an unconstitutional infringement on the right of free speech, one example of the drug lobby's power to influence government to make laws which suppress competition and increase profit at the expense of the constitutional right of free speech.

A Request to Ban Bio-Identical Hormones?

Another example is the "Citizens' Complaint" filed by Wyeth with the FDA, asking the FDA to ban bio-identical hormones. Following the 2002 Women's Health Initiative study, halted early because synthetic hormone pills caused cancer and heart disease, millions of women abandoned the synthetic hormones and switched to the safer bio-identical (natural) human hormones. This massive switch away from synthetic hormones resulted in 4 billion dollar loss for synthetic hormone makers. The drug maker was not happy about the financial loss, so they simply filed a "citizen's complaint" asking the FDA to ban their competition. This outrageous abuse of government was unsuccessful.

The FDA Cannot Protect the American Public

The FDA (Food and Drug Agency) is thought to be guarding and protecting the American Public. Yet upon closer inspection is clearly under the thumb of the pharmaceutical industry. According to the Director of Drug Safety at the FDA, David Graham, the FDA cannot protect the American Public from bad drugs such as chemically altered, synthetic hormones. These are monster hormones which, clearly, should never have been approved nor marketed to the American people.

Bioidentical Hormones Are Safer and More Effective

Over the past 70 years that natural bio-identical hormones have been available, comparison studies have always shown the bioidentical hormones safer and more effective than the chemically altered synthetic hormones, yet these monster hormones are the ones routinely handed out by the "for-profit medical system". As this book is written, deceptive television advertising touting the benefits of synthetic hormones can still be viewed daily. These monster hormones should have been banned from the marketplace years ago.

Basic Medicine 101

One final thought concerns the central aspect of hormones in the health of the individual. A primary care physician's very first concern should be evaluating and balancing hormone levels. But it is not. Instead, the primary care physician has been turned into a vending machine for various synthetic drugs of questionable benefit. American Medicine has lost its way. This book is an attempt to get it back on the right track.

About the Author, Jeffrey Dach MD:

Jeffrey Dach obtained his MD degree from the University of Illinois in Chicago. He was originally trained in clinical medicine and worked as an ER (emergency room) doctor in Illinois. He then trained and earned board certification in Diagnostic and Interventional Radiology, and worked as a hospital based physician for thirty years in the Memorial Hospital System of South Broward, Florida. Because of failing eyesight, Dr. Dach retired from hospital based radiology, and switched back into his original training in outpatient clinical medicine leading to the formation of a new clinic called TrueMedMD, specializing in bioidentical hormones, and natural thyroid. Dr. Dach is author of the book, Natural Medicine 101, and writes a free monthly internet newsletter.

Jeffrey Dach MD, 7450 Griffin Road,
Suite 190, Davie, Florida 33314.
Telephone 954-792-4663
www.jeffreydach.com
www.drdach.com
www.naturalmedicine101.com
www.bioidenticalhormones101.com

FOREWORD

The organization of the book is divided into sections, and starts off with a discussion of thyroid and adrenal issues because the capable bioidentical hormone doctor will first address these preliminary issues before going on to address the other hormones. The low thyroid condition is prevalent in our population. Many low thyroid Northerners report they are cold all the time, and perhaps they have migrated in great numbers here to Florida to seek a warmer climate. Another common condition is "adrenal fatigue", the inability to produce adequate amounts of the hormone called cortisol. This "adrenal fatigue" is especially common in patients on long term SSRI antidepressants which eventually lead to "burn out". A common pitfall to avoid in patients with adrenal fatigue is giving thyroid medication which will worsen the patient's symptoms of fatigue and exhaustion. The adrenal fatigue issues must be addressed before adding in the thyroid medication.

Section four deals with bioidentical hormones, and why we need them, and why they are safer and more effective than synthetic hormones. A chapter deals with the corrupt practice of ghostwriting in the medical literature, specifically designed to "market" synthetic hormones in medical articles and cast doubts on the bioidenticals. Additional chapters deal with menopausal arthritis, anxiety and panic attacks, and dry eye syndrome, all relieved by bioidentical hormones. Another chapter deals with hormone replacement after hysterectomy. Four more chapters deal with the news media, correcting their errors and fallacies in the many newspaper articles on bioidentical hormones. Finally, a chapter deals with "drug litigation" against synthetic hormones with juries punishing drug companies with large monetary awards to the victims of synthetic hormones.

Since breast cancer is a prominent concern in women taking hormone replacement, section five deals with screening mammography, breast cancer detection, and breast cancer prevention. The most important tool for breast cancer prevention is iodine supplementation.

Sections six and seven discuss low testosterone in males, found to be associated with increased mortality and a health risk. Chronic use narcotic pain pills cause profound suppression of hormone levels, especially inducing low testosterone. The question of testosterone's benefit for the heart and the circulation is discussed. The lack of a causative link between testosterone and prostate cancer is discussed. Additionally, PSA screening for prostate cancer detection is discussed as a "failed medical experiment".

Section eight contains four chapters on the essential mineral selenium, how it is important for cancer prevention, the immune system, and useful in the Intensive Care Unit setting. Selenium is also beneficial for reducing antibody levels in Hashimoto's Thyroiditis, a common thyroid condition.

Section nine discusses the problem of "Bad Drugs", which are marginally effective or even harmful. Osteoporosis drugs are intended to make the bones stronger and prevent fractures, yet paradoxically, we find these drugs actually make the bones weaker and cause debilitating femur fractures. The heartburn drugs (proton pump inhibitors—PPI's) work very well at their job of turning off gastric acid. However, we find chronic use of PPI's causes a host of health problems. SSRI Antidepressant drug use is rampant, and touted as safe and effective. However, studies reveal these drugs are no more effective than placebo for the majority of users, and not as safe as originally thought. Statin drugs are also included in the list of "Bad Drugs". The common medical practice of prescribing cholesterol lowering statin drugs is found to be harmful, with the same mortality benefit as a placebo, and yet carries severe adverse side effects.

Heart disease and anti-cholesterol drugs deserve its own Section ten. Statin cholesterol lowering drugs are very effective at lowering cholesterol, but this kind of treatment has no health benefit for women. And for primary prevention of heart disease in healthy people, taking a statin anti-cholesterol drug provides the same mortality benefit as a placebo. The theory that cholesterol causes heart disease is found to be a myth. Patients entering the hospital with heart attacks have low, not high cholesterol, and three years later, follow up studies show patients with lower cholesterol have higher mortality. Heart disease prevention is discussed with lifestyle and diet modification, and supplements such as Vitamin C, tocotrienol Vitamin E, Vitamin D, Vitamin K, Omega 3 oils, Niacin, and various others mentioned by William Davis and Linus Pauling.

Section eleven deals with vitamin therapies with B5 for acne, B6 for carpal tunnel and trigger finger, and the Vitamin E as a heart disease preventive, and a discussion of wheatgrass juice. Section Twelve discusses the dangers of fast food, MSG and aspartame, and GMO genetically modified food. Also included here is a discussion of wheat gluten sensitivity, another food that can make us sick.

Our health is more than a collection of chemical reactions, and atomic particles bouncing off one another. In order to heal our bodies and maintain health, we need a purpose, or a reason to keep ourselves healthy. Section thirteen deals with this spiritual side of healing and medicine with an essay about Steven Meyer's book, Signature in a Cell. Another short essay deals with an unforgettable experience during medical school taking care of a dying patient.

The final section fifteen deals with the future of medicine, with a discussion of low dose naltrexone, medical cannabis, anti-aging breakthroughs with bioidentical hormones, future directions for cancer research, and finally the future of medicine in general. This section deals with the trophoblastic theory of cancer and a final essay discusses what is in store for us in the future of medicine, and what we must do to avoid the "nightmare scenario".

Section One: More Health Care Is Not Necessarily Better Health Care

Chapter 1

Less is More, Mainstream Goes Alternative, and Medical Heresy

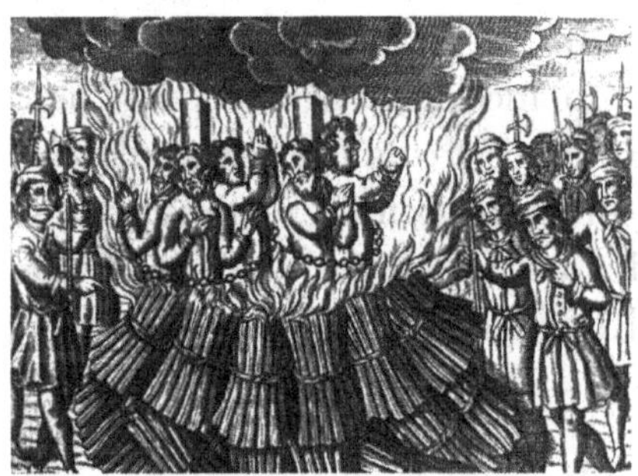

Medieval Heretics Burned At the Stake, 14th to mid-15th Century, courtesy of Wikimedia Commons

A shocking "medical heresy" was quietly stated in a mainstream medical journal.(1) "*Less health care is better than more health care*", says Dr. Deborah Grady in her editorial in the May 10, 2010 Archives of Internal Medicine which is critical of mainstream medicine. We assume and expect that health care should offer some health benefit. And yet, Dr Grady points out that health outcome studies show that more health care leads to worse outcomes. (2,3) This revelation isn't new, and is actually old news, like a worn and familiar old shoe. The real news story is that this "medical heresy" somehow eluded censorship by the editorial board and appeared in print in a mainstream medical journal. Are mainstream doctors getting fed up? Is this the opening salvo of a medical revolution?

Examples of Harmful Medical Care

Dr Grady cites specific examples of treatments that result in harm, with adverse effects outweighing the benefits. The first example is synthetic "monster" hormone therapy used by the mainstream medical system, which was found to cause cancer and heart disease in the famous 2002 Women's Health Initiative study. (4) It seems incredible, but true. The mainstream medical system used synthetic "monster" hormones for years until the WHI (Women's Health Initiative) study finally convinced millions of women to switch to safer and more effective bioidentical human hormones. See the articles on the safety and importance of bioidentical hormones which discusses this at length. (5)(6)

Dr. Grady's second example is the discredited practice of arthroscopic surgery for osteoarthritis. Millions of these useless procedures were performed in the late 90's until it was abandoned after randomized trials showed no benefit.(7) See the article on the power of the placebo which discussed this.(8)

A third example is the case of SSRI antidepressant drugs which have little benefit for patients with mild to moderate depression. These studies show that the benefits of SSRI drugs are equivalent to placebo pills.(9) Dr. Grady points out that in cases of mild depression, the known adverse effects of SSRI antidepressants clearly outweigh the benefits. My previous article on SSRI antidepressants discussed this. (10)

A fourth example is screening mammography. "The adverse effects of mammography—false-positive findings, biopsies, anxiety, and over diagnosis and treatment of latent cancers may overwhelm the benefit." (11) My article on screening mammography discussed this. (12)

Dr Grady's final example is the over-use and misuse of antacid drugs called proton pump inhibitors (PPI's), which have serious adverse effects of increased rates of fractures, Clostridium difficile infection, and increased risk of pneumonia. (13-18)

Reducing Medical Care Opposed as "Rationing"

Dr Grady reminds us that the term "rationing" is frequently misused and abused in health care debates. In politics, those who want more health care oppose those who propose less health care. Less health care is called "rationing", a term originating in the wartime practice of rationing food, fuel and other scarce goods, and services, and may not apply to over use of health services which causes harm rather than benefit.

A False Hope—Bone Marrow Transplantation for Breast Cancer

A perfect example of misuse of the term "rationing' is the discredited bone marrow transplantation for breast cancer. Starting in the 1980's, thousands of procedures were done costing up to 400,000 dollars each. While many women stricken with advanced illness clamored for the "lifesaving" procedure, their health insurance companies balked at paying for an experimental and unproven treatment. A media and legal campaign ensued claiming the insurance companies were cruel tyrants. They were withholding or "rationing" a "lifesaving" treatment. After a couple of decades of harming thousands of severely ill women with an unproven procedure, medical studies were eventually done, and these showed the procedure had no merit, causing it to be discredited and abandoned. Clearly, the term "health care rationing" is misused when applied to a sham procedure that causes more harm than good. This incredible story of bone marrow transplantation for breast cancer can be found in an excellent article by Nicholas Gonzalez MD, and also in a book which documents the story called False Hope. (20-22)

More Examples: Drugs that Don't Work

The misguided use of the term "health care rationing" applies to blockbuster drugs developed over the last few decades that are in fact, **Bad Drugs**. These patented drugs are expensive, yet have marginal effectiveness, and horrendous adverse side effects. In spite of this, thanks to Drug Company advertising, the television viewing audience clamors for these "lifesaving drugs", complaining that high cost and lack of insurance coverage amounts to "health care rationing". See my article on Protect Your Family from Bad Drugs. (26) An excellent book on this topic entitled, "Drugs that Don't Work, Natural Therapies that Do", is available from Dr. David Brownstein.(25)

Solution: Less Health Care

When the health care system is dominated and corrupted by huge corporations that place profit over people, the end result is a health care system that produces more harm than good. Hence, the sage old doctor's advice, "Doing Nothing" is frequently the best treatment plan, and one offered by my medical school advisor, Dr Neil Kurtzman, as the title for his first novel.(23)

Of course, the real solution involves liberating the practice of medicine from the shackles of corporate and government control. Although somewhat draconian, an excellent first step would be the elimination of the entire health insurance industry. Don't hold your breath, as this is unlikely to happen any time soon, judging by the "health care reform" signed into law by President Obama. This latest "health care reform" effort amounts to a giant government subsidy for the health insurance industry with very little in return.

For hyperlinked references, see web site: www.bioidenticalhormones101.com

Chapter One References: Less is More, Mainstream Goes Alternative

(1) http://archinte.ama-assn.org/cgi/content/full/170/9/749
Less Is More, How Less Health Care Can Result in Better Health, Deborah Grady, MD, MPH; Rita F. Redberg, MD, MSc, Editor, Arch Intern Med. 2010;170(9):749-750.

(2) http://www.annals.org/content/138/4/288.abstract
Fisher ES, Wennberg DE, Stukel TA, Gottlieb DJ, Lucas FL, Pinder EL. The implications of regional variations in Medicare spending, part 2: health outcomes and satisfaction with care. Ann Intern Med. 2003;138(4):288-298.

(3) http://www.annals.org/content/138/4/273.abstract
Fisher ES, Wennberg DE, Stukel TA, Gottlieb DJ, Lucas FL, Pinder EL. The implications of regional variations in Medicare spending, part 1: the content, quality, and accessibility of care. Ann Intern Med. 2003;138(4):273-287.

(4) http://jama.ama-assn.org/cgi/content/abstract/288/3/321
Rossouw JE, Anderson GL, Prentice RL; et al, Writing Group for the Women's Health Initiative Investigators. Risks and benefits of estrogen plus progestin in healthy postmenopausal women: principal results

from the Women's Health Initiative randomized controlled trial. JAMA. 2002;288(3):321-333.

(5) http://jeffreydach.com/2008/06/27/the-safety-of-bioidentical-hormones-by-jeffrey-dach-md.aspx The safety of bioidentical Hormones by Jeffrey Dach MD

(6) http://www.drdach.com/BioIdentical_Hormones.html
The Importance of bio-identical Hormones by Jeffrey Dach MD

(7) http://content.nejm.org/cgi/content/abstract/347/2/81
Moseley JB, O'Malley K, Petersen NJ; et al. A controlled trial of arthroscopic surgery for osteoarthritis of the knee. N Engl J Med. 2002;347(2):81-88.

(8) http://jeffreydach.com/2007/05/22/the-power-of-the-placebo—by-jeffrey-dach-md.aspx The Power of the Placebo by Jeffrey Dach MD

(9) http://jama.ama-assn.org/cgi/content/abstract/303/1/47
Fournier JC, DeRubeis RJ, Hollon SD; et al. Antidepressant drug effects and depression severity: a patient-level meta-analysis. JAMA. 2010;303(1):47-53.

(10) http://jeffreydach.com/2010/01/21/jama-says-ssri-antidepressants-are-placebos-by-jeffrey-dach-md.aspx
Antidepressants Found to Be No Better Than Placebo.

(11) http://jama.ama-assn.org/cgi/content/full/303/2/164
Woloshin S, Schwartz LM. The benefits and harms of mammography screening: understanding the trade-offs. JAMA. 2010;303(2):164-165.

(12) http://jeffreydach.com/2009/11/17/mammogram-guideline-reversal-by-jeffrey-dach-md.aspx Mammogram Guideline Reversal by Jeffrey Dach MD

(13) http://archinte.ama-assn.org/cgi/content/abstract/170/9/7659
Gray SL, LaCroix AZ, Larson J; et al. Proton pump inhibitor use, hip fracture, and change in bone mineral density in postmenopausal

women: results from the Women's Health Initiative. Arch Intern Med. 2010;170(9):765-771. FREE FULL TEXT

(14) http://archinte.ama-assn.org/cgi/content/abstract/170/9/784 Howell MD, Novack V, Grgurich P; et al. Iatrogenic gastric acid suppression and the risk of nosocomial Clostridium difficile infection. Arch Intern Med. 2010;170(9):784-790.

(15) http://archinte.ama-assn.org/cgi/content/abstract/170/9/772 Linsky A, Gupta K, Lawler EV, Fonda JR, Hermos JA. Proton pump inhibitors and risk for recurrent Clostridium difficile infection. Arch Intern Med. 2010;170(9):772-778.

(16) http://www.annals.org/content/149/6/391.abstract Sarkar M, Hennessy S, Yang Y-X. Proton-pump inhibitor use and the risk for community-acquired pneumonia. Ann Intern Med. 2008;149(6):391-398.

(17) http://jama.ama-assn.org/cgi/content/abstract/301/20/2120 Herzig SJ, Howell MD, Ngo LH, Marcantonio ER. Acid suppressive medication use and the risk for hospital acquired pneumonia. JAMA. 2009;301(20):2120-2128.

(18) http://archinte.ama-assn.org/cgi/content/full/170/9/747 Katz MH. Failing the acid test: benefits of proton pump inhibitors may not justify the risks for many users. Arch Intern Med. 2010;170(9):747-748.

(19) http://jeffreydach.com/2009/09/14/heartburn-and-acid-blockers-by-jeffrey-dach-md.aspx Heartburn and Acid Blockers by Jeffrey Dach MD

(20) http://www.dr-gonzalez.com/bias.htm Academic Bias and Fraud: The cases of bone marrow transplantation for breast cancer, and HIV-nevirapine By Nicholas J. Gonzalez, M.D.

(21) http://www.amazon.com/False-Hope-Marrow-Transplantation-Breast/dp/0195187768 False Hope: Bone Marrow Transplantation for Breast

Cancer. Richard A. Rettig (Author), Peter D. Jacobson (Author), Cynthia M. Farquhar M.D. (Author), Wade M. Aubry M.D. (Author)

(22) http://www.jcojournal.org/cgi/content/full/26/1/11
Journal of Clinical Oncology, Vol 26, No 1 (January 1), 2008: pp. 11-12 EDITORIAL A Dramatic Story of Hope and Reality Edward A. Stadtmauer

(23) http://medicine-opera.com/doing-nothing-reviews
Neil A Kurtzman MD is the Grover E Murray Professor and University Distinguished Professor, Department of Internal Medicine at Texas Tech University Health Sciences Center in Lubbock. He has combined careers in clinical medicine, education, basic research, and administration for more than 30 years. Dr Kurtzman was my research advisor in medical school.

(24) http://whcrc.ucsf.edu/people/bios/grady_deborah.html
Deborah Grady, MD, MPH is Professor of Medicine, Associate Dean for Clinical and Translational Research and Director of the UCSF Women's Health Clinical Research Center. Dr. Grady is an international expert on menopause and the risks and benefits of postmenopausal hormone therapy. Dr. Grady has trained and mentored over 40 young researchers interested in women's health and received the Chancellor's Award for the Advancement of Women and the UCSF Mentor of the Year award.

(25) https://www.drbrownstein.com/bookstore_NaturalT.php
Drugs that Don't Work, Natural Therapies that Do, is available from Dr David Brownstein

(26) http://jeffreydach.com/2007/08/26/protect-your-family-from-bad-drugs-by-jeffrey-dach-md.aspx Protect Your Family from Bad Drugs by Jeffrey Dach MD

Section Two: Low Thyroid Disorders and Thyroid Nodules

CHAPTER 2

The Unreliable TSH Lab Test

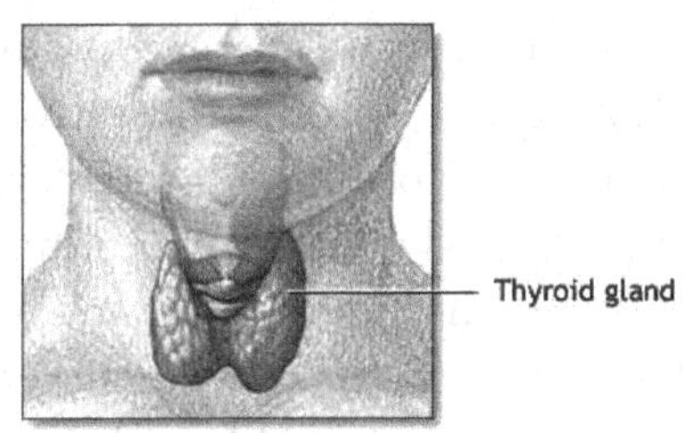

Thyroid Gland Anatomy Diagram, courtesy of National Institute of Health, and wikimedia commons.

Suzy is a 59 year old post menopausal woman with low thyroid function. About three months ago, she started her bio-identicalhormoneprogram which included natural thyroid pills. After starting the program, she was doing well with more energy, better sleep, improved appearance of skin and hair, and resolution of her menopausal symptoms of flashes and sweats. However about 12 weeks into her program, Suzy had a visit with her primary care doctor who did a follow up thyroid panel. Her primary care doctor informed Suzy that her TSH test result was below the lab normal range, and therefore, her thyroid dose was too high, and should be reduced. (Note TSH stands for Thyroid Stimulating Hormone and is made by the pituitary gland)

Too Many Doctors Spoil the Soup

Suzy called me at the office distraught and confused. Two doctors were telling her two different things and she didn't know who to believe. Her primary care doctor was telling her one thing and I was telling her another. I explained to Suzy that her primary care doctor was incorrect in relying slavishly on the TSH test. Even though her TSH test was 0.15 which is below the lab reference range of 0.3, this was perfectly acceptable and indicated her thyroid medicine was suppressing the TSH to a low level which was perfectly fine. This test interpretation means she is taking thyroid pills, and the pills are working. It does not mean she is "hyperthyroid" by any stretch of the imagination.

No Clinical Evidence of Thyrotoxicosis

I also informed Suzy that her Primary Care Doctor is mistakenly relying on the TSH test to determine her thyroid dosage. The TSH test is an indirect measure of thyroid function and can be unreliable to monitor thyroid dosage. A more accurate indicator of thyroid function is the free T3, which in her case was 375, well within the normal range of 240 to 420. The Free T3 lab test together with the absence of any signs or symptoms of thyroid excess indicates she is using the correct dosage of natural thyroid medication. Symptoms of thyroid excess are rapid heartbeat or palpitations, and Suzy reported no such symptoms. In fact, Suzy said she felt fine and now that she understands it, she didn't want to go back to feeling tired and sluggish. Suzy was relieved to find out that the low TSH result was perfectly acceptable and there was nothing to worry about. This TSH scenario is a recurring event at my office.

Conventional Docs Slavishly Rely on the TSH

Conventional primary care doctors use an older thyroid lab panel which does not include the Free T3 test, the most informative thyroid lab test. Instead, mainstream endocrinology relies on the TSH test which is not a direct measure of thyroid function, and can, in fact, be unreliable. Most conventional doctors are unfamiliar with the use of natural thyroid which contains both T3 and T4, and instead use Synthroid which is quite different, containing only T4. Since the Primary care doctors bill the health insurance for the office visit and payment is only a few dollars, the office visit is brief, 3-5 minutes. In this short time, Primary care doctors can provide only the most basic care, which is a quick look at the TSH lab test. If the TSH is below the lab reference range the doctor gives a new prescription for Synthroid with a reduced dosage. If the TSH is above the reference range, the primary care doctor will increase the Synthroid dosage.

The Cleveland Clinic Chimes In

A few months ago, I found myself talking on the phone with an endocrinologist at the Cleveland Clinic explaining why the TSH blood test can be unreliable. He informed me I was wrong, and that he uses the TSH test as the gold standard. We agreed to disagree and parted company as friends. I have found that, in general, endocrinologists and mainstream doctors rely heavily on TSH to make a diagnosis of low thyroid.

Why Thyroid Blood Testing is Unreliable.

I recommend to you a book by Barry Durrant Peatfield, "Your Thyroid and How to Keep It Healthy".(1) A general practitioner in the British National Health Service, Peatfield came to the US to train at the Broda Barnes Institute. He later returned to England and started his own thyroid clinic. His book contains the wisdom of 25 years of diagnosing and treating thyroid conditions. One section of the book is devoted to this question. Here it is:(1)

1) Anxiety in the medical establishment about rules and dogma has led to a slavish reliance on blood tests, such as the TSH, which are often unreliable and can actually produce a false picture.

2) Very few doctors can accept the fact that a normal, or low TSH, may still occur with low thyroid function.

3) As a result of this test (TSH), thousands are denied treatment for low thyroid condition.

Dr. Peatfield's Reward After a LifeTime of Service

After a lifetime of work serving his community, you might imagine the honors and accolades for such a knowledgeable thyroidologist as Dr Peatfield, yet quite the opposite happened. Dr. Peatfield's license was suspended in 2001 at the age of 68 by the General Medical Council of England.(5-6) The GMC ruling was based on "unfavorable testimony" from competing endocrinologists who "slavishly rely on the TSH test" as a measurement of thyroid function to diagnose the low thyroid condition and monitor treatment with thyroxine. Sadly, this is the sort of "Witch Hunt" which has kept medical science in the "Dark Ages" regarding the treatment of the low thyroid condition.(13)

Broda Barnes and the Low Thyroid Condition

Another useful book recommended to you is written by Broda Barnes MD on the low thyroid condition. Broda Barnes MD reported 40 years ago on the same problem of his medical colleagues relying too heavily on thyroid blood tests. The book, "Hypothyroidism the Unsuspected Illness", by Broda Barnes MD, is a medical classic and should be required reading for every medical student and doctor. (2) I have read the book many times. The book contains the condensed wisdom of a lifetime of research and clinical experience with the thyroid, and it rings true today as it did in 1976. Thyroid blood tests come and go, yet human physiology remains the same.

Important Point:
The TSH test is unreliable for determining optimal thyroid dosage. A "below lab range" TSH is routinely encountered when patients are optimally treated with natural thyroid medication and obtain the best clinical results.

Hypothyroidism the Unsuspected Illness, by Broda Barnes MD

Broda Barnes estimated that up to 40% of the population suffers from a low thyroid condition and would benefit from thyroid medication. Of course, Barnes' opinion differed with that of mainstream medicine of his time which relied dogmatically on thyroid blood tests to make the diagnosis of low thyroid. Barnes felt the blood tests were unreliable and instead used the basal temperature, history and physical examination. This medical debate regarding unreliability of thyroid blood testing continues today. (3,4)

Being an astute clinician, Dr. Barnes makes a number of observations about the low thyroid condition. Firstly, low thyroid is associated with a reduced immunity to infectious diseases such as TB (tuberculosis). Before the advent of modern antibiotics in the 1940's, most low thyroid children succumbed to infectious diseases before reaching adulthood. Secondly, low thyroid is associated with a peculiar form of skin thickening called myxedema which causes a characteristic appearance of the face, puffiness around the eyes, fullness under the chin, loss of outer eyebrows, and hair thinning or hair loss.

A third observation by Dr. Barnes is that low thyroid is associated with menstrual irregularities, miscarriages and infertility. Barnes treated thousands of young women with thyroid pills which restored cycle regularity and fertility. In his day, the medical system resorted to the drastic measure of hysterectomy for uncontrolled menstrual bleeding. Although today's use of birth control pills to regulate the cycles is admittedly a far better alternative, Barnes found that the simple administration of desiccated thyroid served quite well. Again, Barnes noted that blood testing was usually normal in these cases which respond to thyroid medication.

A lengthy chapter is devoted to heart attacks and the low thyroid condition. Based on autopsy data from Graz Austria, Barnes concluded that low thyroid patients who previously would have succumbed to infectious diseases in childhood go on years later to develop heart disease. Barnes also found that thyroid treatment was protective in preventing heart attacks, based on his own clinical experience. Likewise for diabetes, Dr. Barnes found that adding thyroid medication was beneficial at preventing the onset of vascular disease in diabetics. Again, blood tests are usually normal.

Important Point:
A low thyroid condition is a serious risk factor for heart disease.

Dr. Barnes devotes separate chapters in the book to discussion of chronic fatigue, migraine headaches and emotional/behavioral disorders all of which respond to treatment with thyroid medication.

The final chapter describes Dr. Barnes work on obesity when he presided over a hospital ward of volunteer obese patients, and monitored everything they ate. He found that the obese patients invariably ate a high carbohydrate diet, and avoided fat. Barnes added fat back into the menu and reduced the refined carbohydrates and found that his obese patients lost 10 pounds a month with no hunger pangs.

Missing from the book are discussions of Iodine supplementation and the role of the Adrenal, both of which are covered in later updated versions of Barnes thyroid book by other authors. See Hypothyroidism Type Two by Mark Starr, and Your Thyroid by Barry Durrant Peatfield. Iodine supplementation is covered by both Derry and Brownstein. The Safe Uses of Cortisol by William McK Jefferies is the companion medical classic devoted to the adrenals and cortisol.

Broda Barnes Institute

Although Broda Barnes has since passed away, his work lives in at the Broda Barnes Institute. Patricia Puglio is the director and a great resource. She is available by phone to answer questions and offer suggestions. Here is her contact information: Patricia A. Puglio, Director, Broda O. Barnes, M.D. Research Foundation, Inc. PO Box 110098 Trumbull, CT 06611.

More on the Unreliability of the TSH Lab Test

Thanks to Jonathan Wright's newsletter for bringing to my attention a recent article in the June 2010 International Journal of Clinical Practice by Dr. O'Reilly which summarizes the medical literature on this question of the reliability of the TSH test. (9) Essentially, Dr O'Reilly reviews the medical literature and the history thyroid medicine and provides all the medical studies and information showing that Dr Barnes and Dr Peatfield were right all along. (7-12). Here are a few quotes from Dr O'Reilly (9):

"The use of the TSH measurement to assess thyroid status in patients on thyroxine (Synthroid) replacement could be considered a classic example of the misapplication of a laboratory test."

Instead of the TSH measurement, Dr. O'Reilly recommends the T3 test for monitoring treatment with thyroid medication.

"The adequacy of thyroxine (Synthroid) replacement should be assessed clinically with the serum T3 being measured, when required, to detect over-replacement." We use the Free T3 measurement which is widely available at any lab.

Still Not Mainstream Medicine

In spite of the obvious need for a better approach to the low thyroid condition, there has been very little movement to rehabilitate mainstream endocrinology which dogmatically clings to the TSH test and synthetic T4 only medications (levothyroxine). Here in the state of Florida, we are fortunate that the state legislature passed a Health Freedom Law in 2001. This "Health Freedom Law" protects doctors and patients from unwarranted abuse or harassment for utilizing "outside of mainstream medical practices", such as correct diagnosis and treatment of the low thyroid condition based on the wisdom of Drs Broda Barnes, Barry Peatfield, DS O'Reilly, Jonathan Wright, David Brownstein and many others. (14)

For References and Links, see my web site: www.bioidenticalhormones101.com

References for Chapter 2. The Unreliable TSH Lab Test

(1) Barry Durrant-Peatfield (2006). Your thyroid and how to keep it healthy. Hammersmith Press, London

(2) Barnes, Broda Otto (1976). Hypothyroidism: The Unsuspected Illness. Harper Collins.

(3) http://ccpd.ucsf.edu/hypothyroidism.shtml Pituitary 101, UCSF California Center for Pituitary Disorders at UCSF. Web Site: "TSH is often an unreliable measure of secondary hypothyroidism and should not be used to assess the adequacy of thyroid replacement in these patients. The inappropriate use of TSH levels to determine hormone replacement is one of the more common mistakes that we see in the

patients we follow, and patients should be cautious if another physician discusses changing their thyroid hormone dose. Many patients have returned for their one-year follow-up visits having had their doses lowered in response to "low TSH levels." Most of them feel poorly, but improve after we increase or restart their medication."

(4) http://www.bmj.com/cgi/content/full/326/7398/1087 BMJ 2003;326:1087 (17 May) Letter—Thyroid function tests and hypothyroidism, A D Toft. "We have long taken the view that most hypothyroid patients are content with a dose of thyroxine that restores serum concentrations of thyroid stimulating hormone to the low normal range. However, some achieve a sense of wellbeing only when serum thyroid stimulating hormone is suppressed, when we take care to ensure that serum tri-iodothyronine is unequivocally normal. Until valid evidence shows that such a policy is detrimental we will continue to treat patients holistically rather than insist on adherence to a biochemical definition of adequacy of thyroxine replacement. The issue of whether a little too much thyroxine is dangerous is likely to evaporate when appropriate preparations become available to allow treat.

(5) http://www.drlowe.com/news/drpeatfield/jclletter.htm In Defense of Dr. Barry Peatfield, letter sent ot General medical council of England as testimony on behalf of Dr. Barry Peatfield. April 17, 2001 by Dr. John C. Lowe

(6) http://news.bbc.co.uk/2/hi/health/1332644.stm Thursday, 17 May, 2001 UK Investigation into thyroid doctor. GP Dr Barry Durrant-Peatfield, 64, who has a practice in Purley, Surrey, has been stopped from working for 18 months so that the GMC can complete its investigation.

(7) http://www.ncbi.nlm.nih.gov/pubmed/8200938 J Clin Endocrinol Metab. 1994 Jun;78(6):1368-71. Comparison of second and third generation methods for measurement of serum thyrotropin in patients with overt hyperthyroidism, patients receiving thyroxine therapy, and those with nonthyroidal illness. Franklyn JA, Black EG, Betteridge J, Sheppard MC. "Undetectable TSH results, even in a third generation

assay, are not diagnostic of overt hyperthyroidism, but are also found in subjects with treated thyroid disease and NTI."

(8) http://www.ncbi.nlm.nih.gov/pmc/articles/PMC1341585/ Br Med J (Clin Res Ed). 1986 September 27; 293(6550): 808-810. Are biochemical tests of thyroid function of any value in monitoring patients receiving thyroxine replacement? W D Fraser, E M Biggart, D S O'Reilly, H W Gray, J H McKillop, and J A Thomson. "These measurements are therefore of little, if any, value in monitoring patients receiving thyroxine replacement."

(9) http://www.ncbi.nlm.nih.gov/pubmed/20584231 Int J Clin Pract. 2010 Jun;64(7):991-4. Thyroid hormone replacement: an iatrogenic problem.O'Reilly DS. "Thyroid hormone replacement is one of the very few medical treatments devised in the 19th century that still survive. It is safe, very effective and hailed as a major success by patients and clinicians. Currently, it is arguably the most contentious issue in clinical endocrinology. The current controversy and patient disquiet began in the early 1970s, when on theoretical grounds and without proper assessment, the serum thyrotropin (TSH) concentration was adopted as the means of assessing the adequacy of thyroxine replacement. The published literature shows that the serum TSH concentration is a poor indicator of clinical status in patients on thyroxine. The adequacy of thyroxine replacement should be assessed clinically with the serum T3 being measured, when required, to detect over-replacement."

(10) http://www.ncbi.nlm.nih.gov/pubmed/3122632 Ann Clin Biochem. 1987 Nov;24 (Pt 6):614-9. Thyroid stimulating hormone measurement by an ultrasensitive assay during thyroxine replacement: comparison with other tests of thyroid function. Wheatley T, Clark PM, Clark JD, Raggatt PR, Edwards OM. "A suppressed serum TSH was found in 65% of patients with a normal serum total thyroxine."

(11) http://www.bmj.com/content/320/7245/1332.extract BMJ 320: 1332 doi: 10.1136/bmj.320.7245.1332 (Published 13 May 2000) Education and debate: Thyroid function tests—time for a reassessment. Denis StJ O'Reilly, consultant clinical biochemist

(12) http://www.bmj.com/content/320/7245/1332.extract/reply#bmj_el_8954 Thyroid function tests—time for a reassessment Denis StJ O'Reilly BMJ 2000;320:1332-1334

(13) http://www.independent.co.uk/life-style/health-and-families/health-news/claims-of-acirciquestiquestwitchhuntacirciquesttrade-as-doctor-is-suspended-for-alternative-thyroid-care-685141.html Claims of witch-hunt as doctor is suspended for alternative thyroid care By Michael Durham Friday, 18 May 2001. Independent UK

(14) http://laws.flrules.org/2001/116 State of Florida Health Freedom Law: CHAPTER 2001-116 Senate Bill No. 1324 An act relating to health care; creating s. 456.41, F.S.; amending s. 381.026, F.S.; Ch. 2001-116 (S.B. 1324) Authorizes provision of and access to complementary or alternative health care treatments; requires specified disclosures by the health care practitioner and the keeping of certain records; conforms the Florida Patient's Bill of Rights. Effective May 31, 2001.

CHAPTER 3

Why Natural Thyroid is Better than Synthetic

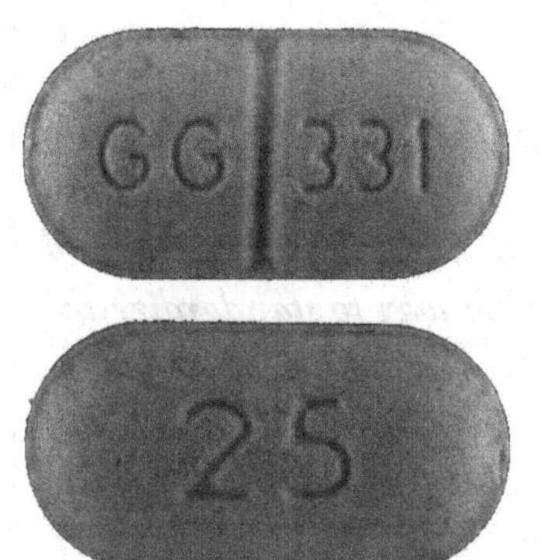

Thyroxine Pill contains T4-only, courtesy of the National Institute of Health and wikimedia commons.

We use exclusively natural thyroid pills in our office, and a few times every day, I find myself explaining why natural thyroid is superior to Synthroid. In this article, we will explain why natural thyroid tablets are better than synthetic T4 only tablets, also called Synthroid.

How Does Synthroid Differ From Natural Thyroid?

Synthroid contains Thyroxine also called T4, which is the same hormone produced by the thyroid gland. Levothyroxine is a generic form of Synthroid. Strictly speaking, Synthroid is bio-identical, even though it is synthetic. Natural Thyroid pills are made from desiccated porcine (pig) thyroid glands which contain Thyroxine (T4), T3, T2, T1 and Calcitonin.

Economics of Thyroid Pills and Synthroid

As of 2005, 10 million people in the U.S. take thyroxine. When one considers that Abbott's Synthroid is the most popular form of thyroxine, and the second-most prescribed drug in the U.S., one starts to understand the financial rivalry between Synthroid and natural thyroid competitors.(4)

What Does Mainstream Medicine Say?

Here is a typical response to a question from a reader on a popular medical information web site called www.Medicine.net. The reader's question is: "*Dear Doctor, what is your feeling regarding natural vs. synthetic replacement therapy in hypothyroid situations? Say for example, Armour vs. Synthroid?*"

The Mainstream Doctor's Answer from Medicine.net:

"While it is reasonable to assume that synthetic medications are less desirable than natural counterparts, in this case—natural thyroid hormone replacement is definitely not an ideal solution for the vast majority of people.

Here's why: *Armour thyroid is derived from desiccated pig (porcine) thyroid gland. A number of years ago, these natural preparations were our only alternative. Replacement with desiccated thyroid creates dosing problems because there is no way to standardize the exact amount of the dose for each batch. As a matter of fact, these preparations do not report their dosage strength in milligrams, but rather, in grains of thyroid. This is because; they don't really know the milligram equivalent in each dose. Dosing is also based on the assumptions that each gland has equal amounts of hormones as the next gland, and that the ratio of T4 and T3 (the more active hormone) are similar and constant in each gland from the pigs. There is no way to be certain of this, and patients on these preparations often have fluctuating hormone levels, which may or may not result in symptoms.*

Regardless of symptoms, the goal of replacement therapy is to keep the hormone levels as stable as possible. This is much easier to achieve with synthetic preparations such as Levoxyl and Synthroid. These preparations come in a vast number of standardized doses, allowing for minute adjustments in hormone dosing. There is another comment that should be made. With all the issues surrounding "mad cow disease" and other ailments, I personally am reluctant to offer animal based therapy to patients when a safe effective well studied synthetic preparation is widely available. I hope this helps answer any questions you may have. Thank you for your question.

From the Medical Author: The Mainstream Doctor M.D.

"Natural Thyroid is Not an Ideal Solution"?!!!!

This nonsense really makes my blood boil and my eyes pop out of head. Let's start by doing a little research. If the above doctor's answer is true, we should expect to find that the FDA **HAS NEVER** recalled Synthroid because of problems with stability or potency, and we would expect that the FDA **HAS** recalled natural thyroid pills because they are unstable, and vary in potency. So let's ask the FDA about this. What do we find? In reality, the FDA says Synthroid is unstable and varies in potency, while natural thyroid from RLC labs HAS NEVER been recalled for instability or variation in potency. (6)

Is Synthroid a Reliable and Stable Drug?

No, Says the FDA. Synthroid was marketed in 1955, but not FDA approved until July 24, 2002 because of a "*history of potency failures . . . which indicates that **Synthroid has not been reliably potent and stable.***"—United States Food and Drug Administration Letter to Synthroid Manufacturer, Knoll Pharmaceuticals, April 26, 2001. (1)

Unstable, not of Consistent Potency from Lot to Lot

FDA document dated August 14, 1997, Docket No. 97N-0314:
"The drug substance levothyroxine sodium (also called Synthroid) is unstable in the presence of light, temperature, air, and humidity. Unless the manufacturing process can be carefully and consistently controlled, orally administered levothyroxine sodium products may not be fully potent through the labeled expiration date, or be of consistent potency from lot to lot. There is evidence from recalls, adverse drug experience reports, and inspection reports that even when a physician consistently prescribes the same brand of orally administered levothyroxine sodium, patients may receive products of variable potency at a given dose. Such variations in product potency present actual safety and effectiveness concerns. However, no currently marketed orally administered levothyroxine sodium product has been shown to demonstrate consistent potency and stability and, thus, no currently marketed orally administered levothyroxine sodium product is generally recognized as safe and effective. "end quote from the FDA. FDA Document [Federal Register: August 14, 1997 (Volume 62, Number 157)][Notices][Page 43535-43538]

Armour Thyroid Pill Recall 2005

To be completely fair, there was a recall of Armour thyroid in 2005. Lots manufactured in 2003 were found to have lost potency 2 years later in 2005, so Forest Labs recalled all tablets made in 2003. Since it was 2 years later, very little product from these lots was still in distribution, so it was actually a small recall. (9-10)

Change in Armour Formulation

Armour changed their thyroid tablet formulation in 2009, and we have seen reports from patients who are not happy with the new formulation. To avoid any questions, we use exclusively Naturethroid from RLC labs. After five years of clinical experience with Naturethroid from RLC labs, I can fully endorse the product as an excellent form of thyroid medication.

Naturethroid Manufacturer Speaks Out: Natural vs. Synthetic

The makers of Naturethroid say this:

> *In contrast to Naturally Desiccated Thyroid (NDT) containing T3 and T4, most synthetic medications contain T4 (or T3) only. In reality, many patients don't start to feel normal again until they switch from synthetic to NDT (Thyroid USP). Natural Desiccated Thyroid hormone replacement has been used since the late 1800s, and it is one of the safest drugs available. It contains a full spectrum of thyroid hormones, T4 and T3 and also T2 and T1 as well."*
>
> *"The typical indication by the proponents of synthetic T4 is that NDT is unstable and inconsistent in its dosage. However, under the full USP monograph of both Thyroid USP as an ingredient and Thyroid USP Tablet as a finished product establishing full prescription status, this conventional argument could not be further from the truth. Unlike Nature-Throid™ and Westhroid™, synthetic medications have often been recalled due to batch inconsistencies. Yet most doctors are led to believe that desiccated thyroid is unstable.*

> *To ensure that Nature-Throid™ and Westhroid™ Thyroid USP tablets are consistently potent from tablet to tablet and lot to lot, analytical tests are performed on the raw material (Thyroid USP powder) and on the actual tablets (finished product) to measure actual T4 and T3 activity." Quoted from RLC Labs Web Site.(3)(11)*

By the way, contrary to the Medicine.net comment above, natural thyroid tablets are labeled in milligrams. One Grain tablets contain 65 mg of desiccated thyroid.

Conversion of T4 to T3

A common problem for many patients who don't feel well on Synthroid is the inability to convert T4 to T3. Synthroid contains T4 which is inactive, and must be converted to T3 by the body for it to work. This conversion is done by a de-iodinase enzyme, which is a selenoprotein. In patients with selenium deficiency, this enzyme is not working properly, and many of these patients have an inability to convert T4 to T3. Selenium supplementation is useful here. In my experience, most patients feel much better, with more energy, and relief of symptoms when switching from Synthroid to a natural thyroid such as Naturethroid.

Important Point:
Natural thyroid medication is clinically superior to T4-only thyroid such as levothyroxine and Synthroid.

Mary Shomon on Natural Thyroid vs. Synthetic

An article by Mary Shomon in the Townsend letter explains why natural thyroid treatment is better, that Synthroid and Levothyroxine are unstable, with dosage varying according to batch, and subjected to multiple recalls. (1) Natural thyroid from RLC labs has never been recalled and is the preferred solution. Mary Shomon's blog is an excellent resource on natural thyroid.(6)(10)(12)

Can I Get Mad Cow Disease from My Pig Thyroid Pill?

Millions of Americans have enjoyed ham sandwiches and pork products for decades without a single case of Mad Cow Disease ever reported. This essentially invalidates the fear of Mad Cow Disease as an argument. However, Mary Shomon advises caution with over-the-counter glandular supplements, which may contain unregulated meat products from areas of Europe known to have mad cow infected livestock. (12)

Stop the Thyroid Madness

Another excellent resource is the Stop Your Thyroid Madness Blog and Book by Janie Bowthorpe. Janie suffered for years with low thyroid symptoms even while on Synthroid, and had a dramatic recovery after converting from Synthroid to natural thyroid. Her book makes a strong statement as an advocate for natural thyroid medication.(14)

Our Program:

For diagnosis of a low thyroid condition, a lengthy questionnaire is used. This reviews over 70 symptoms of the low thyroid condition. In addition, lab testing includes a complete thyroid blood panel with TSH, free T3 and free T4, Thyroid antibodies. Physical examination includes measurement of reflex time. Also included is a basal body temperature chart filled out by the patient at home. We also measure serum selenium and spot urinary iodine levels, and supplement when found low. Both tests are widely available at the larger national labs. Once it has been determined that thyroid hormone is likely to be beneficial, a trial of low dose Nature-Throid from RLC labs is started with a Half Grain (32.5 mg) tablet every other morning.

A log book is kept by the patient describing benefits of increased energy, clarity of mind, etc, or adverse effects such as palpitations, feeling of warmth, anxiety or insomnia. At the end of a week, the log book is reviewed to determine if the thyroid was of benefit.

We have found that monitoring symptoms with a log book, and the Half Grain gradual increments in thyroid dosage every two to three weeks makes this program very safe. In the event of rapid heart rate or palpitations, the patient is instructed to hold the daily dosage of thyroid medication and inform the physician. This program is also excellent for switching patients from Synthroid to Natural Thyroid with patients invariably reporting dramatic improvement afterwards.

Instead of Natural Thyroid, Why Not Use Cytomel and Synthroid Together?

Cytomel is T3 and Synthroid is T4, so why not use the two together? The Cytomel provides the missing T3 to make a combination that is closer to the Natural Thyroid. Some patients arrive at my office having been given this combination from the doctor. The advantage for the prescribing doctor is that both items, Synthroid and Cytomel are available at the corner drugstore, whereas natural thyroid is available from a compounding pharmacy. Natural Thyroid is still the preferred choice. Among other missing ingredients, the Synthroid and Cytomel lacks Calcitonin which is present in natural thyroid, and usually lacking in patients after thyroidectomy. Giving back the missing Calcitonin makes sense, and patients usually feel better.

References for Chapter 3. Why Natural Thyroid is Better than Synthetic

(1) http://findarticles.com/p/articles/mi_m0ISW/is_2002_Feb-March/ai_82881784/?tag=content;col1 Treating hypothyroidism naturally, Townsend Letter for Doctors and Patients, Feb-March, 2002 by Sunny Willmington, Howard Hagglund, and Mary Shomon—Natural vs. Synthetic Thyroid

(2) http://thyroid.about.com/cs/synthroidlawsuit/a/settlement.htm The Synthroid Settlement: Fair Payoff or Patient Ripoff? By Mary Shomon, About.com December 14, 2003

(3) http://www.wes-throid.com/vs.asp Westthroid—Natural vs Synthetic Thyroid

(4) http://pubs.acs.org/cen/coverstory/83/8325/8325thyroxine.html Chemical and Engineering News. The Top Pharmaceuticals That Changed The World Vol. 83, Issue 25 (6/20/05) Today, more than 10 million people in the U.S. take thyroxine. Synthroid, manufactured by Abbott Laboratories and the most popular brand of thyroxine, is the second-most prescribed drug in the U.S.

(5) http://www.thecompounder.com/alternative-treatments/hormone-imbalance/thyroid/armour-thyroid-synthroid-a-thyroid-madness Larry Frieders, the compounder, THYROID MADNESS DEFINITION:

(6) http://www.thyroid-info.com/articles/synthroidproblems.htm Synthroid Has a Long History of Problems, Says FDA In Denying Synthroid's Request for Special Approval Status, FDA's Scathing Letter Outlines History of Subpotent Product, Inconsistency and Poor Stability by Mary Shomon

(7) http://www.medicinenet.com/script/main/art.asp?articlekey=17253 Medicine net web site

(8) http://www.naturalthyroidchoices.com/FDANT.html What's up with desiccated thyroid & the FDA?

(9) http://www.life-enhancement.com/article_template.asp?id=907 Between 1991 and 1997, there were ten recalls of synthetic T4, involving over 100 million tablets.9 In nine of these recalls, the tablets had been found to be subpotent, or they were losing their potency before their expiration date; in the tenth recall, the tablets were found to be too potent. Source: Federal Register 62, No. 157, 14 August 1997, pp. 43535-8.

(10) http://thyroid.about.com/od/thyroiddrugstreatments/a/recall2005.htm What Forest found in recent sample testing was that there were several lots of Armour Thyroid that were not maintaining full potency.

(11) http://www.nature-throid.com/vs.asp Unlike Nature-Throid™ and Westhroid™, synthetic medications have often been recalled due to batch inconsistencies.

(12) http://www.thyroid-info.com/articles/madcow.htm Is There A Real Risk of Mad Cow Disease from Armour Thyroid? An Update on Armour Thyroid and Glandulars by Mary Shomon

(13) http://www.altsupportthyroid.org/dt/dtrefs.php Desiccated Thyroid References

(14) Stop the Thyroid Madness: A Patient Revolution Against Decades of Inferior Treatment. Janie A. Bowthorpe. Grape Publishing (2008)

CHAPTER 4

Why Natural Thyroid is Better than Synthroid, Part Two

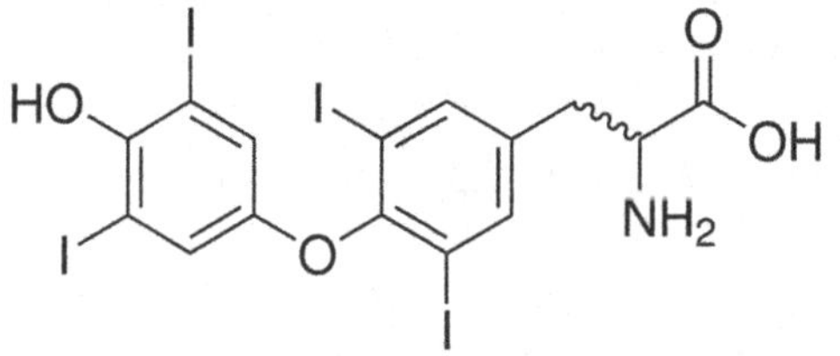

Thyroxine Chemical structure, courtesy of Wikimedia commons

Will Thyroid Medication Give Me Osteoporosis?

New concerns were raised by Dr. Marci Turner in the April 2011 British Medical Journal reporting elderly women on Synthroid(tm) have increased fracture risk.(13) Note: Synthroid is a T4-only medication, also called thyroxine or levothyroxine. A 2010 report by Murphy looked at thyroid function and fracture risk in normal postmenopausal women, and they found a 35% increase in fracture risk in women with lower TSH values (TSH=thyroid stimulating hormone). (1) Higher TSH was protective of fracture.

No Real Consensus on The Issue

To add confusion to the issue, a 2003 meta-analysis by Schneider reviewed 63 studies looking at the effect of thyroid medication (T4-only) on bone mineral density, finding no real consensus and concluding that, "*currently debate still exists about the effects of thyroid hormone therapy on skeletal integrity, that is the safety of levothyroxine use with respect to bone mineral density.*" (14)(15) Let us take a look at this issue and try to come up with some real answers.

The Calcitonin Connection

The thyroid gland not only makes thyroid hormone. It also makes Calcitonin, a hormone manufactured by the parafollicular cells (C cells) imbedded in the thyroid tissue. (24) Calcitonin is involved in calcium metabolism, bone maintenance and prevents osteoporosis.

Thyroid Disorders Cause Destruction of Calcitonin Cells

Hashimoto's Thyroiditis is a common cause of hypothyroidism and is associated with destruction of the C-cells with loss of Calcitonin production. (2-4) The resulting Calcitonin deficiency is a potential cause of bone resorption and osteoporosis. (7-12) On the other hand, treatment with Calcitonin nasal spray is an FDA approved treatment for osteoporosis and is shown to increase bone density. (16)

Hashimoto's, Radio-Iodine and Surgery all Destroy Calcitonin Cells

All three, the autoimmune process of Hashimoto's Thyroiditis, Radioactive Iodine ablation and Thyroid surgical ablation, serve to reduce or eliminate thyroid function, and the C-cells which make Calcitonin get knocked out as well. Synthroid, levothyroxine, and T4-only medications do not provide the missing Calcitonin. One would expect the Calcitonin deficient patient to be at greater risk for osteoporosis and fracture. Unlike Synthroid and T4-only medications which **DO NOT** contain Calcitonin, natural desiccated thyroid pills **DO CONTAIN** Calcitonin, providing the missing hormone, and is the preferred form of thyroid medication.

Oral Absorption of Porcine Calcitonin

Since Calcitonin is a small peptide, it is subject to degradation and digestion when taken by the oral route. To avoid the oral route, Porcine Calcitonin is given as intramuscular injection, and salmon Calcitonin which is 25 times more potent is given as intranasal spray. Newer Calcitonin formulations use some type of carrier to allow for oral dosing. Studies show that oral absorption of Calcitonin is a small fraction of the ingested dose, about 0.022%, yet even this small amount has a physiologic effect with a drop in serum calcium observed.(41) How much Calcitonin is in a One Grain natural thyroid pill? We don't know the exact amount. Obviously, further medical research in this area is needed.

None of the Studies Used Natural Desiccated Thyroid

Unfortunately, all of the medical studies of the bone density-thyroid connection used T4-only medication, none used desiccated natural thyroid, so we don't have any studies to evaluate the long term lack of osteoporosis from natural desiccated thyroid. NIH funded research is needed to evaluate bone density and fracture risk for natural desiccated thyroid compared to T4-only medications. Will this ever take place? Don't hold your breath. The NIH is a government agency, and the government is influenced by Big Pharma dollars, so natural is out and synthetic is in. We may never see NIH funding for research on natural desiccated thyroid.

The TSH Connection, TSH is Protective and Prevents Bone Resorption

Advances in our understanding of physiology and animal research have revealed TSH hormone (thyroid stimulating hormone) has a direct effect on bone cells, preventing degradation of bone and bone resorption, and therefore protective of bone density.(17-19) This could explain the many studies that find a correlation between higher TSH and improved bone density. The problem with using TSH as a treatment for osteoporosis is that higher TSH is associated with increased heart disease (see the HUNT study), as well as a host of low thyroid symptoms of fatigue, malaise, muscle aches and pains etc.(25) Patients feel better with a lower TSH and higher thyroid function, so cutting back on thyroid medication to let the TSH drift up may be good for bone density, but it is not good for the patient.

Good News About Bioidentical Hormones

The good news is that the TSH effect on bone density is relatively modest and is offset by the addition of estrogen, a bioidentical hormone, which increases bone density. (20) In addition, we routinely employ a natural bone building program. One of the interventions is to measure and optimize vitamin D levels which protects and maintains bone density. In my experience with our TrueMedMD clinic patients using natural thyroid and bioidentical hormones, we have seen only benefits with increasing bone density, and no observed cases of osteoporosis.

In conclusion, an excellent reason to switch from T4-only thyroid medication to natural desiccated thyroid is because it contains Calcitonin, protective of bone density and preventive of osteoporosis. T4-only medication does not contain Calcitonin and is associated with loss of bone density and increased fracture risk. We have found good clinical results with a natural desiccated thyroid product called Naturethroid from RLC labs. Dosage range is from one to four Grains per day depending on underlying thyroid function and body weight. We pay close attention to clinical symptom resolution during the follow up period. For lab monitoring, we follow the advice of Jonathan Wright MD who advocates the use of the serum Free T3 test, as more useful than the TSH test.

References for Chapter 4, Why Natural Thyroid is Better than Synthetic Part Two

(1) http://www.ncbi.nlm.nih.gov/pubmed/20410228
J Clin Endocrinol Metab. 2010 Jul;95(7):3173-81. Epub 2010 Apr 21. Thyroid function within the upper normal range is associated with reduced bone mineral density and an increased risk of nonvertebral fractures in healthy euthyroid postmenopausal women. Murphy E et al.

(2) http://www.ncbi.nlm.nih.gov/pubmed/9669288
Thyroid. 1998 Jun;8(6):505-9. Quantitative analysis of C cells in Hashimoto's thyroiditis. Lima MA, Santos BM, Borges MF. Brazil.

(3) http://www.ncbi.nlm.nih.gov/pubmed/9797849
Calcitonin deficiency in early stages of chronic autoimmune thyroiditis Borges MF, Abelin NM, Menezes FO, Dahia PL, Toledo SP. Department of Medicine, Federal School of Medicine of Triângulo Mineiro, Uberaba, Brazil.

(4) http://www.ncbi.nlm.nih.gov/pubmed/10646660
Thyroid. 1999 Dec;9(12):1211-4. Calcitonin reserve in different

stages of atrophic autoimmune thyroiditis. Poppe K, Verbruggen LA, Velkeniers B, Finné E, Body JJ, Vanhaelst L.

(5) http://www.ncbi.nlm.nih.gov/pubmed/11327616
Thyroid. 2001 Mar;11(3):249-55. One-year prophylactic treatment of euthyroid Hashimoto's thyroiditis patients with levothyroxine: is there a benefit? Padberg S et al.

(6) http://www.ncbi.nlm.nih.gov/pubmed/16006728
Endocr J. 2005 Jun;52(3):337-43. Effects of prophylactic thyroid hormone replacement in euthyroid Hashimoto's thyroiditis. Aksoy DY, Kerimoglu U, Okur H, Canpinar H, Karaagaoglu E, Yetgin S, Kansu E, Gedik O. Source Section of Endocrinology and Metabolism, Department of Internal Medicine, Hacettepe University, Ankara, Turkey.

(7) http://endo.endojournals.org/cgi/content/full/147/9/4007
Endocrinology Vol. 147, No. 9 4007-4009 Calcitonin—Guardian of the Mammalian Skeleton or Is It Just a Fish Story? Scott Miller

(8) http://endo.endojournals.org/cgi/content/abstract/147/9/4010?ijkey=bd61473312d62e7a5ef50cedc6ef1baa19c21cf3&keytype2=tf_ipsecsha
Endocrinology Vol. 147, No. 9 4010-4021 Calcitonin Plays a Critical Role in Regulating Skeletal Mineral Metabolism during Lactation. Janine P. Woodrow, Christopher J. Sharpe, Neva J. Fudge, Ana O. Hoff, Robert F. Gagel and Christopher S. Kovacs

(9) http://www.ncbi.nlm.nih.gov/pmc/articles/PMC2680171/
J Bone Miner Res. 2008 August; 23(8): 1182-1193. Calcitonin Receptor Plays a Physiological Role to Protect Against Hypercalcemia in Mice. Rachel A Davey et al.

(10) http://www.ncbi.nlm.nih.gov/pubmed/10230474
Acta Med Austriaca. 1999;26(1):29-31. Possible effect of calcitonin deficiency on bone mass after subtotal thyroidectomy. Mirzaei S, Krotla G, Knoll P, Koriska K, Köhn H.

(11) http://www.ncbi.nlm.nih.gov/pubmed/15258552
Minerva Endocrinol. 2004 Mar;29(1):1-10. [Bone density and mineral metabolism in calcitonin-deficiency patients]. CONCLUSION: The results of this study show that the chronic lack of calcitonin in total thyroidectomized patients may play a role in increased bone degradation and osteopenia with a higher risk of bone fracture.

(12) http://www.ncbi.nlm.nih.gov/pubmed/1929193
Ann Endocrinol (Paris). 1991;52(2):109-12. [Chronic autoimmune thyroiditis and C-cell hyperplasia. Study of calcitonin secretion in 24 patients].[Article in French]Barbot N, Guyetant S, Beldent V, Akrass A, Cerf I, Perdrisot R, Bigorgne JC.

(13) http://www.bmj.com/content/342/bmj.d2238.full
BMJ 2011; 342:d2238 Levothyroxine dose and risk of fractures in older adults: nested case-control study. Marci R Turner et al.

(14) http://www.ncbi.nlm.nih.gov/pubmed/14714266
Exp Clin Endocrinol Diabetes. 2003 Dec;111(8):455-70. The effect of levothyroxine therapy on bone mineral density: a systematic review of the literature. Schneider R, Reiners C.

(15) http://thyroid.about.com/cs/osteoporosis/a/osteoporosis_2.htm Is Thyroid Medication Going to Give You Osteoporosis? Experts Evaluate the Risks
What Does this Mean for Patients? Mary J. Shomon and Dr. William Cline March 2004

(16) http://www.ncbi.nlm.nih.gov/pubmed/11874243
J Bone Miner Res. 2002 Mar;17(3):521-7. A randomized trial of nasal spray salmon calcitonin in men with idiopathic osteoporosis: effects on bone mineral density and bone markers. Trovas GP, Lyritis GP, Galanos A, Raptou P, Constantelou E.

(17) http://www.ncbi.nlm.nih.gov/pubmed/20151763
Endocr Regul. 2010 Jan;44(1):9-15. The level of TSH appeared favourable in maintaining bone mineral density in postmenopausal

women. Baqi L, Payer J, Killinger Z, Susienkova K, Jackuliak P, Cierny D, Langer P.

(18) http://www.ncbi.nlm.nih.gov/pubmed/15746993
J Bone Miner Res. 2005 Mar;20(3):480-6. Epub 2004 Nov 29. Recombinant human TSH modulates in vivo C-telopeptides of type-1 collagen and bone alkaline phosphatase, but not osteoprotegerin production in postmenopausal women monitored for differentiated thyroid carcinoma. Mazziotti G, Sorvillo F, Piscopo M, Cioffi M, Pilla P, Biondi B, Iorio S, Giustina A, Amato G,

(19) http://www.ncbi.nlm.nih.gov/pubmed/19548061
J Bone Miner Metab. 2010;28(1):35-41. The effects of recombinant human TSH on bone turnover in patients after thyroidectomy. Karga H, Papaioannou G, Polymeris A, Papamichael K, Karpouza A, Samouilidou E, Papaioannou P.

(20) http://www.ncbi.nlm.nih.gov/pubmed/8563472
Thyroid. 1995 Oct;5(5):359-63. Effect of estrogen replacement therapy upon bone mineral density in thyroxine-treated postmenopausal women with a past history of thyrotoxicosis. Franklyn JA, Betteridge J, Holder R, Sheppard MC.

(21) http://www.ncbi.nlm.nih.gov/pubmed/2375563
Accelerated Bone Loss in Hypothyroid Patients Overtreated with L-Thyroxine Annals of Internal Medicine August 15, 1990 vol. 113 no. 4 265-269 Glenn M. Stall, MD; Susan Harris, MS; Lori J. Sokoll, MCC; and Bess Dawson-Hughes, MD

(22) http://www.ncbi.nlm.nih.gov/pubmed/14727010
Osteoporos Int. 2004 Mar;15(3):209-16. Epub 2004 Jan 16. Restoration of euthyroidism accelerates bone turnover in patients with subclinical hypothyroidism: a randomized controlled trial.

(23) http://www.ncbi.nlm.nih.gov/pubmed/9156039
Clin Endocrinol (Oxf). 1997 Mar;46(3):301-7. Longitudinal changes of bone mineral density and bone turnover in postmenopausal women on thyroxine. Guo CY, Weetman AP, Eastell R.

(24) http://vet.sagepub.com/content/27/6/445.long
Veterinary Pathology November 1990 vol. 27 no. 6 445-452
Immunocytochemistry of Thyroid C-Cell Complexes in Dogs B. LEBLANCG, PAULUSM, ANDREUA, ND M. C. BONNET

(25) http://jeffreydach.com/2008/10/12/hunt-study-shows-thyroid-prevents-heart-attacks-by-jeffrey-dach-md.aspx
Hunt Study Shows Thyroid Prevents Heart Attacks by Jeffrey Dach MD

(26) http://www.ncbi.nlm.nih.gov/pubmed/20429634
Endocr Regul. 2010 Apr;44(2):57-63. Thyrotropin versus thyroid hormone in regulating bone density and turnover in premenopausal women. Baqi L, Payer J, Killinger Z, Hruzikova P, Cierny D, Susienkova K, Langer P.

(27) http://www.ncbi.nlm.nih.gov/pubmed/20688622
Hormones (Athens). 2010 Jul-Sep;9(3):245-52. Combined therapy with L-thyroxine and L-triiodothyronine compared to L-thyroxine alone in the treatment of primary hypothyroidism. Fadeyev VV, Morgunova TB, Melnichenko GA, Dedov II.

(28) http://www.ncbi.nlm.nih.gov/pubmed/11095447
J Clin Endocrinol Metab. 2000 Nov;85(11):4157-61.
Persistent increase in bone turnover in Graves' patients with subclinical hyperthyroidism.
Kumeda Y, Inaba M, Tahara H, Kurioka Y, Ishikawa T, Morii H, Nishizawa Y.

(29) http://www.ncbi.nlm.nih.gov/pubmed/15278189
J Formos Med Assoc. 2004 Jun;103(6):442-7. Bone mineral density in women receiving thyroxine suppressive therapy for differentiated thyroid carcinoma. Chen CH et al.

(30) http://www.ncbi.nlm.nih.gov/pubmed/16834835
Curr Med Res Opin. 2006 Jul;22(7):1369-73. Changes of bone mineral density in pre-menopausal women with differentiated thyroid cancer receiving L-thyroxine suppressive therapy. Mazokopakis EE, Starakis IK, Papadomanolaki MG, Batistakis AG, Papadakis JA.

(31) http://www.ncbi.nlm.nih.gov/pubmed/12803168
Ann Intern Med. 2001 Apr 3;134(7):561-8. Risk for fracture in women with low serum levels of thyroid-stimulating hormone. Bauer DC, Ettinger B, Nevitt MC, Stone KL

(32) http://www.ncbi.nlm.nih.gov/pubmed/19892039?dopt=Abstract
Bone. 2010 Mar;46(3):747-51. Epub 2009 Nov 3.
Serum TSH values and risk of vertebral fractures in euthyroid post-menopausal women with low bone mineral density. Mazziotti G, Porcelli T, Patelli I, Vescovi PP, Giustina A.
SourceDepartment of Medical and Surgical Sciences, University of Brescia, Italy.

(33) http://www.ncbi.nlm.nih.gov/pubmed/7891045?dopt=Abstract
J Intern Med. 1995 Mar;237(3):241-7. Hip fractures and the thyroid: a case-control study. Wejda B, Hintze G, Katschinski B, Olbricht T, Benker G.

(34) http://www.ncbi.nlm.nih.gov/pubmed/9579237
Clin Endocrinol (Oxf). 1998 Feb;48(2):229-34. Effect of replacement doses of thyroxine on bone mineral density. Hanna FW, Pettit RJ, Ammari F, Evans WD, Sandeman D, Lazarus JH.

(35) http://www.ncbi.nlm.nih.gov/pubmed/15555712
J Affect Disord. 2004 Dec;83(2-3):183-90. Bone mineral density during maintenance treatment with supraphysiological doses of levothyroxine in affective disorders: a longitudinal study.
Bauer M et al.

(36) http://www.ncbi.nlm.nih.gov/pubmed/11578671
J Affect Disord. 2001 Oct;66(2-3):185-91. Bone mineral density in pre-and post-menopausal women with affective disorder treated with long-term L-thyroxine augmentation. Gyulai L, Bauer Metal.

(37) http://www.ncbi.nlm.nih.gov/pubmed/14748891
J Clin Pharm Ther. 2004 Feb;29(1):1-5. Effects of levothyroxine suppressive therapy on bone mineral density in premenopausal women.

Larijani B, Gharibdoost F, Pajouhi M, Sadjadi A, Aghakhani S, Eshraghian R, Akrami SM, Maalouf G.

(38) http://www.ncbi.nlm.nih.gov/pubmed/7647577
Thyroid. 1995 Apr;5(2):81-7. Possible limited bone loss with suppressive thyroxine therapy is unlikely to have clinical relevance. Müller CG, Bayley TA, Harrison JE, Tsang R.

(39) http://www.ncbi.nlm.nih.gov/pubmed/16322336
Endocr Relat Cancer. 2005 Dec;12(4):973-81. Lack of deleterious effect on bone mineral density of long-term thyroxine suppressive therapy for differentiated thyroid carcinoma. Reverter JL, Holgado S, Alonso N, Salinas I, Granada ML,

(40) http://www.ncbi.nlm.nih.gov/pubmed/11698925
Medscape Womens Health. 2001 Oct;6(5):3. Bone loss in premenopausal women on long-term suppressive therapy with thyroid hormone. Sijanovic S, Karner I.

(41) http://www.ncbi.nlm.nih.gov/pubmed/8587058
Utility of pharmacodynamic measures for assessing the oral bioavailability of peptides. 1. Administration of recombinant salmon calcitonin in rats. Patrick J. Sinko1 et al. J Pharm Sci. 1995 Nov;84(11):1374-8. The absorption of rsCT after id. (Duodenal) administration was low (0.022%); however, a significant lowering of serum calcium concentrations was observed.

CHAPTER 5

The Thyroid Nodule Epidemic

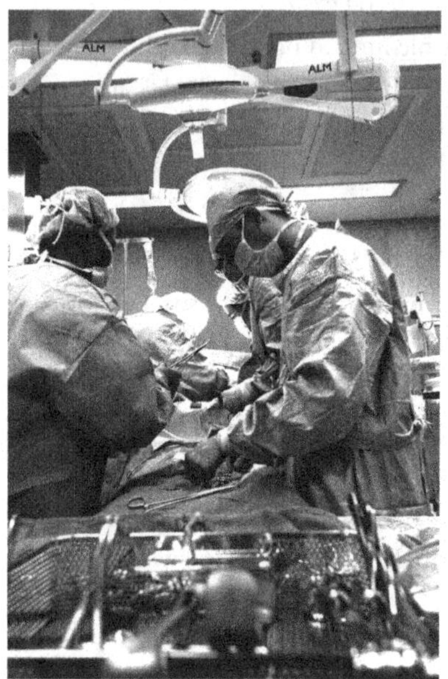
Thyroid Surgery, U.S. Navy photo by Journalist Seaman Joseph Caballero, courtesy of Wikimedia Commons

A 36 Year Old Female With Hypothyroidism After Thyroidectomy For Thyroid Cancer

Lisa, a 36 year old model and actress, arrived in my office and told me her story. Ever since her thyroidectomy for cancer, she has had symptoms of severe fatigue, muscle pain, hair loss, and dry skin. The small dose of Synthroid prescribed by her endocrinologist doesn't seem to be helping. Four years ago, Lisa's family doctor palpated her thyroid gland, thought he felt a nodule and sent her for thyroid ultrasound, "just to be sure". The thyroid ultrasound images showed a small nodule about 9 mm in size, and the doctors recommended ultrasound guided needle biopsy, "just to be sure". About a week after the biopsy, the pathology report came back with a diagnosis of "papillary carcinoma of the thyroid".

Lisa is Told She Has Thyroid Cancer—Undergoes Thyroidectomy

As you can imagine, Lisa became upset and distraught when she learned from the doctor that she had thyroid cancer. "*Not to worry*", said her doctor, "*You have an excellent prognosis and a high likelihood for cure after surgery followed by radioactive Iodine treatment.*" Grateful that she had a treatable cancer with a good prognosis, Lisa underwent the surgery and radiation. Since the surgery completely removed her thyroid gland, she later required thyroid medication every day. She also needed periodic screening tests to check for cancer recurrence.

Unfortunately, Lisa was not spared the adverse effects of her treatment. The surgery had disturbed her recurrent laryngeal nerve leaving her with a chronic hoarseness, cough and voice change. The surgery also removed the parathyroid glands leaving her at risk for osteoporosis. The radioactive iodine treatment caused salivary gland damage, leaving her with a chronic dry mouth and bad taste. The radioactive Iodine also carried an increased generalized cancer risk over her lifetime, and of course, detrimental effect on fertility in the future when Lisa decides to have a family.

Switching from Synthroid to Natural Thyroid

I explained to Lisa that her symptoms of hypothyroidism were due to the miniscule dose of Synthroid, which was not enough to relieve her low thyroid symptoms. In addition, Synthroid, which contains only T4, does not completely replace the function of her missing thyroid gland. A natural thyroid medication made from desiccated porcine thyroid gland containing T3, T4 and Calcitonin is a far better alternative. Lisa was switched over to her natural thyroid medication, called NatureThroid from RLC labs, along with Iodine supplementation, and 3 weeks later called the office to report a dramatic improvement with relief of chronic fatigue and improved energy levels.

A Cancer with No Biological Significance

For twenty years as an interventional radiologist, my job was to perform ultrasound needle biopsies of small thyroid nodules sent into the hospital by primary care doctors. The vast majority of thyroid cancers found with ultrasound scanning and needle biopsy are the small papillary carcinoma, a relatively benign tumor with excellent prognosis (30 year survival rate 95%). (1)

A Frustrated Radiologist Says: Turn Off the Ultrasound Machines

An exasperated radiologist, John J. Cronan, MD says in the June 2008 issue of Radiology, "*we should turn off the ultrasound machines*". Dr. Cronan questions this entire medical enterprise of detecting thyroid nodules, and small cancers with ultrasound guided biopsy. "*From the patient perspective, we have hung the psychological stigma of cancer on these patients and the dependency for daily thyroid supplementation . . . We accept all these consequences to control a cancer with a 99% 10-year survival.*" (1-7)

A Normal Finding in Finland

Dr Harach says occult papillary carcinoma of the thyroid is a "normal" finding in Finland, and does not cause biologically significant disease. (8) Dr. Louise Davies agrees with Dr Harach, and says in JAMA, "*papillary cancers smaller than 1 cm could be classified as a normal finding*".(4)

Our Quixotic Approach to Thyroid Nodules

Keith Heller, MD, a neck surgeon who operated on 1,000 cases of thyroid cancer over a 28 year career, addressed his colleagues in a medical meeting saying: "*I do not believe that this epidemic of (thyroid cancer) is real. It is due to . . . the increasing use of ultrasound-guided needle biopsy of thyroid nodules. We may be diagnosing and treating cancers that have no clinical significance . . . We have embarked on a quixotic quest to rid our patients of microscopic and probably clinically unimportant thyroid cancer . . . . We are performing far too many unnecessary thyroidectomies.* "(3)

Important Point
Our current epidemic of thyroid cancer is not real. It is due to the use of thyroid ultrasound to diagnose and treat small, clinically unimportant "cancers".

Japan to the Rescue—Watchful Waiting

A thyroid cancer expert, Dr. Yasuhiro Ito of Kobe, Japan, has come up with a "watchful waiting" approach for papillary thyroid cancer. Dr Ito published this statement in the 2003 Thyroid Journal: "*Our preliminary data suggest that papillary microcarcinomas do not frequently become clinically apparent, and that patients can choose observation while their tumors are not progressing, although they are pathologically multifocal and involve lymph nodes in high incidence.*" Dr Ito observed 162 patients with papillary thyroid microcarcinoma (< 10 mm) over 8 years. 70% of tumors either remained stable or decreased in size. Only 10% enlarged by more than 10 mm. Only 1.2% of patients developed neck node metastasis over the 8 years observation. (26) Because of this study, Dr. Ito says the patient can opt for watchful waiting with serial ultrasound follow up studies. Dr Ito says that if follow up ultrasound shows enlarging tumor, or enlarging metastatic neck nodes, then more aggressive surgical treatment is indicated with an excellent prognosis. In another study of 52 cases, Dr Ito found when the papillary thyroid cancer is resected as a benign nodule (by mistake), even this is sufficient treatment and no further immediate surgery is needed. (28)

It's the Pathologist's Fault—Just Stop Calling It Cancer

Perhaps this whole problem is caused by incorrect terminology used by the pathologist who reviews the biopsy slide and uses the word "cancer", a word that strikes fear and creates undue stress. Once a pathology report with the word "cancer" is placed on the desk, rationality gets thrown out the window, and the patient demands aggressive treatment, usually out of proportion to the actual pathology.

In the 2003 issue of the International Journal of Surgical Pathology, Dr Rosai presented the Porto Proposal, in which he proposed a change in terminology. (23)(24) Instead of the word, "cancer", he suggested the terminology, papillary microtumor. Others (Hazard et al.) proposed "*nonencapsulated thyroid tumor*" because "*the surgeon may become unduly alarmed when the pathologist reports the presence of carcinoma.*" (46) Harach et al. proposed the term occult papillary tumor, "in order to avoid unnecessary operations and serious psychologic effects on patients." (45)

Important Point
Most young women with "thyroid cancer" have a slow growing relatively non-aggressive type called "papillary thyroid cancer", yet receive overtreatment with thyroidectomy and radioactive iodine.

Is Treatment of Papillary Micro-Carcinoma Overly Aggressive?

Over the years, we have seen surgical treatment for breast cancer evolve from the overly aggressive and debilitating radical mastectomy procedure, to the current day simple lumpectomy for many small breast cancers. Perhaps treatment for thyroid cancer is going in this same direction, and is playing "catch-up" with the more limited breast cancer treatments.

Dr Ian Hay's 2008 study published in Endocrine Abstracts followed 900 patients with papillary thyroid microcarcinoma over 54 years. Dr Ian Hay says, "*neither total thyroidectomy, nor Postoperative Radioactive Iodine Ablation, improved long term outcome during 40 years, in terms of either tumor recurrence or cause-specific mortality.*" (17) Dr Hay advocates removal of the tumor with unilateral lobectomy, saying that it was **unnecessary** to perform total thyroidectomy or radioactive iodine treatment, since they did not improve prognosis compared to unilateral thyroid lobectomy alone. (17) In the future, I predict initial treatment for small papillary cancer of the thyroid gland will evolve into a simpler procedure, namely, unilateral thyroid lobectomy, or removal or the nodule alone, without the additional treatment with radioactive iodine.

The Role of Iodine Supplementation

You might ask the obvious question, "Thyroid nodules are found in 67% of the population. What is causing this?" I would suggest that the most likely explanation is subclinical iodine deficiency in the population. Iodine deficiency causes thyroid enlargement (goiter), thyroid nodules, and thyroid cancer. Thyroid cancer appears linked to Iodine deficiency in both animal models and humans. (12) Studies have shown that iodine deficiency is associated with increased anaplastic thyroid cancer, the aggressive type unresponsive to treatment and associated with high mortality rate. (15) Population studies in which iodine supplementation was given showed reduction in mortality from thyroid cancer. (11)

References for Chapter 5. The Thyroid Nodule Epidemic

(1) http://radiology.rsnajnls.org/cgi/content/full/247/3/602
Editorials—Thyroid Nodules: Is It Time to Turn Off the US Machines? by John J. Cronan, MD June 2008 Radiology, 247, 602-604.

(2) http://jcem.endojournals.org/cgi/content/full/87/5/1938
The Journal of Clinical Endocrinology & Metabolism Vol. 87, No. 5 1938-1940. Nonpalpable Thyroid Nodules—Managing an Epidemic by Douglas S. Ross

(3) http://archotol.ama-assn.org/cgi/content/full/133/7/639
Do All Cancers Need to Be Treated? The Role of Thyroglobulin in the Management of Thyroid Cancer—The 2006 Hayes Martin Lecture—Keith S. Heller, MD. Arch Otolaryngol Head Neck Surg. 2007;133(7):639-643.

(4) http://jama.ama-assn.org/cgi/content/full/295/18/2164
Increasing Incidence of Thyroid Cancer in the United States, 1973-2002 by Louise Davies, MD, MS; H. Gilbert Welch, MD, MPH. JAMA. 2006;295:2164-2167.

(5) http://www.aafp.org/afp/20030201/559.html
Thyroid Nodules by MARY JO WELKER, M.D., and DIANE ORLOV, M.S., C.N.P. AAFP Magazine

(6) http://www.cmaj.ca/cgi/content/full/177/11/1383
CMAJ • November 20, 2007; 177 (11) Explaining the increasing incidence of differentiated thyroid cancer by Jacques How, MB ChB and Roger Tabah, MD Jacques How is with the Division of Endocrinology and Roger Tabah is with the Department of Surgery, Montreal General Hospital, McGill University Health Centre, Montréal, Que.

(7) http://jama.ama-assn.org/cgi/content/full/295/18/2179
Managing Small Thyroid Cancers by Ernest L. Mazzaferri, MD. JAMA. 2006;295:2179-2182.

(8) http://www.ncbi.nlm.nih.gov/pubmed/2408737
Cancer. 1985 Aug 1;56(3):531-8. Occult papillary carcinoma of the thyroid. A "normal" finding in Finland. A systematic autopsy study. by Harach HR, Franssila KO, Wasenius VM.

(9) http://ije.oxfordjournals.org/cgi/content/full/32/4/584
Cancer—Iodine deficiency, radiation dose, and the risk of thyroid cancer among children and adolescents in the Bryansk region of Russia following the Chernobyl power station accident by V Shakhtarin et al.

(10) http://www.ncbi.nlm.nih.gov/pubmed/12762644
Influence of iodine deficiency and iodine prophylaxis on thyroid cancer histotypes and incidence in endemic goiter area. Huszno B, Szybinski Z, Przybylik-Mazurek E, Stachura J, Trofimiuk M, Buziak-Bereza M, Golkowski F, Pantoflinski J.

(11) http://www.ncbi.nlm.nih.gov/pubmed/9349576
Thyroid. 1997 Oct;7(5):733-41. Incidence and clinical characteristics of thyroid carcinoma after iodine prophylaxis in an endemic goiter country. Bacher-Stier C et al.

(12) http://findarticles.com/p/articles/mi_m0FDN/is_2_13/ai_n27943644/
Iodine: deficiency and therapeutic considerations—Alternative Medicine Review, June, 2008 by Lyn Patrick

(13) http://www3.interscience.wiley.com/journal/112684400/abstract
The frequency of cold thyroid nodules and thyroid malignancies in patients from an iodine-deficient area by Antonino Belfiore, MD

(14) http://www.ncbi.nlm.nih.gov/pubmed/17891233
Arq Bras Endocrinol Metab vol.51 no.5 São Paulo July 2007. Relevance of iodine intake as a reputed predisposing factor for thyroid cancer

(15) http://www.ncbi.nlm.nih.gov/pubmed/18018554
Nippon Rinsho. 2007 Nov;65(11):1953-8. Epidemiology of thyroid tumors: effect of environmental iodine intake. Kasagi K. et al.

(16) http://www.ncbi.nlm.nih.gov/pubmed/19655332
Laryngoscope. 2009 Aug 4. Survival impact of treatment options for papillary microcarcinoma of the thyroid. Lin HW, Bhattacharyya N.

(17) http://www.endocrine-abstracts.org/ea/0016/ea0016P685.htm
Endocrine Abstracts (2008) 16 P685 European Congress of Endocrinology 2008 Berlin, Germany 03 May 2008—07 May 2008. Neither total thyroidectomy nor radioiodine remnant ablation improved long-term outcome in 900 patients with papillary thyroid microcarcinoma treated during 1945 through 2004. Ian Hay, Maeve Hutchinson, Megan Reinalda, Clive Grant, Bryan McIver & Geoffrey Thompson. Mayo Clinic, Rochester, Minnesota, USA.

(18) http://www.cancernetwork.com/cme/article/10165/1421632
June 11, 2009 ONCOLOGY. Vol. 23 No. 7 Areas of Confusion in Oncology. What Is the Optimal Initial Treatment of Low-Risk Papillary Thyroid Cancer (and Why Is It Controversial)? Ernest L. Mazzaferri, MD, MACP

(19) http://emedicine.medscape.com/article/849000-overview
Papillary thyroid carcinoma

(20) http://www.medscape.com/viewarticle/707327
Radioiodine for Most Papillary Thyroid Cancers Is Overtreatment, Says Expert, Zosia Chustecka Medscape Today

(21) http://cancerology.blogspot.com/2009/08/radioiodine-probably-overtreatment-for.html RADIOIODINE PROBABLY OVERTREATMENT FOR MOST THYROID CANCER PATIENTS

(22) http://www.bmj.com/cgi/eletters/338/mar13_1/b733#210607
Radiological and Cytological Burden, Dr Steve Colley, reply to Investigating the thyroid nodule by H M Mehanna,

(23) http://www.redorbit.com/news/science/34848/renaming_papillary_microcarcinoma_of_the_thyroid_gland_the_porto_proposal/ Renaming papillary microcarcinoma of the thyroid gland: The Porto proposal.

(24) http://ijs.sagepub.com/content/11/4/249.extract
Renaming Papillary Microcarcinoma of the Thyroid Gland: The Porto Proposal. Rosai et al. Int J Surg Pathol.2003; 11: 249-251.

(25) http://www.annals.org/cgi/content/full/126/3/226
Thyroid Incidentalomas: Management Approaches to Nonpalpable Nodules Discovered Incidentally on Thyroid Imaging Gerry H. Tan, MD, and Hossein Gharib, MD Annals of Internal Medicine February 1, 1997, Volume 126, Issue 3, Pages 226-231

(26) http://www.ncbi.nlm.nih.gov/pubmed/12804106
Thyroid. 2003 Apr;13(4):381-7. An observation trial without surgical treatment in patients with papillary microcarcinoma of the thyroid. Ito Y, Uruno T, Nakano K, Takamura Y, Miya A, Kobayashi K, Yokozawa T, Matsuzuka F, Kuma S, Kuma K, Miyauchi A.

(27) http://www.ncbi.nlm.nih.gov/pubmed/15490053
World J Surg. 2004 Nov;28(11):1115-21. Papillary microcarcinoma of the thyroid: how should it be treated? Ito Y et al.

(28) http://www.ncbi.nlm.nih.gov/pubmed/17465240
Anticancer Res. 2007 Mar-Apr;27(2):1039-43. Long-term follow-up for patients with papillary thyroid carcinoma treated as benign nodules. Ito Y et al.

(29) http://www.pubmedcentral.nih.gov/articlerender.fcgi?artid=1770442
J Clin Pathol. 2004 October; 57(10): 1041-1046. Papillary carcinoma of the thyroid in Japan: subclassification of common type and identification of low risk group—K Kakudo,1 W Tang,1 Y Ito et al.

(30) http://www.jpgmonline.com/article.asp?issn=0022-3859;year=2007;volume=53;issue=1;spage=23;epage=26;aulast=Sakorafas. PGM 2007, Volume: 53, Issue: 1, Page: 23-26, Post Graduate Medicine. Microscopic papillary thyroid cancer as an incidental finding in patients treated surgically for presumably benign thyroid disease. GH Sakorafas et al.

(31) http://www.ncbi.nlm.nih.gov/pubmed/17786355
Comparative genomic hybridization, BRAF, RAS, RET, and oligo-array analysis in aneuploid papillary thyroid carcinomas. Rodrigues R et al.

(32) http://www.ncbi.nlm.nih.gov/pubmed/15880523
Evidence that one subset of anaplastic thyroid carcinomas are derived from papillary carcinomas due to BRAF and p53 mutations. Quiros RM, Ding HG, Gattuso P, Prinz RA, Xu X. Department of General Surgery, Rush University Medical Center, Chicago, Illinois 60612, USA.

(33) http://www.springerlink.com/content/unl9e830025jrlwa/
Anaplastic Thyroid Carcinoma Survival. Petri E. Voutilainen1, Markku Multanen1, Reijo K. Haapiainen1, Ari K. Leppäniemi1 and Arto H. Sivula1 Second Department of Surgery, Helsinki University Central Hospital, Box 260, FIN-00029 HUCH, Helsinki, Finland, FI

(34) http://www.ncbi.nlm.nih.gov/pubmed/11742333
Surgery. 2001 Dec;130(6):1028-34. Anaplastic thyroid carcinoma: a 50-year experience at a single institution. McIver B, Hay ID, Giuffrida DF, Dvorak CE, Grant CS, Thompson GB, van Heerden JA, Goellner JR. Department of Medicine, Mayo Clinic & Foundation, Rochester, MN 55905, USA.

(35) http://www.thyroid.org/professionals/publications/news/07_10_05_kuffner.html ATA News Release 2007. Small Papillary Thyroid Cancer Is More Common and Not Without Risk than Previously Believed

(36) http://thyroid.about.com/od/thyroidcancer/a/microcarcinoma.htm
Papillary Thyroid Microcarcinoma—Do Total Thyroidectomy and/or Postoperative Radioiodine Improve the Outcome? By Mary Shomon, About.com Updated: May 09, 2008

(37) http://www.bcm.edu/oto/grand/12_04_03.htm
Papillary Thyroid Carcinoma—Grand Rounds Christopher Prichard, M.D. December 4, 2003

(38) http://www.snm.org/index.cfm?PageID=6730&RPID=7320
September 11, 2007 Thyroid Cancer Treatment May Be Overly Aggressive Reuters Health

(39) http://www.ncbi.nlm.nih.gov/pubmed/16780882
J Surg Res. 2006 Aug;134(2):160-2. Epub 2006 Jun 14. What is the biology and optimal treatment for papillary microcarcinoma of the thyroid? Cheema Y, Olson S, Elson D, Chen H.

(40) http://www.ncbi.nlm.nih.gov/pubmed/18035964
Expert Opin Pharmacother. 2007 Dec;8(18):3205-15. Appropriate treatment for asymptomatic papillary microcarcinoma of the thyroid. Ito Y

(41) http://www.ncbi.nlm.nih.gov/pubmed/17315032?
Nat Clin Pract Endocrinol Metab. 2007 Mar;3(3):240-8. A therapeutic strategy for incidentally detected papillary microcarcinoma of the thyroid. Ito Y, Miyauchi A.Department of Surgery, Kuma Hospital, Kobe, Japan.

(42) http://www.trnres.com/ebook/uploads/itocontents.pdf
Recent Advances in Thyroid Cancer Research 2006 Editors Yasuhiro Ito Akira Miyauchi Nobuyuki

(43) http://www.springerlink.com/content/uuecjwpd8tdgmxq8/fulltext.pdf?page=1 Preoperative Ultrasonographic Examination for Lymph Node Metastasis: Usefulness when Designing Lymph Node Dissection for Papillary Microcarcinoma of the Thyroid. Yasuhiro Ito April 2004

(44) http://www.springerlink.com/content/6khwgm0h98wh2h0h/
Papillary Microcarcinoma of the Thyroid: How Should It Be Treated? Yasuhiro Ito Department of Surgery, Kuma Hospital, 8-2-35 Shimoyamate-dori, Chuo-ku, 650-0011 Kobe City, Japan October 2004

(45) http://www.pubmedcentral.nih.gov/articlerender.fcgi?artid=502418
J Clin Pathol. 1991 March; 44(3): 205-207. Occult papillary

microcarcinoma of the thyroid—a potential pitfall of fine needle aspiration cytology? H R Harach, E Saravia Day, and S B Zusman

(46) http://www.ncbi.nlm.nih.gov/pubmed/15395984
J Clin Endocrinol Metab. 1949 Nov;9(11):1216-31. Nonencapsulated sclerosing tumors of the thyroid. Hazard JB, et al.

CHAPTER 6

Hunt Study Shows Thyroid Prevents Heart Attacks

In 1976, an endocrinologist named Broda Barnes MD was the first to connect low thyroid function with heart disease with his book, Hypothyroidism, the Unsuspected Illness. How did Broda Barnes discover the connection between low thyroid and heart disease? Dr. Barnes took summer vacations in Graz, Austria every year to study the autopsy files. The town of Graz had a high prevalence of thyroid disorders, and anyone in Graz who died over the past 100 years required an autopsy to determine cause of death, as mandated by the authorities. The Graz autopsy data showed that low thyroid patients survived the usual childhood infectious diseases thanks to the invention of antibiotics, yet years later, develop heart disease instead. Barnes also found that thyroid treatment was protective in preventing heart attacks, based on his own clinical experience. Likewise for diabetes, Dr. Barnes found that adding thyroid medication was beneficial at preventing the onset of vascular disease in diabetics. Again, blood tests are usually normal. New research like the Hunt Study confirms that Broda Barnes was right all along, creating a paradigm shift in thyroid treatment.

The Hunt Study—Thyroid Function and Mortality from Heart Disease

TSH is short for thyroid stimulating hormone, made by the pituitary gland. TSH actually stimulates the thyroid gland to make more thyroid hormone, and can therefore be used as a barometer of thyroid function. If thyroid function is low, the pituitary sends out more TSH to stimulate the thyroid to make more thyroid hormone. Mainstream Medicine regards the TSH as the single most important test for determining thyroid function. High TSH means low thyroid function, and a Low TSH means normal or high thyroid function.

What Did The Hunt Study Find?

The Hunt Study from the April 2008 Archives of Internal Medicine examined mortality from coronary heart disease (CHD) and TSH level.

(1-2) The authors conclude, "*The results indicate that relatively low but clinically normal thyroid function may increase the risk of fatal CHD.*" (CHD=coronary heart disease). The Hunt Study measured thyroid function with the TSH test in 17,000 women and 8,000 men with no known thyroid disease or heart disease. All patients had "normal TSH" levels meaning the TSH values were in the lab reference range of 0.5 to 3.5. The women were stratified into three groups, lower TSH, intermediate and upper TSH levels, and mortality from heart disease was recorded over an 8 year observation period.

70% Increase in Heart Disease Mortality for TSH in Upper Normal Range

The Hunt study found that group with the higher TSH had 70% increased mortality from heart disease compared to the lower TSH group. Remember all these TSH vales were in the normal lab range.

Results of the Hunt Study below:

Group	TSH range	Risk of Death from Heart Disease
Group 1	0.50-1.4	Baseline Risk
Group 2	1.5-2.4	40% Higher than Baseline
Group 3	2.5-3.5	70% Higher than Baseline

This Finding is Earthshaking!!

This means that merely by taking natural thyroid pills to reduce TSH to the low end of "normal" (0.5), one can reduce death from cardiovascular disease by 70 percent. This mortality benefit is mind boggling and far exceeds any drug intervention available. Another report from the Hunt Study published in 2007 showed that LDL cholesterol was linearly associated with TSH level. (2)

The Conclusion is Clear

The best way to normalize lipoprotein profile and reduce mortality from heart disease is to reduce TSH to the lower end of the normal range with thyroid medication. A TSH in the upper end of the normal range is associated with increased cardiovascular mortality and elevations in LDL lipo-protein measurements. A TSH at the lower end of the normal range is associated with protection from heart disease.

Important Point:
A low thyroid condition, and high TSH, dramatically increases risk for heart disease.

Statin Drugs or Thyroid to Prevent Heart Disease in Women?

Another chapter of this book discusses the issue of statin drugs for women. Decades of published statin drug studies show that statin drugs simply don't work for women, and don't reduce mortality from heart disease in women. But on the other hand, the HUNT study shows that TSH levels in the lower normal range provide a 70% reduction in heart disease mortality for women. This can be accomplished safely with inexpensive thyroid medication under a physician's supervision. So for women concerned about preventing heart disease, this is good news.

Natural Thyroid is Better

Rather than Synthroid, we prefer to use natural thyroid which is a desiccated porcine thyroid gland from RLC Labs or Armour Thyroid. The reason for this is that we have seen better clinical results with the natural thyroid preparations compared to Synthroid.

Natural Thyroid is Safer, but can Cause Adverse Effects of Palpitations

Although natural thyroid is safe, there is always the possibility of adverse effects from thyroid excess, defined as too much thyroid medication. The first sign of thyroid excess is usually a rapid heart rate at rest or perhaps palpitations at rest. We spend time with each patient discussing the adverse effects before starting patients on thyroid medication. Usually, patients will notice the heart rate going up or the heart beat sounding louder than usual as the first sign that can be easily recognized. Once recognized, the patient is instructed to stop the thyroid medication, and symptoms usually resolve within 6 hours (for natural thyroid). It is perfectly safe to stop the thyroid medication at any time, as there will be no acute changes, merely a gradual reversion to the original state that existed before starting the thyroid pills.

Some patients are very sensitive to thyroid medication and will have thyroid excess symptoms such as rapid heart rate and palpitations from small amounts of thyroid medication. These are usually the elderly with underlying heart disease and/or magnesium deficiency. Thyroid medication should be avoided in these cases. Measuring magnesium levels and magnesium supplementation is very important in patients contemplating thyroid in order to reduce the risk of cardiac excitability.

A small subset of patients initially starting thyroid will notice symptoms of thyroid excess with a rapid heart rate, and they will stop the medication for a day or two and restart at a lower dosage with no further problems. This is more common in Hashimoto's patients whose own production of thyroid hormones may fluctuate from month to month. Patients with magnesium deficiency or adrenal fatigue with low cortisol output on salivary testing will also tend to be more sensitive to small amounts of thyroid medication, so caution is advised in these groups as well.

Thyroid Excess Can Rarely Cause Atrial Fibrillation

Atrial fibrillation is a common type of cardiac arrhythmia which is more common in elderly males with underlying heart disease. However, it can happen to anyone as a result of severe thyroid excess from excessive thyroid medication. However, atrial fibrillation and thyroid excess can be avoided by spending time with the patient discussing the symptoms of thyroid excess, and the importance of stopping the thyroid medication when symptoms are first noted. Patients are instructed to monitor their heart rate and to stop the thyroid medication at the first sign of thyroid excess.

Warning:
Excessive thyroid medication can cause rapid heart rate, palpitations and in severe excess, cardiac arrhythmia such as atrial fibrillation. Magnesium deficiency can predispose to cardiac irritability. Best to avoid thyroid excess by maintaining dosage in the proper range.

Mainstream Doctors Don't Have Time To Discuss Adverse Effects

One of the reasons the mainstream conventional docs will give only a minuscule amount of Synthroid to the low thyroid patient is that they simply don't have the time to discuss thyroid excess, which is more likely if the patient is not alerted to the symptoms to watch for. In addition, mainstream medical docs don't recognize the syndromes of adrenal fatigue and magnesium deficiency, so they can run into problems with thyroid excess without understanding why, producing caution and tendency to under treat.

In patients with underlying heart disease who are prone to cardiac arrhythmias, thyroid excess can cause atrial fibrillation with characteristic EKG appearance. Atrial fibrillation can be a problem, because if it becomes chronic and doesn't go away on its own, the cardiologist will try a maneuver called cardioversion, the application of an electrical shock to restart a normal cardiac rhythm, or blood thinners, all of which is not without risk. So it is better to avoid atrial fibrillation altogether by simply stopping the thyroid pills whenever symptoms of rapid heart rate or palpitations are noted while at rest. Exercise induced rapid heart rate, of course, doesn't count since that is normal cardiovascular response to exercise.

How To Design A Better Hunt Study

How would I design an even better Hunt Study? That's easy. Include another group of patients with TSH levels above and below the study group, namely, below 0.5, and above 3.5. I would also include data on annual CAT coronary calcium scores. I would predict that the lower TSH group (below 0.5) would have even less heart disease than the higher TSH group, and that coronary calcium score, indicating plaque burden, would go up as TSH went up.

Thanks and credit goes to William Davis MD and Jacob Teitelbaum MD. Their articles on the Hunt study brought this to my attention. (3)(4)

For references see the web site www.bioidenticalhormones101.com

References for Chapter 6. Hunt Study Shows Thyroid Prevents Heart Attacks

(1) http://archinte.ama-assn.org/cgi/content/abstract/168/8/855 Arch Intern Med. 2008;168(8):855-860. Thyrotropin Levels and Risk of Fatal Coronary Heart Disease, The HUNT Study. Arch Intern Med. 2008;168(8):855-860.

(2) http://www.eje-online.org/cgi/content/full/156/2/181 European Journal of Endocrinology, Vol 156, Issue 2, 181-186, 2007 The association between TSH within the reference range and serum lipid concentrations in a population-based study. The HUNT Study. Bjørn O Åsvold1,2, Lars J Vatten1, Tom I L Nilsen1 and Trine Bjøro.

(3) http://www.endfatigue.com/health_articles_f-n/Heart-low_thyroid_major_cause_heart_attacks.html Jacob Teitelbaum, MD. Low Thyroid (Even if Tests are Normal) is a Major Cause of Heart Attacks,

(4) http://heartscanblog.blogspot.com/2008/06/is-normal-tsh-too-high.html William Davis MD, on the Hunt Study at the Heart Scan Blog.

(5) http://www.intlhormonesociety.org/ref_cons/Ref_cons_9_thryoid_treatment_of_clinically_hypothyroid_b iochemically_hypothyroid_patients.pdf International Hormone Society, lab references, clinically hypothyroid, lab euthyrroid

Section Three: Adrenal Fatigue the Ignored Epidemic of Modern Civilization

CHAPTER 7

Adrenal Fatigue

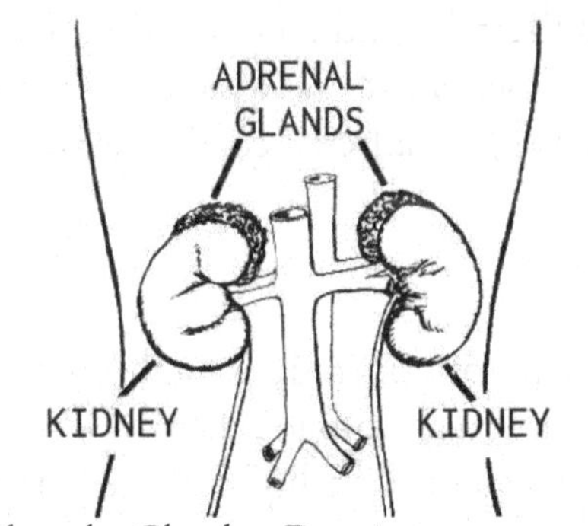

Adrenal Glands Drawing, courtesy of Pearson Scott Foresman, and the Wikimedia Foundation

Ignored by mainstream medicine, adrenal fatigue is a common problem seen routinely every day at any busy medical office. The paramount symptom is fatigue unrelieved by sleep. Other symptoms include craving for salty foods, hypoglycemic episodes, decreased libido, stress intolerance, light headed upon standing, depression, loss of memory and cognitive decline, allergies, sinus problems, and prolonged recovery from flu-like illnesses. The basic underlying cause is low cortisol output by the adrenal glands.

A Self-Help Book for Chronic Burn-Out called Adrenal Fatigue

The definitive book on this topic is entitled, "Adrenal Fatigue", by James L Wilson, PhD, a self-help guide for all of us chronically stressed out members of the "rat race" suffering from this new 21st century epidemic. (1) In his book, Wilson outlines how to diagnose and treat adrenal fatigue, a syndrome not yet recognized by mainstream medicine and it should be. I found Chapter 10 on physical signs of adrenal fatigue the most useful. This chapter describes the findings on physical examination such as the unstable pupil, blood pressure reduction upon standing, and Sergent's white line test.

Cortisol Testing

Chapter eleven of Wilson's book covers the different cortisol testing methods available for cortisol in saliva, blood, and urine, as well as the ACTH stimulation test. Wilson favors the four sample salivary cortisol test as the easiest and most convenient method; with the added advantage that salivary testing can be done at home without a doctor's prescription.

Another chapter in the book covers treatment and recovery from adrenal fatigue with modification of diet and lifestyle, and diet, avoiding food allergies, and the use of hormone supplements and dietary supplements. He also weighs the use of Cortef (cortisol) vs. adrenal cortical extracts.

Results from Years of Chronic Stress

Adrenal fatigue is the net result of years of continuous high cortisol output by the adrenals caused by chronic stress from job, family, illness, injury, and poor diet and lifestyle associated with high-tech modern living. After years of chronic stress, the two small triangular supra-renal glands poop out, and we become another casualty of adrenal fatigue, the 21st century epidemic. Since mainstream doctors can't seem to help, either ignoring the syndrome, or prescribing SSRI anti-depressants for it, this self-help book may be a life-saver.

Definition of Adrenal Fatigue:
"Adrenal Fatigue is a collection of signs and symptoms that results from low function of the adrenal glands. The paramount symptom is fatigue that is not relieved by sleep. The syndrome may be caused by intense or prolonged stress, or after acute or chronic infections, especially respiratory infections such as influenza, bronchitis or pneumonia . . . . People suffering from Adrenal Fatigue often have to use coffee, colas and other stimulants to get going in the morning and to prop themselves up during the day." Quoted from James L. Wilson, Adrenal Fatigue.(1)

Symptoms and Conditions Associated with Adrenal Fatigue
Anxiety Asthenia—lack of, or loss of strength, generalized weakness Asthma Autoimmune problems Bronchitis—recurrent, chronic or slow recovery from Burnout Chemical Sensitivity Chronic fatigue syndrome (CFS) Chronic infections, Chronically run down—with early morning fatigue and low blood pressure Chronic mental and/or physical exhaustion Cravings for carbohydrates, sweets or salt Depression Fatigue—severe, disabling early morning fatigue Feeling tired despite sufficient hours of sleep Fibromyalgia Hair loss Hypoglycemia Immune System dysfunction—frequent illnesses Insomnia—or non-restful sleep Low Blood Pressure Nervous breakdown (nervous exhaustion) Pneumonia Respiratory infections—recurrent, chronic or slow recovery from Rheumatoid arthritis Reliance on stimulants like caffeine Slow recovery following acute infectious diseases, especially influenza, pneumonia, or other respiratory Infections Weight gain

Why is Cortisol Important?

Cortisol is the stress hormone, and is produced in response to stress. Cortisol is important for blood sugar regulation. Cortisol mobilizes glycogen in the liver to maintain blood glucose levels. Symptoms of hypoglycemia are common in low cortisol adrenal fatigue. Also low blood pressure or inability to maintain blood pressure upon standing is also a common symptom. Another physical exam finding is an unstable pupil response to light. The pupil at first contracts and then after a few seconds opens and closes.

The Adrenal Glands Make the Cortisol

The two small triangular adrenal glands are located just above the kidneys and secrete the hormone cortisol in response to stress, physical, emotional, or traumatic stress. The adrenal glands make the hormone cortisol.

What is Cortisol? It's the Stress Hormone

Cortisol is a steroid hormone, and like all the others it is made from cholesterol. Cholesterol, in turn, is made from Vitamin B5 and Acetyl CoA. The manufacture of steroidal hormones can be best understood by referring to a steroidal pathway chart.

Salivary Cortisol Test:

Although cortisol can be measured in a blood sample, the best way to measure cortisol levels is with 4 saliva samples taken throughout the day. There are literally hundreds of medical research studies validating the usefulness of salivary cortisol measurements. A recent study showed that low early morning salivary cortisol is associated with chronic fatigue syndrome in women.(8) We use a 4 sample salivary kit that has a cotton cylinder that is placed under the tongue to collect the sample. Collecting a sample with this kit is much easier than the older method of spitting into the tube.

Nutritional Supplement Program for Adrenal Fatigue and Recovery

The keystone of the treatment program is a nutritional supplement program to restore adrenal function that includes vitamin C, B5, magnesium, biotin and adaptogenic herbs. Recovery takes about 6 weeks.

Cortef for Severe Cases of Adrenal Fatigue

In very severe cases of adrenal failure, Cortef tablets are available and produce a dramatic improvement in clinical condition. For more information, see the classic book, Safe Use of Cortisol by William Mck Jefferies. (41) Cortef is the name for bio-identical cortisol which is widely available at the local drug store. Synthetic forms of cortisol such as prednisone and dexamethasone are not recommended as they can be associated with adverse side effects.

Other Useful Interventions For Adrenal Fatigue:

Avoid excess caffeine, refined carbohydrates, alcohol and sugar.
Get plenty of sleep.
Take steps to reduce stress with gentle exercise, meditation, and yoga.
Bioidentical hormones as determined by lab profile.

Warning:
Paradoxically, thyroid medication may worsen symptoms when given to a patient with adrenal fatigue. Salivary cortisol testing and treatment of adrenal fatigue is mandatory prior to beginning thyroid medication to avoid this pitfall.

Cortisol's Relation to Thyroid Function—Avoiding A Common Pitfall

Low cortisol level adrenal fatigue will induce a protective state in which the body's metabolic rate is reduced in order to cope with low cortisol levels. The body compensates by reducing thyroid function by shunting thyroid hormone production into the reverse T3 pathway, the inactive form of thyroid hormone. This creates a functional low thyroid state which will show up on thyroid labs. Treating the patient with thyroid hormone under this scenario is a common error and a pitfall to be avoided. Giving thyroid hormone to a patient with low cortisol adrenal fatigue will only make the patient feel worse. The low adrenal function must be addressed first before attempting to raise thyroid levels. This is done with a salivary cortisol test and a nutritional supplement program over 6 weeks as described above. In the event the patient is already taking thyroid hormone medication which doesn't seem to be working or is not tolerated, this is a red flag that most likely cause is low cortisol adrenal fatigue. Once this is addressed, the patient will do well with thyroid medication.

For More Reading:

Another excellent book on adrenal fatigue is, "From Fatigued to Fantastic", by Jacob Teitelbaum MD.(43) Also recommended is the article, "Diagnosis and Treatment of Hypothalamic-Pituitary-Adrenal (HPA) Axis Dysfunction in Patients with Chronic Fatigue Syndrome (CFS) and Fibromyalgia" by Kent Holtorf M.D. (44)

For references and links, see my web site: www.bioidenticalhormones101.com

References for Chapter 7. Adrenal Fatigue

(1) http://www.adrenalfatigue.org/
Adrenal Fatigue by James Wilson, Smart Publications; January 25, 2002.

(2) http://coastherbal.com/web_standard/adrenal_stress.html
THE STANDARD Adrenal Stress: Measuring and Treating Thomas G. Guilliams Ph.D.

(3) http://www.spinelife.com/pdf/AdrenalStress.pdf
THE STANDARD Adrenal Stress: Measuring and Treating Thomas G. Guilliams Ph.D.

(4) http://www.medaus.com/p/200,516.html
Saliva Reference Summary ZRT Laboratory (3-12-01) METHOD VALIDATION.

(5) http://advan.physiology.org/cgi/content/full/31/1/110
ADV PHYSIOL EDUC 31:110-115, 2007 TEACHING IN THE LABORATORY A laboratory exercise to illustrate increased salivary cortisol in response to three stressful conditions using competitive ELISA
Mark F. Haussmann, Carol M. Vleck and Eugenia S. Farrar

(6) http://www.biovit.hr/ibl/saliva/cortisol_e.pdf
Cortisol Physiology/Effects of Cortisol

(7) http://www.jacemedical.com/store/low_cortisol.html
The Medical Evidence for Low Cortisol in Chronic Fatigue Syndrome!

(8) http://www.cdc.gov/cfs/publications/clinical_10.htm
Attenuated morning salivary cortisol concentrations in a population-based sample of cases with chronic fatigue syndrome and well controls. Nater UM, Maloney E, Boneva RS, Jones JF, Reeves WC, Heim C.
Journal of Clinical Endocrinology & Metabolism 26 December 2007

(9) http://ajp.psychiatryonline.org/cgi/content/full/162/4/807
Am J Psychiatry 162:807-809, April 2005 Brief Report Enhanced Early Morning Salivary Cortisol in Neuroticism. Maria J. Portella et al

(10) http://archpsyc.ama-assn.org/cgi/content/full/57/1/38
Low Salivary Cortisol and Persistent Aggression in Boys Referred for Disruptive Behavior Keith McBurnett, PhD; Benjamin B. Lahey, PhD; Paul J. Rathouz, PhD; Rolf Loeber, PhD Arch Gen Psychiatry. 2000;57:38-43.

(11) http://www.sav.sk/journals/endo/full/er0298f.pdf
Iatrogenic Adrenal Cortex Failure in Patients woth Steroid Dependent Asthma in Relation to Different Methods of Glucocorticoid Treatment, B. KOS-KUDLA, Endocrine Regulations, Vol. 32, 99.106, 1998

(12) http://bbh.hhdev.psu.edu/labs/bbhsl/PDF%20files/klein%20et%20al.%20cortisol%20and%20naltrexone.pdf
Sex Differences in Salivary Cortisol Levels Following Naltrexone Administration LAURA COUSINO LARRY D. JAMNER, JANEL ALBERTS, MATTHEW

(13) http://bjp.rcpsych.org/cgi/content/full/184/2/136
Salivary cortisol response to awakening in chronic fatigue syndrome Amanda D. L. Roberts, PhD. The British Journal of Psychiatry (2004) 184: 136-141

(14) http://www.virginiahopkinstestkits.com/cortisolzava.html
Cortisol Levels, Thyroid Function and Aging HOW CORTISOL LEVELS AFFECT THYROID FUNCTION AND AGING Interview with David Zava, Ph.D. Originally published in the John R. Lee, M.D. Medical Letter

(15) http://www.drmyhill.co.uk/article.cfm?id=266
Common Hormonal Problems in CFS—Adrenal Underactive adrenal gland (DHEA and cortisol) If the pituitary gland is underfunctioning then the adrenal gland will also underfunction. However the gland itself may fail as a result of chronic stress.

(16) http://www.adrenalfatigue.org/qa.php
James Wilson Questionnaires on Adrenal Fatigue.

(17) http://www.jacemedical.com/store/low_cortisol.html
The Medical Evidence for Low Cortisol in Chronic Fatigue Syndrome! Jace Medical

(18) http://www.cdc.gov/cfs/publications/clinical_10.htm
Attenuated morning salivary cortisol concentrations in a population-based sample of cases with chronic fatigue syndrome and well controls. Nater UM, Maloney E, Boneva RS, Jones JF, Reeves WC, Heim C. Journal of Clinical Endocrinology & Metabolism 26 December 2007

(19) http://ajp.psychiatryonline.org/cgi/content/full/162/4/807
Am J Psychiatry 162:807-809, April 2005. Brief Report Enhanced Early Morning Salivary Cortisol in Neuroticism. Maria J. Portella et al.

(20) http://www.intlhormonesociety.org/ref_cons/Ref_cons_3_mild_glucocorticoid_deficiency.pdf International Hormone Society. Uses of Cortisol references.

(21) http://archpsyc.ama-assn.org/cgi/content/full/57/1/38
Low Salivary Cortisol and Persistent Aggression in Boys Referred for Disruptive Behavior Keith McBurnett, PhD; Benjamin B. Lahey, PhD; Paul J. Rathouz, PhD; Rolf Loeber, PhD Arch Gen Psychiatry. 2000;57:38-43.

(22) http://www.drmyhill.co.uk/article.cfm?id=266
Common Hormonal Problems in CFS

(23) http://www.drpressman.com/library/view.html?id=78
The Use Of Adrenal Cortical Extracts In Adrenal Fatigue by James L. Wilson DC, ND, PhDWhat Is Hypoadrenia and Adrenal Fatigue?Wilson, James L. ND, DC, PhD. Adrenal Fatigue: The 21st Century Stress Syndrome Smart Publications, Petaluma CA, 2001

(24) http://www.ncbi.nlm.nih.gov/pubmed/12377295
Tsigos C, Chrousos GP.Hypothalamic-pituitary-adrenal axis, neuroendocrine factors and stress. J Psychosom Res. 2002 Oct;53(4):865-71.

(25) http://ajp.psychiatryonline.org/cgi/content/full/160/9/1554
Raison CL, Miller AH. When not enough is too much: the role of insufficient glucocorticoid signaling in the pathophysiology of stress-related disorders. Am J Psychiatry. 2003 Sep;160(9):1554-65.

(26) http://www.biodia.com/TechnicalCharts/ChronicStresschart.pdf
Chronic Stress Response Chart

(27) http://www.biodia.com/TechnicalCharts/SteroidalHormonechart.pdf Steroidal Hormone Principle Pathways. (Understanding Pregnenolone Steal, the Preferential Pathway Under Chronic Stress)

(28) http://www.drlam.com/A3R_brief_in_doc_format/adrenal_fatigue.cfm Cortisol (The Hormone of Death), Dr. Lam.

(29) http://meeting.chestjournal.org/cgi/content/abstract/132/4/555 Chest 2007, Critical Care Sepsis: Markers. Wednesday, October 24, 2007. SALIVARY CORTISOL IN CRITICAL CARE PATIENTS. Eduardo F. Sad et al.

(30) http://www.ncbi.nlm.nih.gov/pubmed/6316831 Salivary cortisol: a better measure of adrenal cortical function than serum cortisol.Vining RF, McGinley RA, Maksvytis JJ, Ho KY. Ann Clin Biochem. 1983 Nov;20 (Pt 6):329-35.

(31) http://www.ncbi.nlm.nih.gov/pubmed/2828410 Salivary cortisol measurement: a practical approach to assess pituitary-adrenal function. J Clin Endocrinol Metab. 1988 Feb;66(2):343-8. Laudat MH, Cerdas S, Fournier C, Guiban D, Guilhaume B, Luton JP.

(32) http://www.ncbi.nlm.nih.gov/pubmed/11164057 Salivary cortisol patterns in vital exhaustion. Nicolson NA, van Diest R. J Psychosom Res. 2000 Nov;49(5):335-42.

(33) http://bjp.rcpsych.org/cgi/content/full/184/2/136 Salivary cortisol response to awakening in chronic fatigue syndrome. Roberts AD, Wessely S, Chalder T, Papadopoulos A, Cleare AJ. Br J Psychiatry. 2004 Feb;184:136-41. (FULL TEXT)

(34) http://jcem.endojournals.org/cgi/content/full/86/8/3545 Hypothalamo-Pituitary-Adrenal Axis Dysfunction in Chronic Fatigue Syndrome, and the Effects of Low-Dose Hydrocortisone Therapy. The Journal of Clinical Endocrinology & Metabolism Vol. 86, No. 8 3545-3554 A. J. Cleare et al.

(35) http://www.annalsnyas.org/cgi/content/abstract/1057/1/466
Stress-Induced Hypocortisolemia Diagnosed as Psychiatric Disorders Responsive to Hydrocortisone Replacement, SUZIE E. SCHUDER Ann. N.Y. Acad. Sci. 1057: 466-478 (2005).

(36) http://edrv.endojournals.org/cgi/content/full/24/2/236
The Neuroendocrinology of Chronic Fatigue Syndrome. Anthony J. Cleare. Endocrine Reviews 24 (2): 236-252, 2003, Full Text.

(37) http://crobm.iadrjournals.org/cgi/content/full/13/2/197
THE DIAGNOSTIC APPLICATIONS OF SALIVA—A REVIEW, The Monitoring of Hormone Levels, Eliaz Kaufman,Ira B. Lamster. Crit Rev Oral Biol Med 13(2):197-212 (2002)

(38) http://www.biodia.com/TechnicalCharts/SALIVARY_REFERENCES.pdf Listing of about one hundred medical references on salivary hormone testing with hyperlinks.

(39) http://coastherbal.com/web_standard/adrenal_stress.html
Adrenal Stress: Measuring and Treating, by Thomas G. Guilliams Ph.D. The Standard, Volume 3, No. 1. Excellent review article on diagnosis, treatment of adrenal fatigue with salivary cortisol testing.

(40) http://www.amazon.com/review/R1QNDLO1R9EX3U/ref=cm_cr_rdp_perm Adrenal Fatigue by James L Wilson D.C., N.D., Ph.D. The 21st Century Syndrome reviewed by Jeffrey Dach MD.

(41) http://www.amazon.com/review/R2IPB7XGMO20NE/ref=cm_cr_rdp_perm Safe Uses of Cortisol (Cortisone, Hydrocortisone) by William McK., M.D. Jefferies (Author) reviewed by Jeffrey Dach MD.

(42) http://jcem.endojournals.org/cgi/content/abstract/93/3/703
The Journal of Clinical Endocrinology & Metabolism Vol. 93, No. 3 703-709. Attenuated Morning Salivary Cortisol Concentrations in a Population-Based Study of Persons with Chronic Fatigue Syndrome and Well Controls Urs M. Nater, Elizabeth Maloney, Roumiana S. Boneva, B

(43) From Fatigued to Fantastic by Jacob Teitelbaum MD, Avery Trade; 3rd edition (October 4, 2007).

(44) http://jeffreydach.com/files/80618-70584/JOURNAL_CFSF_6_(2).pdf Diagnosis and Treatment of Hypothalamic-Pituitary-Adrenal (HPA) Axis Dysfunction in Patients with Chronic Fatigue Syndrome (CFS) and Fibromyalgia (FM) Kent Holtorf M.D. J of Chronic Fatigue Syndrome, V 14:3. (pub) 2008.

Section Four: Bioidentical Hormones

Safer and More Effective than Synthetic Hormones

CHAPTER 8

Abandoning the Synthetic Hormone Ship

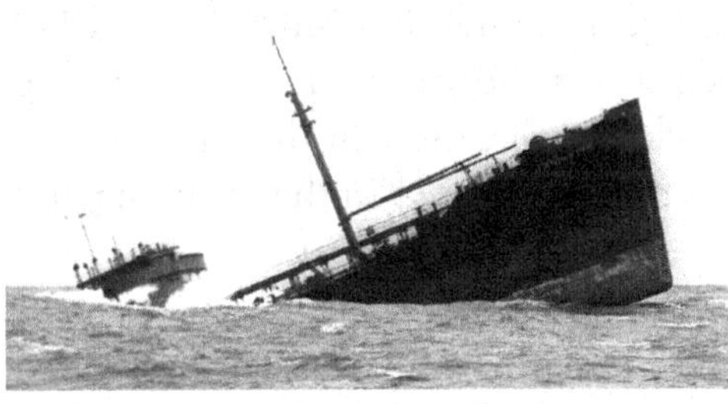

Abandon Ship, Sinking Ship: Bow section of tanker SS Pendleton grounded near Pollock Rib lightship six miles off Chatham, Mass on the morning of Feb. 19, 1952." Courtesy of Wikimedia Commons.

Shirley is 52, and suffering from menopausal symptoms of hot flashes, night sweats, insomnia and mood disturbance. The first chance she had, Shirley asked her doctor for bioidentical hormones. Instead, her doctor offered a prescription for Lexapro™, an SSRI antidepressant. Shirley declined the prescription and ran out the door crying all the way home. A few days later, Shirley was sitting in my office asking, "*Why won't my doctor give me what I want, bioidentical hormones?*"

Ghost Writing—A Shocking Medical Scandal

I explained to Shirley that her doctor's opinion is shaped by misleading information in medical journals corrupted by a technique called medical ghostwriting, a shocking scandal uncovered by Senator Grassley's Committee.(1) In this sinister practice, the prestigious name of an academic MD "opinion leader" appears as author. However, unknown to the reader, the article is actually written by the drug company's paid-for-hire writers. Grassley discovered that sixty articles on women's hormones were ghostwritten, downplaying the adverse effects of synthetic hormones, and casting doubts about bioidentical hormones. Medical ghostwriting is scientific misconduct and fraud which harms society and corrupts the medical literature.

A Brief History of Synthetic Hormones—Re-Living the Nightmare

The following is a short history of synthetic hormone replacement as brought to you by the Drug Industry. (2) Many people have forgotten about the disaster of DES, Diethylstilbestrol, the first synthetic hormone invented in 1938. This carcinogenic, monster hormone was approved by the FDA and given to millions of women from 1940 until it was banned in 1975 when it was shown carcinogenic, causing cervical cancer. The first reports of cervical cancer in the daughters of DES treated women were published in April 1971 in the New England Journal of Medicine.(3-4)

Next, the Drug Industry invented Premarin, a horse estrogen isolated from the urine of pregnant horses. Available since FDA approval in 1942, Premarin has caused an estimated 15,000 cases of endometrial cancer, representing the largest epidemic of serious iatrogenic disease ever reported.(5-8) One might think this would be the end of any drug. However Premarin was promptly rehabilitated with the addition of another synthetic hormone, a progestin, to prevent endometrial cancer. Thus, in 1995, Prempro was born, a synthetic hormone pill containing both Premarin (the horse estrogen) and Provera (the progestin). Again, this was FDA approved, thought safe and handed out freely to millions of women.

However, storm clouds soon appeared on the horizon when four large scale studies showed increased breast cancer and heart disease from this estrogen-progestin combination pill. The Breast Cancer Detection Demonstration Project, published in 2000, showed an eight fold increase in breast cancer for estrogen-progestin users.(9) The Swedish Record Review, published in 1996, had a fourfold increase in breast cancer with progestin use.(10) The Million Woman study, published in Lancet in 2003, had a fourfold increase in breast cancer for estrogen-progestin combination users compared to estrogen alone users.(11) The brakes came on to this synthetic hormone experiment in 2002 with the JAMA publication of the Women's Health Initiative (WHI), an NIH funded study terminated early because of increased breast cancer and heart disease in the estrogen-progestin users.(12)

Abandoning the Synthetic Hormone Ship

Two important things happened after this 2002 WHI study was published. Smart women abandoned synthetic hormones and switched in large number to bioidentical hormones, producing an immediate decline in breast cancer rates of about nine per cent.(13,14) A second important thing happened. Apparently, women have decided to turn to lawyers to protect them, since the FDA has been unable to do so. Thirteen thousand women have filed cases in court claiming synthetic hormones caused their breast cancer. These cases are slowly working their way through the court system, and the jury is still out, so stay tuned.(15)

Dispelling the Myths and Misconceptions

Over the years, I have compiled a list of myths and misinformation commonly encountered about bioidentical hormones in newspapers and magazines. Here are a few of them, followed by the corrections. The misinformation is in italics, with the correct information to follow.

Myth Number One: "*The term bioidentical hormone is undefined and has no meaning.*"

This is incorrect. Bioidentical is a term which is defined as having the exact same chemical structure as hormones found naturally in the human body. Bioidentical Hormones are the ones circulating in your blood stream right now.

Myth Number Two: "*There is no proof that Bioidentical Hormones are safer and more effective than synthetic hormones . . . All of the evidence that we have suggests that all of these hormones should be painted with the same brush,*"

This is incorrect and misleading. As we have seen in the above short history of synthetic hormones, there exists a large body of science showing that synthetic chemically altered hormones cause cancer and heart disease.(9-14) On the other hand, medical studies have found bioidentical hormones are safe with no increase in breast cancer or heart disease compared to non-hormone users. (33-41) An excellent review of this medical science can be found in a 2009 article by Kent Holtorf MD in Postgraduate Medicine. (16)

Myth Number Three: *"Bioidentical Hormones are not FDA approved."*

This is blatantly incorrect. There are twenty or so FDA approved bioidentical hormone preparations widely available at corner drug stores. Here are a few examples: Vivelle-Dot™, Estrace™, Climara™, Prometrium™, Androgel™, etc.

Myth Number Four: *"Bioidentical Hormones made by compounding pharmacies are Non-FDA approved."*

This is not only incorrect, it is misleading and deceptive. Compounding pharmacies are regulated at the state level, and do not fall under FDA jurisdiction. So, of course compounding is not FDA approved. No FDA approval is required or even desired. Your local hospital pharmacy is a compounding pharmacy that makes up life saving medication such as IV antibiotics with no FDA oversight or "approval". The FDA approval process is designed for manufactured capsules and tablets, and is impractical and unnecessary for compounded medications prepared to order by hand. Are we going to reject IV antibiotics from the hospital pharmacy because these are non-FDA approved compounded medication? Of course not. Compounding is here to stay.

Myth Number Five: *"Unless a woman has symptoms of hot flashes and night sweats, she doesn't need hormones."*

This is incorrect. In addition to night sweats and hot flashes, there are many other valid symptoms of hormone deficiency such as insomnia, cognitive dysfunction, menopausal arthritis, evaporative dry eye, anxiety, panic, mood disorder, vaginal dryness, and decreased libido and post hysterectomy. These are all good indications for prescribing bioidentical hormones. (17-25)

Myth Number Six: *"The idea that Menopause is a Hormone Deficiency Disease was disproven, and the idea that hormone replacement rejuvenates youth, or prevents degenerative diseases is also disproven . . . . Hormones decline with age, and is normal and does not require treatment."*

This is incorrect. There is no question that hormonal decline is a health risk. Three separate studies have shown low testosterone in males carries a 40% increase in mortality.(26-28) Studies in females show the same findings, with low hormone levels in women after hysterectomy associated with increased mortality. (29-30) Hormonal decline is a direct cause of degenerative diseases of aging, all of which may be prevented or partially reversed by replenishing hormone levels, a vastly more effective treatment which competes directly with the Drug Industry.(42-46)

Myth Number Seven: *"Hot flashes and sweats in menopausal women can be treated with SSRI antidepressants. They don't need to use hormones."*

This is not only wrong, it is criminal. The use of SSRI antidepressants for menopausal symptoms is NOT FDA approved, and is a cruel mistreatment and medical victimization of women. This practice should be halted immediately. Studies of SSRI drugs show they are no better than placebo for most cases of depression(31), and they are not much better than placebo for menopausal hot flashes. (32) Synthetic hormones are bad enough, they cause cancer and heart disease. SSRI drugs like Lexepro™, Effexor™ and Pristiq™ are even worse; they are chemically addictive with horrendous withdrawal effects. Avoid becoming a medical victim. Stay away.

In Conclusion:

It is time to **awaken** from the nightmare of synthetic hormones, known for decades to cause cancer and heart disease. You can put lipstick on a pig, and it is still a pig. The drug industry can spin, deceive, and misleading the medical journals and media. Yet, after all the lies and propaganda, synthetic hormones remain monsters that should be avoided. Smart women have made the switch to safer and more effective bioidentical hormones. The future of medicine is your choice to make. It is recommended you work closely with a knowledgeable physician before making any decisions regarding hormone treatment. Please feel free to share this chapter with your doctor.

References for Chapter 8, Abandoning the Synthetic Hormone Ship.

(1) http://grassley.senate.gov/about/upload/Senator-Grassley-Report.pdf Ghostwriting in Medical Literature Minority Staff Report 111th Congress United States Senate Committee on Finance Sen. Charles E. Grassley, Ranking Member June 24, 2010

(2) http://www.nytimes.com/2009/12/13/business/13drug.html Menopause, as Brought to You by Big Pharma By NATASHA SINGER and DUFF WILSON Published: December 12, 2009

(3) http://www.nejm.org/doi/pdf/10.1056/NEJM197104222841604 Adenocarcinoma of the Vagina—Association of Maternal Stilbestrol Therapy with Tumor Appearance in Young Women. Arthur L. Herbst, M.D., Howard Ulfelder, M.D., and David C. Poskanzer, M.D. N Engl J Med 1971; 284:878-881April 22, 1971

(4) http://www.jstor.org/pss/2683841 Epidemiologic Evidence for Adverse Effects of DES Exposure during Pregnancy Theodore Colton and E. Robert Greenberg The American Statistician Vol. 36, No. 3, Part 2: Proceedings of the Sixth Symposium on Statistics and the Environment (Aug., 1982), pp. 268-272

(5) http://ajph.aphapublications.org/cgi/reprint/70/3/264.pdf The Epidemic of Endometrial Cancer:A Commentary Hershel Jick et al.Am J Public Health 70:264-267, 1980.

(6) http://www.nejm.org/doi/full/10.1056/NEJM197512042932303 Increased Risk of Endometrial Carcinoma among Users of Conjugated

Estrogens. Harry K. Ziel, M.D., and William D. Finkle, Ph.D. N Engl J Med 1975; 293:1167-1170 December 4, 1975

(7) http://www.ncbi.nlm.nih.gov/pubmed/213722
N Engl J Med. 1979 Jan 4;300(1):9-13. Endometrial cancer and estrogen use. Report of a large case-control study. Antunes CM, Strolley PD, Rosenshein NB, Davies JL, Tonascia JA, Brown C, Burnett L, Rutledge A, Pokempner M, Garcia R.

(8) http://www.ncbi.nlm.nih.gov/pubmed/3358913
The dose-effect relationship between 'unopposed' oestrogens and endometrial mitotic rate: its central role in explaining and predicting endometrial cancer risk.Key TJ, Pike MC.
Br J Cancer. 1988 Feb;57(2):205-12.

(9) http://jama.ama-assn.org/content/283/4/485.abstract
Menopausal Estrogen and Estrogen-Progestin Replacement Therapy and Breast Cancer Risk. Catherine Schairer, PhD et al. JAMA. 2000;283(4):485-491.

(10) http://onlinelibrary.wiley.com/doi/10.1002/(SICI)1097-0215(19960729)67:3%3C327::AID-IJC4%3E3.0.CO;2-T/pdf see also http://www.ncbi.nlm.nih.gov/pubmed/8707404 Cancer incidence and mortality in women receiving estrogen and estrogen-progestin replacement therapy—long-term follow-up of a Swedish cohort. Ingemar Persson et al. International Journal of Cancer Volume 67, Issue 3, pages 327-332, 29 July 1996

(11) http://www.ncbi.nlm.nih.gov/pubmed/12927427
Lancet. 2003 Aug 9;362(9382):419-27. Breast cancer and hormone-replacement therapy in the Million Women Study. Beral V; Million Women Study Collaborators.

(12) http://jama.ama-assn.org/cgi/content/abstract/288/3/321
Risks and Benefits of Estrogen Plus Progestin in Healthy Postmenopausal Women Principal Results From the Women's Health Initiative Randomized Controlled Trial Writing Group for the Women's Health Initiative Investigators JAMA. 2002;288:321-333.

(13) http://www.nejm.org/doi/full/10.1056/NEJMsr070105 The Decrease in Breast-Cancer Incidence in 2003 in the United States. Peter M. Ravdin, Ph.D., M.D et al. N Engl J Med 2007; 356:1670-1674 April 19, 2007. A comparison of incidence rates in 2001 with those in 2004 (omitting the years in which the incidence was changing) showed that the decrease in annual age-adjusted incidence was 8.6%.

(14) http://jnci.oxfordjournals.org/content/early/2010/09/23/jnci.djq345.abstract Breast Cancer Incidence and Hormone Replacement Therapy in Canada by Prithwish De, C. Ineke Neutel, Ivo Olivotto and Howard Morrison. JNCI J Natl Cancer Inst (2010). This drop occurred concurrently with a 9.6% decline in the incidence rate of breast cancer

(15) http://www.bloomberg.com/news/2010-08-27/pfizer-settles-arkansas-prempro-case-before-retrial-over-punitive-damages.html Pfizer Said to Pay $330 Million to Settle Prempro Lawsuits Claiming Cancer By Jef Feeley—Feb 9, 2011 4:42 PM ET

(16) http://jeffreydach.com/files/80618-70584/The_Bioidentical_Hormone_Debate_Ken_Holtorf_MD.pdf Postgraduate Medicine: Volume 121: No.1 January 2009. The Bioidentical Hormone Debate:Are Bioidentical Hormones (Estradiol, Estriol, and Progesterone) Safer or More Efficacious than Commonly Used Synthetic Versions in Hormone Replacement Therapy? Kent Holtorf, MD

(17) http://www.ncbi.nlm.nih.gov/pubmed/11386980 Arch Gen Psychiatry. 2001 Jun;58(6):529-34. Efficacy of estradiol for the treatment of depressive disorders in perimenopausal women: a double-blind, randomized, placebo-controlled trial. by Soares CN et al.

(18) http://www.neurology.org/cgi/content/abstract/57/4/605 Neurology 2001;57:605-612, 2001 American Academy of Neurology High-dose estradiol improves cognition for women with AD Results of a randomized study by S. Asthana, MD et al.

(19) http://www.ncbi.nlm.nih.gov/pubmed/19804793
Estradiol reduces anxiety—and depression-like behavior of aged female mice by Alicia A. Walf and Cheryl A. Frye Neuroscience

(20) http://www.ncbi.nlm.nih.gov/pubmed/16142740
Arthritis Rheum. 2005 Sep;52(9):2594-8. Aromatase inhibitors and the syndrome of arthralgias with estrogen deprivation. Felson DT, Cummings SR.

(21) http://www.ncbi.nlm.nih.gov/pubmed/9609575
Am J Obstet Gynecol. 1998 May;178(5):1002-9.When does estrogen replacement therapy improve sleep quality? Polo-Kantola P et al.

(22) http://cme.medscape.com/viewarticle/512093
"Menopausal Arthritis" May Develop in Women Receiving Estrogen-Depleting Treatments News Author: Laurie Barclay, MD CME Author: Désirée Lie, MD, MSEd

(23) http://www.emaxhealth.com/70/3606.html
Women treated with aromatase inhibitors often experience joint pain and musculoskeletal aching: severe enough, in some cases, to make them stop the treatment.

(24) http://www.ncbi.nlm.nih.gov/pubmed/11173183
Maturitas. 2001 Jan 31;37(3):209-12. Treatment of keratoconjunctivitis sicca with topical androgen. by Worda C et al.

(25) http://abstracts.iovs.org/cgi/content/abstract/44/5/2450
Invest Ophthalmol Vis Sci 2003;44: E-Abstract 2450. Treatment of Dry Eye with a Transdermal 3% Testosterone Cream by C.G. Connor.

(26) http://eurheartj.oxfordjournals.org/content/31/12/1494.abstract
Eur Heart J (2010) 31 (12): 1494-1501. Low serum testosterone levels are associated with increased risk of mortality in a population-based cohort of men aged 20-79, Robin Haring et al.

(27) http://circ.ahajournals.org/cgi/content/abstract/116/23/2694
Endogenous Testosterone and Mortality Due to All Causes,

Cardiovascular Disease, and Cancer in Men European Prospective Investigation Into Cancer in Norfolk (EPIC-Norfolk) Prospective Population Study (Circulation. 2007;116:2694-2701.)

(28) http://archinte.ama-assn.org/cgi/content/abstract/166/15/1660
Vol. 166 No. 15, Aug 14/28, 2006 Low Serum Testosterone and Mortality in Male Veterans Molly M. Shores, MD et al. Arch Intern Med. 2006;166:1660-1665.

(29) http://www.ncbi.nlm.nih.gov/pmc/articles/PMC2755630
Menopause. 2009 Jan-Feb; 16(1): 15-23. Increased cardiovascular mortality following early bilateral oophorectomy. Cathleen M. Rivera, MD et al.

(30) http://www.ncbi.nlm.nih.gov/pubmed/19384117
Obstet Gynecol. 2009 May;113(5):1027-37.Ovarian conservation at the time of hysterectomy and long-term health outcomes in the nurses' health study. Parker WH et al.

(31) http://jama.ama-assn.org/content/303/1/47
Antidepressant Drug Effects and Depression Severity A Patient-Level Meta-analysis. Jay C. Fournier et al. JAMA. 2010;303(1):47-53.

(32) http://jama.ama-assn.org/content/305/3/267
Efficacy of Escitalopram for Hot Flashes in Healthy Menopausal Women A Randomized Controlled Trial Ellen W. Freeman, PhD; JAMA. 2011;305(3):267-274

(33) http://www.ncbi.nlm.nih.gov/pubmed/15551359
Int J Cancer. 2005 Apr 10;114(3):448-54. Breast cancer risk in relation to different types of hormone replacement therapy in the E3N-EPIC cohort. Fournier A et al.

(34) http://www.ncbi.nlm.nih.gov/pmc/articles/PMC2211383/
Breast Cancer Res Treat. 2008 January; 107(1): 103-111. Unequal risks for breast cancer associated with different hormone replacement therapies: results from the E3N cohort study. Agnès Fournier et al.

(35) http://www.ncbi.nlm.nih.gov/pubmed/19752341
J Clin Oncol. 2009 Nov 1;27(31):5138-43. Estrogen-progestagen menopausal hormone therapy and breast cancer: does delay from menopause onset to treatment initiation influence risks? Fournier A et al.

(36) http://www.ncbi.nlm.nih.gov/pubmed/17651686
Ann Endocrinol (Paris). 2007 Sep;68(4):241-50. Epub 2007 Jul 24. Hormonal replacement therapy (HRT) in postmenopause: a reappraisal. Caufriez A.

(37) http://jeffreydach.com/files/80618-70584/Hormones_in_wellness_and_disease_prevention_common_practices_current_state_evidence_Erika_Schwartz_Kent_Holtorf.pdf Prim Care. 2008 Dec;35(4):669-705. Hormones in wellness and disease prevention: common practices, current state of the evidence, and questions for the future. Schwartz ET, Holtorf K.

(38) http://www.jpands.org/vol13no2/hotze.pdf
Point/Counterpoint:The Case for Bioidentical Hormones by Steven F. Hotze, M.D. Donald P. Ellsworth, M.D. Journal of American Physicians and Surgeons Volume 13 Number 2 Summer 2008 p43.

(39) http://www.ncbi.nlm.nih.gov/pubmed/18775609
Could transdermal estradiol + progesterone be a safer postmenopausal HRT? A review. L'hermite M, Simoncini T, Fuller S, Genazzani AR. Maturitas. 2008 Jul-Aug;60(3-4):185-201.

(40) http://www.thorne.com/altmedrev/.fulltext/11/3/208.pdf
A Comprehensive Review of the Safety and Efficacy of Bioidentical Hormones for the Management of Menopause and Related Health Risks Deborah Moskowitz, ND Altern Med Rev 2006;11(3):208-223

(41) http://online.wsj.com/article/SB123717056802137143.html
March 16, 2009 The Truth About Hormone Therapy Wall Street Journal By Erika Schwartz, Kent Holtorf, and David Brownstein

(42) http://www.tasciences.com/pdf/Harley_CMM_final.pdf Current Molecular Medicine 2005, 5, 29-38 205 Telomerase Therapeutics for Degenerative Diseases. By Calvin B. Harley.

(43) http://mcb.asm.org/cgi/content/full/20/11/3764 Molecular and Cellular Biology, June 2000, p. 3764-3771, Vol. 20, No. 11 Induction of hTERT Expression and Telomerase Activity by Estrogens in Human Ovary Epithelium Cells. Silvia Misiti, et al.,

(44) http://cancerres.aacrjournals.org/content/59/23/5917.full Estrogen Activates Telomerase. Satoru Kyo et al. Cancer Res December 1, 1999 59; 5917

(45) http://www.ncbi.nlm.nih.gov/pmc/articles/PMC120798/ Microbiol Mol Biol Rev. 2002 September; 66(3): 407-425. Human Telomerase and Its Regulation. Yu-Sheng Cong et al.

(46) http://www.nature.com/nature/journal/vaop/ncurrent/full/nature09603.html Telomerase reactivation reverses tissue degeneration in aged telomerase-deficient mice by Ronald A. DePinho et al. Nature November 2010.

CHAPTER 9

The Importance of Bioidentical Hormones

What is a Bioidentical Hormone, and How Do They Differ From Synthetic Hormones?

First of all, let us look at the definition and meaning of "bioidentical hormones". How do bioidentical hormones differ from the synthetic hormones offered by the mainstream medical system? Bioidentical hormones are the hormones that exist in the human body naturally. Synthetic hormones are these very same human hormones that are chemically altered. Here, we are referring to the chemical structure of the molecule. Bioidentical hormones have the naturally occurring chemical structure, so it cannot be patented. Synthetic hormones have been chemically altered so they CAN BE patented. This is the key distinction.

Why Chemically Alter a Human Hormone?

You might ask, "Why Chemically Alter a Human Hormone"? This is done in order to obtain a patent. The drug company hires chemists to alter the structure of human hormones in the laboratory so the drug company can obtain a patent on the new chemical structure, which is a new drug. The patent grants exclusive marketing rights to the drug company, and is necessary to protect profits. Because of a quirk in our patent laws, only chemically altered substances can be patented. Natural substances like human hormones cannot be patented, and are therefore generally not profitable to manufacture.

Chemically Altered Hormones are Monster Hormones

The reality is that it is not a good idea to alter the chemical structure of a human hormone. Hormones fit onto their receptors just like a "lock and key", so any slight alteration of their chemical structure creates a "monster hormone" with unintended effects. These resulting "monster hormones" are never found in the human body or anywhere else in nature. The reality is that these synthetically altered monster hormones should never have been approved for marketing and sale to the American People, and yet that is exactly what your mainstream medical doctor will offer you if you ask for hormones.

Why do we use the word bio-identical to describe natural human hormones?

You are probably wondering why we use the word, "bioidentical"? That's an excellent question. I can remember back when I was in first year medical school learning biochemistry at the University of Illinois in Chicago. Our class used Lehninger's classic textbook of biochemistry which is still in use today.(5) Dr. Lehninger never uses the word, "bio-identical hormones", because all human hormones are by definition, "bioidentical hormones". Dr Lehninger's biochemistry book simply used the word, "hormone". Using a word like "bioidentical" was simply redundant and unnecessary for biochemistry textbooks, as it should be today.

Important Point:
Synthetic Hormones are chemically altered versions of natural human hormones. This alteration is required in order to obtain a patent. However, this chemical alteration creates a "monster" which causes cancer and heart disease.

The Medical Information War and Terminology

Years ago, after the invention of synthetic monster hormones, an information war was launched by the drug industry creating confusion in the public and even among medical professionals about the difference between natural human hormones and synthetic monster hormones. Because of this medical information war, we must use the terminology, "bioidentical hormones", which really means human hormones, in order to differentiate them from synthetic hormones. In reality, it is an embarrassment to medical science that we use the word "bio-identical" for natural hormones found in the human body. We shouldn't feel that we are forced to do this. It should be sufficient to use the same old names in the biochemistry text books. The simple word "hormone" should suffice. Yet here we are again finding ourselves using the word "bio-identical hormone" thanks to the "Information War" going on between natural medicine and the drug industry.

How do Hormones Work? They Turn on Protein Production

Hormones are messengers that attach directly to the DNA of trillions of our cells and influence gene expression. Once bound to the DNA, the hormone messenger turns on DNA expression of protein synthesis. DNA contains the source code for the manufacture of proteins. The Hormone is a messenger that tells the DNA to produce these proteins. You might ask, "Why Are Proteins Important?" Proteins are the major building block for the human body, and all life for that matter. Proteins serve a variety of functions. For example, "structural" proteins make up the structural elements of the body such as bones, skin, arteries, hair, connective tissue, ligaments, tendons, muscles. Other proteins called enzymes are involved in energy production. There are proteins involved in communication, neurological function, and cognition called neurotransmitters. There are proteins involved in the immune system called antibodies, and the list goes on. The various types of proteins are used to make the cells in every organ in the body.

Regenerative and Reparative Proteins

We need a constant supply of proteins to repair the body's wear and tear. A marathon runner, for example, suffers wear and tear on the tendons, ligaments and muscles used in the marathon run. Recovery time after a marathon depends on the speed of repair of these injuries. During recovery, new proteins and new cells are manufactured and used for repair.

Important Point:
All life, including ours, is based on the ability to regenerate new cell layers made of proteins. Protein production, in turn, is controlled by DNA in the cell nucleus. Hormones attach to receptors on the DNA and control protein production. Low hormone levels mean low protein production and reduced ability to repair and regenerate tissues.

New Cell Layers Are Needed for Life

In order to live, we need to make new cells. As our older cells and cell layers age and eventually die, we must have the ability to manufacture new cells. Examples are blood cells that must be replaced by the bone marrow every 90 days, the skin cells that slough off as the outer layer to be replaced by new layers of cells underneath. The gastrointestinal lining is generated at the basal cell layer. These basal cells mature as they migrate to the surface where they eventually live out their life span, die and slough off. All organ systems in our body require new cells to replace old ones. These new cells are made of proteins, so regeneration of new cell layers requires the DNA to be "turned on" to make these new proteins and cells.

Hormone Levels Decline with Age

We know from observational studies that hormones levels decline with age. Starting around age 50, the abrupt hormone decline in women is called menopause with cessation of ovulation. In men, hormonal decline after age 50 is called Andropause, with a gradual decline in testosterone levels.

Increase in Human Life Span

Starting around the year 1820, which marks the beginning of the Industrial Revolution, there has been an increase in the human life span. (1) I suspect this is due to improved living standards, mass production of goods and services, and better nutrition. Before 1900, most people did not live past 50 years, so hormonal decline was not an really an issue in the population. However, after the year 1900, people are living beyond the age of 50, with the onset of hormonal decline called menopause in women, and andropause in men. This trend has increased to the point that we now have more people over fifty than ever before, creating a huge population of people with hormonal decline.

Lack of Reparative Proteins Leads to Degenerative Diseases of Aging

Without this hormone message which turns on DNA expression of protein synthesis, we lack the reparative and regenerative proteins needed to prevent the degenerative diseases of aging. A Natural Medicine approach provides bioidentical hormone replacement which prevents (and in some cases reverses) these degenerative diseases of aging. Here is a list with the mainstream drug treatment offered.

List of the Degenerative Diseases	Drugs Used
Osteoarthritis	Naprosyn™, Ibuprofen™
Osteoporosis	Fosamax™, Actonel™
Atherosclerotic Vascular Disease	Lipitor™, Statins
Cognitive Dysfunction	Aricept™
Immune System Dysfunction	Cipro, Z-pack
Loss of Libido	Viagra™, Cialis™
Depression	Prozac™, Zoloft™, SSRI's

Degenerative Disease Means Great Profits for Drug Companies

The major drug companies make most of their profits on blockbuster drugs aimed at one of the above degenerative diseases of aging. Since all of these degenerative diseases are directly caused by hormonal decline, they can be prevented or reversed (at least partially reversed) with the use of bio-identical hormones, representing direct economic competition with the drug industry which sells a drug for each degenerative disease (see above chart).

Important Point:
Bioidentical Hormones prevent or reverse the degenerative diseases of aging, directly competing with the profits of the drug industry, thereby explaining the animosity and information warfare between the drug industry and bioidentical hormones.

Natural Medicine Means Lost Profits for the Drug Industry

If bio-identical hormones were widely used, this would mean massive lost sales and lost profits for the drug industry. It is not difficult to understand why there is animosity and competition between the drug industry and natural medicine, and especially between the drug industry and natural bioidentical hormones, with a raging medical information war going on.

For references and links, see my web site: www.bioidenticalhormones101.com

References for Chapter 9. The Importance of BioIdentical Hormones

(1) http://www.demogr.mpg.de/publications/files/brokenlimits.htm Broken Limits to Life Expectancy Jim Oeppen and James W.Vaupel. also see: http://www.prb.org/pdf06/nia_futureoflifeexpectancy.pdf

(2) http://www.postgradmed.com/index.php?article=1949 Postgraduate Medicine: Volume 121: No.1 January 2009. The Bioidentical Hormone Debate:Are Bioidentical Hormones (Estradiol, Estriol, and Progesterone) Safer or More Efficacious than Commonly Used Synthetic Versions in Hormone Replacement Therapy?Kent Holtorf, MD

(3) http://online.wsj.com/article/SB123717056802137143.html March 16, 2009 The Truth About Hormone Therapy Wall Street Journal by Erika Schwartz, Kent Holtorf, and David Brownstein,

(4) http://www.ncbi.nlm.nih.gov/pubmed/18928825 Prim Care. 2008 Dec;35(4):669-705. Hormones in wellness and disease prevention: common practices, current state of the evidence, and questions for the future. By Schwartz ET, Holtorf K.

(5) Lehninger Principles of Biochemistry by Albert Lehninger, David L. Nelson, Michael M. Cox. W. H. Freeman; Fifth Edition edition (June 15, 2008)

CHAPTER 10

The Safety of Bioidentical Hormones

Bioidentical Hormones are safer and more effective than synthetic hormones. (1-2)

Do You Have Hormone Excess or Hormone Deficiency?

A deficiency or an excess of women's bio-identical hormones can produce adverse symptoms. This is called estrogen deficiency/excess, and progesterone deficiency/excess, and they each have typical signs and symptoms easily recognized.(3)

Common Signs of Estrogen Deficiency (4)
Insomnia, Difficulty Falling Asleep
Hot flashes
Night sweats
Mental Fogginess
Forgetfulness
Depression
Anxiety
Mood Disturbance
Fatigue, Reduced stamina
Decreased sense of sexuality
Lessened self-image and attention to appearance
Dry eyes, skin, and vagina
Sagging breasts and loss of fullness
Vaginal Dryness, Pain with sexual activity
Weight gain
Menopausal Arthritis, back and joint pain
Headaches and migraines
Gastrointestinal discomfort, bloating

Common Signs of Excess Estrogen:
Breast enlargement, tenderness or pain
Water retention, fingers, legs
Impatient, snappy behavior, but with clear mind

Common Signs of Progesterone Deficiency
No periods at all (no ovulation)
The period comes infrequently (every few months)
Heavy and frequent periods (large clots, due to buildup in the uterus)
Spotting a few days before the period. (Progesterone level is dropping)
PMS
Cystic breasts
Painful breasts
Breasts with lumps (fibrocystic)
Most cases of endometriosis, adenomyosis, and fibroids.
Anxiety, irritability, nervousness and water retention.

Above list courtesy of Uzzi Reiss MD from his book, Natural Hormone Balance for Women: Look Younger, Feel Stronger, and Live Life with Exuberance. and also see Dr. Reiss's book, "The Natural SuperWoman", by Uzzi Reiss MD and Yfat Reiss Gendell. (4)(42)

No Adverse Events from Bio-Identical Hormones Reported to the FDA: NONE

Over-the-counter pain pills (NSAIDs) such as aspirin, naproxen™ and ibuprofen™ are considered fairly safe. After all, you don't need a prescription to buy them, yet they cause an estimated 16,500 deaths in the US annually, mostly from gastric bleeding.(5) Compare this to no reported adverse events from bio-identical hormones in 2008, according to an FDA press conference January 2008.(6) Bioidentical hormones must be considered safer when compared to commonly available over the counter pain remedies. However, one must remember that hormonal excess or deficiency is associated with the adverse events and the symptoms listed above.

FDA Admits No Adverse Reports: Transcript of FDA Press Conference Jan 9, 2008:

Anna Matthews: Hi. Couple of questions; one is have you guys (the FDA) received any reports of adverse events or other harm to patients from these products (bioidentical hormone products)?

Kathy Anderson (of the FDA): With your respect to your question about whether we received any adverse event reports, ***we have not.***

Quoted from: Transcript of FDA Press Conference on FDA Actions on Bio-Identical Hormones. Moderator: Susan Cruzan, January 9, 2008 Edited for brevity.(6)

Do Hormones Cause Breast Cancer? (7)

The 2002 WHI (Women's Health Initiative) study revealed that synthetic hormones increase the risk of breast cancer. However, Bioidentical Hormones do not. How do we know this? The French Cohort Study showed there was no increased risk of breast cancer in women using bio-identical hormones.(8)(43) Rather, the 2008 French Cohort Study by Fournier showed that in women using hormone replacement combination drugs, increased breast cancer was associated with synthetic progestin use, while women using bioidentical progesterone had no increased breast cancer (compared to non-hormone users).(43) Remember, in addition to avoiding synthetic hormones, the addition of Iodine supplementation is our most useful tool for prevention of breast cancer. See the chapter on breast cancer prevention with iodine supplementation for more on this.(10)

Do Bio-Identical Hormones Cause Heart Disease?

Again, we know from the 2002 WHI study that synthetic hormones cause heart disease, and bioidentical hormones do not. Calcium score is an accepted measure of heart disease risk. A study of CAT calcium scores by JoAnn E. Manson in the June 2007 JAMA actually lower scores, and less heart disease in the women taking estrogen (they had hysterectomies and were not given the synthetic progestins).(11) These same results had already been published 2 years previously in a calcium score study by Budoff in J Women's Health 2005. (12) Clearly the data shows that bioidentical hormones are protective and prevent heart disease, while synthetic hormones increase heart disease risk.

What Was the Women's Health Initiative—WHI Study

The WHI study was the large NIH sponsored medical study in which synthetic hormones were given to women. The WHI study consisted of two arms. The first arm used the combined synthetic hormones Premarin™ and Provera™, and the second arm used Premarin™ alone. The WHI results were published in JAMA in 2002 and 2004.(13-14)

What is Premarin and Provera?

Premarin™ and Provera™ are not bio-identical hormones. Premarin™ is a hormone obtained from pregnant horses, which contains Equilin, a horse hormone not found in humans.(15) Provera™ is a synthetic hormone which is not found anywhere in the natural world. (16) The Premarin™ and Provera combination is called PremPro™, a synthetic hormone pill commonly prescribed by mainstream medicine. Prempro™ was the hormone preparation used in the first arm of the WHI study. (13) Prempro™ is currently in litigation in drug court. Women are seeking damages from the PremPro™ manufacturer claiming Prempro™ caused their breast cancer.

WHI study First Arm:

The WHI study (first arm published in JAMA 2002) was terminated early because the combination of premarin™ and provera™ (Prempro™) caused increased breast cancer and heart disease.(13) Immediately after this WHI study was published in JAMA in 2002, there was a massive switch by women to bio-identical hormones which resulted in a 4 billion dollar loss for Wyeth, the maker of Prempro™.

WHI Study (Second Arm):

All the women in the second arm of the WHI study had prior hysterectomies (uterus absent), so they did not need the synthetic progestin, called Provera, which is required to prevent the endometrial cancer caused by Premarin alone. Rather, this post-hysterectomy group was given Premarin alone (the horse hormone, also called CEE, for Conjugated Equine Estrogen). Unlike the first arm of the study, these women had no increased risk of breast cancer. (18) Premarin causes endometrial cancer, so the mainstream medical system always gives Provera (progestins) to prevent endometrial cancer, unless of course, the uterus is absent from prior hysterectomy.(20)(56)(57)

The WHI Culprit was the Synthetic Progestin (an altered form of Progesterone)

Back to the first arm of the WHI which used Prempro, it is clear from the data that the culprit which caused breast cancer and heart disease was Provera™, a synthetic monster hormone. This is nothing new. For years, Provera™ has been known to cause heart disease and breast cancer.(21-22)(39) Three previous large scale human studies revealed increased breast cancer with progestin use. The Breast Cancer Detection Demonstration Project published in JAMA in 2000 showed an eight fold increase in breast cancer for estrogen-progestin users compared to estrogen alone users. (53) The Swedish Record Review published in 1996 had a four fold increase in breast cancer with progestin use. (54) The Million Woman study published in Lancet in 2003 had a fourfold increase in breast cancer for estrogen-progestin combination users compared to estrogen alone users.(55) A 2007 animal study with primates treated with either bioidentical progesterone or a progestin (Provera™) showed that the progestin drug (Provera™) worsens breast cancer biomarkers, while the bioidentical progesterone provides a beneficial effect on breast tissue and reduces cancer markers.(22)

Monster Hormones are Chemically Altered

Chemically altered hormones were used in the WHI study, and are routinely handed out by the medical system. These altered hormones are **monsters** that should never have been approved for marketing to the American people. They should be banned.

The Media Says Hormones Cause Cancer and Heart Disease

If bio-identical hormones are so safe, then why do the newspapers say that women's hormones cause breast cancer and heart disease?(23) The answer is that the media and the medical profession routinely confuse synthetic chemically altered monster hormones with the bio-identical hormones. The drug companies intentionally create this confusion because they want to hide the fact that synthetic hormones are monsters that should be banned.

Chemically altered hormones were made because of a quirk in our legal system which grants patent protection for chemically altered versions of a natural substance. The natural hormones were chemically altered so that they could be patented to protect profits from competition. Naturally occurring bio-identical hormones by law cannot be patented. Examples of monster synthetic hormones are provera, all progestins, and birth control pills which are never found in nature. These are the monster hormones.

A Listing of a Few Monster Hormones: Chemically Altered
Chemically Altered Progesterone: Dienogest, Desogestrel, Drospirenone, Dydrogesterone, Ethisterone, Etonogestrel, Ethynodiol diacetate, Gestodene, Gestonorone, Levonorgestrel, Lynestrenol, Medroxyprogesterone, Megestrol, Norelgestromin, Norethisterone, Norethynodrel, Norgestimate, Norgestrel, Norgestrienone, Tibolone
Chemically Altered Estrogen: Dienestrol, Diethylstilbestrol, Ethinylestradiol, Fosfestrol, Mestranol
Chemically Altered Hormones in Birth Control Pills: levonorgestrel and ethinyl estradiol [oral contraceptive] (Alesse 28, Aviane, Nordette, Seasonale, Triphasil, Trivora-28); norethindrone and ethinyl estradiol (Combi Patch, Loestrin FE 1/20, Neocon 1/35, Ortho-Novum 7/7/7, Ovcon 35); norgestimate and ethinyl estradiol (Ortho-Cyclen, Orthotri-Cyclen, Trinessa); norgestrel and ethinyl estradiol (LO/OVRAL 28, Low-Ogestrel), desogestrel and ethinyl estradiol (Desogen, Miracette, Ortho-Cept), drospirenone and ethinyl estradiol (Yasmin)

Chemically Altered Testosterone: Androstanolone, Fluoxymesterone, Mesterolone, Methyltestosterone

An Illustration Explaining the Problem of Synthetic Drugs

Supposing a biochemist working for a drug company has an idea to alter the chemical structure of vitamin C so a patent can be obtained. The biochemist adds a chlorine molecule to the vitamin C carbon ring, and gives is a new name "super-Vitamin C", which is really a chlorinated version of vitamin C. Next they do a one year medical study with 5,000 people taking the chlorinated vitamin C tablet every day, and another 5000 people taking a placebo. After the year is up, they count a 0.5 per cent incidence of heart disease events in the Super Vitamin C group and a 1.0 percent in the placebo group. FDA approval is easily obtained based on reduction in heart disease events by 50 per cent (0.5 per cent is 50% of 1.0 %). The drug company is at liberty to spend million dollars on television advertising designed to rake in millions more for the new heart prevention miracle drug. This absurd scenario is now the norm for our medical system. Why would anyone want to spend money for a monster version of vitamin C when the real thing is available for pennies? Why use a monster hormone when human hormones are available? Compared to their monster counterparts, Bio-Identical Hormones are more effective, have fewer adverse side effects, and are less costly.

High Hormone Levels of Early Pregnancy Confer Protection from Breast Cancer.

During the 16th century in Italy, breast cancer was quite rare. An Italian doctor, Bernardino Ramazzini, noted in 1713 the relatively high incidence of breast cancer in nuns and wondered whether this was related to celibate lifestyle.(24) Recent studies confirm that early pregnancy and multiple pregnancies confer protection from breast cancer, while no pregnancies (as in the nuns) leads to increased risk of breast cancer.(25) This protection is thought to be conferred by high levels of progesterone. This was confirmed in a 2007 study by Rajkumar showing hormone treatment protected genetically engineered mice from developing breast cancer. (26)

Progesterone, the Great Protector

Progesterone is so safe, it is available over the counter without a prescription. In addition, a deficiency of progesterone is associated with an increase in breast cancer risk.(27) Progesterone is known to be protective and prevents breast cancer.(28)

Why Don't Birth Control Pills use Natural Progesterone?

Birth Control Pills, BCP's, are very effective at preventing pregnancy by suppressing ovulation. However, BCP's contain synthetic hormones which have adverse side effects.(29-31) To avoid these monster hormones, the IUD (intra-uterine device) is available. Make sure you ask the doctor for a plain IUD, without the implanted hormones. In the future, BCP's will be made from natural progesterone which is available in highly absorbable micronized oral capsules.

Warning About IUD's With Synthetic Hormones
Avoid synthetic hormones in IUDs. If you plan on using an IUD, ask for a **PLAIN** IUD without synthetic hormones implanted in it. (IUD=Intra-uterine device)

For More Reading, See These Recommended Articles:

1) The Bioidentical Hormone Debate: Are Bioidentical Hormones (Estradiol, Estriol, and Progesterone) Safer or More Efficacious than Commonly Used Synthetic Versions in Hormone Replacement Therapy? Kent Holtorf, MD1 Postgraduate Medicine, Volume 121, Issue 1, January 2009. (1)

2) Hormones inWellness and Disease Prevention: Common Practices, Current State of the Evidence, and Questions for the Future. Erika T. Schwartz, MD, Kent Holtorf, MD Prim Care Clin Office Pract 35 (2008) 669-705. (2)

3) The Case for Bioidentical Hormones Steven F Hotze MD. 2008.(33)

4) The Safety of Bioidentical Hormones—the Data vs. the Hype by Jacob Teitelbaum, MD From the Townsend Letter June 2007.(34)

5) Bioidentical vs. Synthetic HRT, A Review of the Literature by the Bio-Identical Hormone Initiative, Erika Schwartz MD, David Brownstein MD, Kent Holtorf MD.(40)(41)

Books on Bioidentical Progesterone by John R Lee MD (35)

What Your Doctor May Not Tell You About Menopause: The Breakthrough Book on Natural Progesterone, by John R Lee MD, (Warner Books, 1996)(35)

What Your Doctor May Not Tell You About Premenopause: Balance Your Hormones and Your Life from Thirty to Fifty, by John R Lee, (Warner Books, 1999)(35)

References for Chapter 10, The Safety of Bioidentical Hormones

(1) http://jeffreydach.com/files/80618-70584/The_Bioidentical_Hormone_Debate_Ken_Holtorf_MD.pdf
The Bioidentical Hormone Debate: Are Bioidentical Hormones (Estradiol, Estriol, and Progesterone) Safer or More Efficacious than Commonly Used Synthetic Versions in Hormone Replacement Therapy? Kent Holtorf, MD1 Postgraduate Medicine, Volume 121, Issue 1, January 2009

(2) http://jeffreydach.com/files/80618-70584/Hormones__in_wellness_and_disease_prevention_common_practices_current_state_evidence_Erika_Schwartz_Kent_Holtorf.pdf
Hormones inWellness and Disease Prevention: Common Practices, Current State of the Evidence, and Questions for the Future. Erika T. Schwartz, MDa,*, Kent Holtorf, MDb Prim Care Clin Office Pract 35 (2008) 669-705

(3) http://www.johnleemd.com/store/premenstrual_syndrome.html
Excerpted From: WHAT YOUR DOCTOR MAY NOT TELL YOU

ABOUT BREAST CANCER: Balance Your Hormones and Your Life from Thirty to Fifty. PHYSIOLOGICAL EFFECTS OF ESTROGEN AND PROGESTERONE. How Hormone Balance Can Help Save Your Life. by John R. Lee, M.D., David Zava, Ph.D. and Virginia Hopkins. Warner Books 2002

(4) http://www.uzzireissmd.com/book_naturalhormone.html
Natural Hormone Balance for Women: Look Younger, Feel Stronger, and Live Life with Exuberance. by Uzzi Reiss MD

(5) http://www.drtheo.com/news/NSAIDs.pdf
Medical Progress. p 1888. June 17, 1999 The New England Journal of Medicine
Gastrointestinal Toxicity of NonSteroidal Anti-inflammatory Drugs by M. Michael Wolfe et al.

(6) http://www.fda.gov/downloads/NewsEvents/Newsroom/MediaTranscripts/ucm122174.pdf
Transcript of FDA Press Conference on FDA Actions on Bio-Identical Hormones
FTS HHS FDA Susan Cruzan January 9, 2008

(7) http://www.womentowomen.com/breasthealth/estrogenbreastcancer.aspx Causes of Breast Cancer—the Estrogen Controversy, Dixie Mills MD

(8) http://www.ncbi.nlm.nih.gov/pubmed/12626212
Climacteric. 2002 Dec;5(4):332-40. Combined hormone replacement therapy and risk of breast cancer in a French cohort study of 3175 women.de Lignières B et al. French Cohort Study.

(9) http://www.johnleemd.com/store/cancer_progest.html
Breast Cancer Book Intro. WHAT YOUR DOCTOR MAY NOT TELL YOU ABOUT BREAST CANCER. How Hormone Balance Can Help Save Your Life

By John R. Lee, M.D., David Zava Ph.D., and Virginia Hopkins
INTRODUCTION

(10) http://jeffreydach.com/2007/05/05/jeffreydachdrdachiodine.aspx
Breast Cancer Prevention and Iodine Supplementation by Jeffrey Dach MD

(11) http://content.nejm.org/cgi/content/short/356/25/2591
Estrogen Therapy and Coronary-Artery Calcification. NEJM Volume 356:2591-2602 June 21, 2007 Number 25. JoAnn E. Manson, M.D., et al.

(12) http://www.ncbi.nlm.nih.gov/pubmed/15989413
J Women's Health (Larchmt). 2005 Jun;14(5):410-7. Effects of hormone replacement on progression of coronary calcium as measured by electron beam tomography.Budoff MJ, et al.

(13) http://jama.ama-assn.org/cgi/content/abstract/288/3/321
Risks and Benefits of Estrogen Plus Progestin in Healthy Postmenopausal Women
Principal Results From the Women's Health Initiative Randomized Controlled Trial
Writing Group for the Women's Health Initiative Investigators JAMA. 2002;288:321-333. First Arm.

(14) http://jama.ama-assn.org/cgi/content/full/291/14/1701
Effects of Conjugated Equine Estrogen in Postmenopausal Women With Hysterectomy
The Women's Health Initiative Randomized Controlled Trial. JAMA. 2004;291:1701-1712. Second Arm. This is the Second Arm of the Study. Premarin Only.

(15) http://en.wikipedia.org/wiki/Premarin
Premarin From Wikipedia, the free encyclopedia

(16) http://en.wikipedia.org/wiki/Medroxyprogesterone
Provera, Medroxyprogesterone,

(17) http://homecoalition.org/TakeAction
Take Action. Write a letter to your elected officials using our online advocacy tool. Act now to defend your right to bio-identical hormones!

(18) http://jama.ama-assn.org/cgi/content/full/295/14/1647
Effects of Conjugated Equine Estrogens on Breast Cancer and Mammography Screening in Postmenopausal Women With Hysterectomy. Marcia L. Stefanick, PhD et al. for the WHI Investigators. JAMA. 2006;295:1647-1657. Conclusions Treatment with CEE alone for 7.1 years does not increase breast cancer incidence in postmenopausal women with prior hysterectomy.

(19) http://courses.washington.edu/bonephys/opestrogen.html#WHI
Osteoporosis and Bone Physiology, Susan Ott, MD, Associate Professor, Department of Medicine, University of Washington. A Review of the results from the Women's Health Initiative.

(20) http://www.ncbi.nlm.nih.gov/pubmed/3358913
The dose-effect relationship between 'unopposed' oestrogens and endometrial mitotic rate: its central role in explaining and predicting endometrial cancer risk.Key TJ, Pike MC.
Br J Cancer. 1988 Feb;57(2):205-12.

(21) http://atvb.ahajournals.org/cgi/content/full/24/7/1171
Should Progestins Be Blamed for the Failure of Hormone Replacement Therapy to Reduce Cardiovascular Events in Randomized Controlled Trials? Kwang Kon Koh; Ichiro Sakuma. Arteriosclerosis, Thrombosis, and Vascular Biology. 2004;24:1171.

(22) http://www.ncbi.nlm.nih.gov/pubmed/16841178
Effects of estradiol with micronized progesterone or medroxyprogesterone acetate on risk markers for breast cancer in postmenopausal monkeys.Wood CE et al. Breast Cancer Res Treat. 2007 Jan;101(2):125-34.

(23) http://www.time.com/time/magazine/article/0,9171,1002897,00.html The Truth About Hormones Monday, Jul. 22, 2002 Time Magazine. By CHRISTINE GORMAN AND ALICE PARK

(24) http://www.ama-assn.org/amednews/2006/04/17/hlsa0417.htm AMA Medical News. Collecting clues: Cancer registries might have an answer. By Kathleen Phalen Tomaselli, AM News correspondent. April 17, 2006.

(25) http://breast-cancer-research.com/content/7/3/131 The protective role of pregnancy in breast cancer. Jose Russo et al. Breast Cancer Research 2005, 7:131-142doi:10.1186/bcr1029

(26) http://www.pubmedcentral.nih.gov/articlerender.fcgi?tool=pubmed&pubmedid=17257424 Hormone-induced protection of mammary tumorigenesis in genetically engineered mouse models Lakshmanaswamy Rajkumar et al.Breast Cancer Res. 2007; 9(1): R12.

(27) http://aje.oxfordjournals.org/cgi/content/abstract/114/2/209 BREAST CANCER INCIDENCE IN WOMEN WITH A HISTORY OF PROGESTERONE DEFICIENCY LINDA D. COWAN et al. American Journal of Epidemiology Vol. 114, No. 2: 209-217

(28) http://www.annclinlabsci.org/cgi/content/abstract/28/6/360 Progesterone inhibits growth and induces apoptosis in breast cancer cells: inverse effects on Bcl-2 and p53. B Formby and TS Wiley. Annals of Clinical and Laboratory Science, Vol 28, Issue 6, 360-369

(29) http://en.wikipedia.org/wiki/Birth_control_pill Combined oral contraceptive pill. From Wikipedia, the free encyclopedia. (Redirected from Birth control pill)

(30) http://www.worstpills.org/results.cfm?disease_id=26 Oral Contraceptives on Worst Pills.org. The pill can cause many adverse effects.

(31) http://www.jeffreywarber.com/hc%20pages/pillsideeffects.html
Birth Control Pill Adverse Side Effects by Jeffrey Warber MD

(32) http://www.quickoverview.com/reproductive/birth-control-pill.html
History and Development of an effective combined oral contraceptive. People Involved.

(33) http://www.jpands.org/vol13no2/hotze.pdf
Point/Counterpoint: The Case for Bioidentical Hormones Steven F. Hotze, M.D.Donald P. Ellsworth, M.D.Journal of American Physicians and Surgeons Volume 13 Number 2 Summer 2008

(34) http://www.townsendletter.com/June2007/painfree0607.htm
The Safety of Bioidentical Hormones—the Data vs. the Hype by Jacob Teitelbaum, MD

(35) http://www.johnleemd.com/store/main_books.html
John Lee Web Site: Books by John R Lee MD

(36) http//:naturalnews.com/022595.html
FDA's Assault of Bioidentical Hormones Demonstrates Pro-Pharma Loyalties, Disregard for Consumer Choice Tuesday, February 05, 2008 by: Mike Adams

(37) http://www.drerika.com/blog?action=viewBlog&blogID=-7512711561726201l3 February 16, 2008. Women, Doctors Wage Crucial Battle With FDA To Save Bioidentical Hormones From Wyeth's Wrath. A major coalition of informed women and their doctors have launched an all out war on the Federal Drug Administration's (FDA) cynical and corrupt decision to ban compounded hormones containing Estriol.

(38) http://jeffreydach.com/2008/01/11/fda-declares-war-on-bioidentical-hormones-by-jeffrey-dach-md.aspx
FDA Declares War on BioIdentical Hormones by Jeffrey Dach MD

(39) http://atvb.ahajournals.org/cgi/content/full/17/1/217
Medroxyprogesterone Acetate Antagonizes Inhibitory Effects of Conjugated Equine Estrogens on Coronary Artery Atherosclerosis. Michael R. Adams et al. Arteriosclerosis, Thrombosis, and Vascular Biology. 1997;17:217-221.

(40) http://www.drerika.com/pg/jsp/bhi/bioidentical_vs_synthetic.pdf
Bioidentical vs. Synthetic HRT, A review of the literature

(41) http://www.bioidenticalhormoneinitiative.org/
Bio-Identical Hormone Initiative, Erika Schwartz MD, David Brownstein MD, Kent Holtorf MD

(42) The Natural Superwoman: The Scientifically Backed Program for Feeling Great, Looking Younger, and Enjoying Amazing Energy at Any Age, Uzzi Reiss, Yfat Reiss Gendell, Avery (November 8, 2007)

(43) http://jeffreydach.com/files/80618-70584/Unequal_Risks_Breast_Cancer_hormone_replacement_E3N_cohort_study_Fournier.pdf Breast Cancer Res Treat. 2008 January; 107(1): 103-111.Unequal risks for breast cancer associated with different hormone replacement therapies: results from the E3N cohort study. Agnès Fournier et al.

(44) Menapause-safety_effectiveness_bioidentical_hormones.html
The Safety and Effectiveness of Bio-Identical Hormones: Natural (Bio-Identical) vs. Synthetic HRT. Kent Holtorf, M.D.

(45) http://www.thorne.com/media/hormones11-3.pdf
A Comprehensive Review of the Safety and Efficacy of Bioidentical Hormones for the Management of Menopause and Related Health Risks Deborah Moskowitz, ND. Altern Med Rev 2006;11(3):208-223)

(46) http://www.drcranton.com/hrt/hrt_references.htm
Hormone Replacement References. Most references below are linked to the National Library of Medicine (MEDLINE)

(47) http://www.medscape.com/viewarticle/408096_print Addressing Postmenopausal Estrogen Deficiency: A Position Paper. January 26, 2001 Sander Shapiro, MD Medscape General Medicine 3(1), 2001.

(48) http://www.drerika.com/pg/jsp/general/scientificarchive.jsp Scientific Literature on Hormones on Dr Erika.com

(49) http://www.womeninbalance.org/research/ research available women in balance.

(50) http://www.fimdefelice.org/archives/arc.promise.html The Promise and Problems of Natural Substances in Medicine Stephen L. DeFelice, M.D.

(51) http://www.nwhn.org/healthinfo/detail.cfm?info_id=9&topic=Fact%20Sheets Menopause Hormone Therapy and Breast Cancer. National Women's Health Network

(52) http://www.bmj.com/cgi/content/full/310/6979/598/b BMJ 1995;310:598 (4 March) Letters Risk factors for breast cancer, BMJ

(53) http://jama.ama-assn.org/content/283/4/485.abstract Menopausal Estrogen and Estrogen-Progestin Replacement Therapy and Breast Cancer Risk. Catherine Schairer, PhD et al. JAMA. 2000;283(4):485-491.

(54) http://onlinelibrary.wiley.com/doi/10.1002/(SICI)1097-0215(19960729)67:3%3C327::AID-IJC4%3E3.0.CO;2-T/pdf see also http://www.ncbi.nlm.nih.gov/pubmed/8707404 Cancer incidence and mortality in women receiving estrogen and estrogen-progestin replacement therapy—long-term follow-up of a Swedish cohort. Ingemar Persson et al. International Journal of Cancer Volume 67, Issue 3, pages 327-332, 29 July 1996

(55) http://www.ncbi.nlm.nih.gov/pubmed/12927427
Lancet. 2003 Aug 9;362(9382):419-27. Breast cancer and hormone-replacement therapy in the Million Women Study. Beral V; Million Women Study Collaborators.

(56) http://www.nejm.org/doi/full/10.1056/NEJM197512042932303
Increased Risk of Endometrial Carcinoma among Users of Conjugated Estrogens. Harry K. Ziel, M.D., and William D. Finkle, Ph.D. N Engl J Med 1975; 293:1167-1170 December 4, 1975

(57) http://www.ncbi.nlm.nih.gov/pubmed/213722
N Engl J Med. 1979 Jan 4;300(1):9-13. Endometrial cancer and estrogen use. Report of a large case-control study. Antunes CM, Strolley PD, Rosenshein NB, Davies JL, Tonascia JA, Brown C, Burnett L, Rutledge A, Pokempner M, Garcia R.

CHAPTER 11

Bioidentical Hormones and Medical Ghost Writing, the Latest Scandal

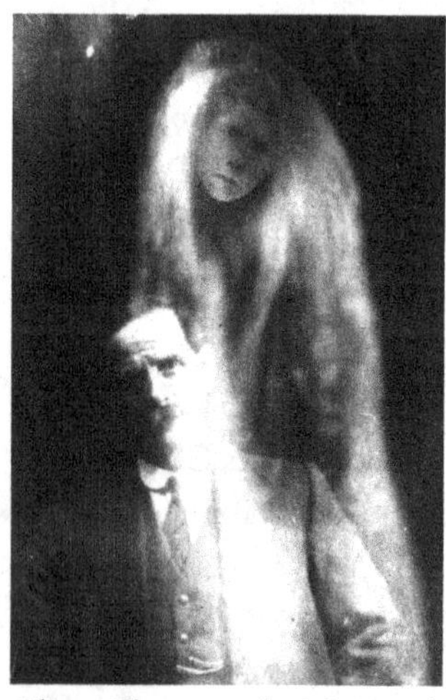

Ghost Photograph, Man with the spirit of his second wife, by William Hope (1863-1933), Courtesy of National Media Museum and Wikimedia Commons

Why is My Doctor Opposed to Bioidentical Hormones?

Linda is 53, and suffering from menopausal symptoms of hot flashes, night sweats, insomnia and mood disturbance. While at the hair salon, a friend told her she needed hormone therapy, so she went on the internet to read up on it. Linda learned about the Women's Health Initiative Study that showed synthetic hormones are unsafe, causing breast cancer and heart disease. Once she learned this information, she felt confident her OB Gyne doctor would prescribe the safer bioidentical hormones. She cheerfully called the office to make an appointment to see her OB Gyne doctor, thinking he would gladly prescribe bioidentical hormones. To her dismay, Linda's doctor was not at all pleased when she raised the topic. Her doctor scowled and said, "*Those aren't any good*", and besides, "*there is no evidence that bioidentical hormones are any safer than synthetics*". Linda ran out the door crying all the way home. A few days later, Linda was sitting in my office asking, "*Why is my doctor opposed to bioidentical hormones?*"

Your Doctor is Reading Ghost Written Articles Biased Against Bioidenticals

I explained to Linda that her doctor reads medical journals containing ghost written articles from the synthetic hormone makers, Wyeth and Pfizer. Ghost written is a term which means the real author is not the doctor listed at the top of the article. The real author of the article is a ghost writer hired by the pharmaceutical company. The two companies, DesignWrite and PharmaWrite provide the medical writers for hire, with instructions to downplay the adverse effects of synthetic hormones, and raise doubts about bioidentical hormones. Medical ghostwriting is marketing, rather than science. As such, it is a form of plagiarism, scientific misconduct and fraud. The invited "author" is usually an academic professor in a university medical center serving as opinion leader who lends his name to the article.

Shocking Revelations from Drug Litigation, Medical Ghostwriting

8,000 women have filed court claims against Wyeth-Pfizer, claiming that their synthetic hormone pill, Prempro, caused breast cancer. During the discovery process, internal company documents were made public revealing the extent of the medical ghost writing. About 44 articles in the women's health medical literature are ghost written by Wyeth in a marketing program to convince doctors to prescribe their synthetic hormones, and not to prescribe bioidentical hormones. These documents are publicly available in a document database.

An Example of Medical Ghost Writing in the Women's Hormone Literature

Here is an example of biased pro-industry medical ghostwriting. The article is entitled, "Bioidentical Hormone Therapy: A Review of the Evidence", by Michael Cirigliano, an Internist at the University of Pennsylvania School of Medicine, published in the Journal of Women's Health. (2007 Jun;16(5):600-31. (10) Michael Cirigliano is Associate Professor of Medicine at the University of Pennsylvania Medical center. At the very end of the article (page 625), you will find this acknowledgement written by Dr. Cirigliano:

> ***ACKNOWLEDGEMENTS—***
> *I received editorial assistance from Eugene R. Tombler, Ph.D., Florencia Schapiro, Ph.D., and Monica Ramchandani, Ph.D., of PharmaWrite,LLC.*

Pharmawrite, also called Designwrite, is the medical ghostwriting company paid by Wyeth to ghostwrite medical articles on women's hormones.

They have been under investigation by Grassley's senate committee for writing about 44 such articles. (11)(12) Dr. Cirigliano acknowledges three PHD medical ghost writers from Pharmawrite. I would assume an unnamed drug company paid these three PhD's from Pharmawrite for a pro-synthetic hormone article biased against bioidentical hormones. The name of the drug company that hired Designwrite is not disclosed. I leave that to your own investigation. The resulting medical article is a literature review to establish if sufficient scientific evidence supports the claim that bioidentical hormones are safer and more effective than chemically altered synthetic hormones. And as you could have guessed, the author's conclusion is: "*There is **No Scientific Evidence** to support this (claim)*". (Quote from Dr. Cirigliano's article.)

In case you were thinking this is OK, the University Of Pennsylvania School Of Medicine (Penn Medicine) has policies against plagiarism, and considers ghostwriting to be the equivalent of plagiarism. Plagiarism is a serious academic infraction, and a deviation from academic norms. Worse, ghostwriting harms society because it convinces doctors and patients to use harmful drugs that should be avoided.

Important Point:
Ghostwriting is a form of plagiarism, and grounds for dismissal from most universities. Medical ghostwriting is especially pernicious because it is fraudulent, unethical, and harmful to society. The practice should be banned.

Comparison with Non-Biased Review

For comparison, let's look at a very different review of the medical literature, this time not ghost written by the synthetic hormone industry. This review article is entitled, "The Bioidentical Hormone Debate: Are Bioidentical Hormones Safer or More Efficacious than Synthetic Hormone Replacement Therapy?", by Kent Holtorf, MD, published in Postgraduate Medicine: Volume 121: No.1 January 2009. (1-2) The doctor's conclusion after reviewing the medical literature is: **YES, There IS Evidence** to support the claim that bioidentical hormones are safer and more effective than synthetics. Dr. Holtorf's conclusion is quoted here:

> *"Bioidentical hormones have lower risk of breast cancer and heart disease, and are more efficacious than synthetic counterparts. Until evidence is found to the contrary, bioidentical hormones remain the preferred method of HRT."*

Dr. Holtorf cites 196 medical studies to support his conclusion. I invite you to read his article for yourself by clicking on the hyperlinked reference for the internet version of this chapter.(1) You are probably wondering, how is it possible for two smart doctors to come to the exact opposite conclusion? Dr. Cirigliano says **NO** they are not, and Dr. Holtorf says **YES** they are.

The answer is simple; none of the medical studies that Holtorf cites are mentioned in Dr. Cirigliano's article. The two articles review the medical literature to answer the same question, yet they come up with two sets of totally different medical studies. Why is that? This is another use of medical sampling, a commonly used gimmick to slant or spin a medical study to get the intended results.

The ghost written Cirigliano article selectively accepts only RCT studies as evidence. RCT means randomized controlled trial. This is a drug trial with two groups of patients, a drug group and a placebo group. Randomized means the patients are randomly selected for each group. RCT trials are large and very expensive drug studies funded by drug companies for FDA approval of a new drug. Since bioidentical hormones are not a new drug, (they are natural substances that cannot be patented), drug companies will not spend money funding such a controlled trial.

Important Point: Using The RCT Gimmick
The Randomized Controlled Trial (RCT) argument is a commonly used gimmick to claim there is "no evidence" for a natural substance. Basic science lab studies, animal studies, and epidemiological studies account for the vast majority of medical research and represent "medical evidence" as well. When convenient, the drug companies ignore this mountain of evidence favoring a natural substance competitor such as bioidentical hormones. They will then plant into the medical literature a series of biased, ghostwritten articles restricting discussion to RCTs as the only acceptable form of "evidence".

Since there are no large RCT studies of bioidentical hormones, Dr. Holtorf cites other types of medical studies that are equally valid, such as observational studies like the French Cohort Study and others. Many of his cited studies are epidemiological studies, which are not the gold standard, but are still published and accepted as medical evidence. Dr. Holtorf's article also includes basic science and animal studies. If you search the medical literature, you will find no privately funded Randomized Controlled Trials (RCT) for Bioidentical Hormones because they are natural and cannot be patented. A drug company would **NEVER** invest the millions for a RCT for a drug without the patent protection to insure a profit. In any event, with the information currently available, it would be a breach of medical ethics to do a randomized controlled study comparing progesterone to the chemically altered progestins. The adverse effects of progestins, which cause breast cancer and heart disease, are well known. Inflicting these adverse effects on a test group would be unethical.

Medical Ghost Writing Should Be Banned

Medical ghost writing, as we have seen in the women's hormone literature, is a form of plagiarism, scientific misconduct and fraud. It is harmful to the public and should be banned.

For references and links, see my web site: www.bioidenticalhormones101.com

Chapter 11. Bioidentical Hormones and Medical GhostWriting

(1) http://www.postgradmed.com/index.php?article=1949 see also

(2) http://jeffreydach.com/files/80618-70584/The_Bioidentical_Hormone_Debate_Ken_Holtorf_MD.pdf
Postgraduate Medicine: Volume 121: No.1 January 2009. The Bioidentical Hormone Debate: Are Bioidentical Hormones (Estradiol, Estriol, and Progesterone) Safer or More Efficacious than Commonly Used Synthetic Versions in Hormone Replacement Therapy? Kent Holtorf, MD

(3) http://online.wsj.com/article/SB123717056802137143.html
MARCH 16, 2009 The Truth About Hormone Therapy Wall Street Journal By ERIKA SCHWARTZ, KENT HOLTORF, and DAVID BROWNSTEIN

(4) http://www.ncbi.nlm.nih.gov/pubmed/18928825 see also http://jeffreydach.com/files/80618-70584/Hormones_in_wellness_and_disease_prevention_common_practices_current_state_evidence_Erika_Schwartz_Kent_Holtorf.pdf
Prim Care. 2008 Dec;35(4):669-705. Hormones in wellness and disease prevention: common practices, current state of the evidence, and questions for the future. Schwartz ET, Holtorf K.

(5) http://www.jpands.org/vol13no2/hotze.pdf
Point/Counterpoint: The Case for Bioidentical Hormones by Steven F. Hotze, M.D. Donald P. Ellsworth, M.D. Journal of American Physicians and Surgeons Volume 13 Number 2 Summer 2008 p43.

(6) http://www.ncbi.nlm.nih.gov/pubmed/18775609
Could transdermal estradiol + progesterone be a safer postmenopausal HRT? A review. L'hermite M, Simoncini T, Fuller S, Genazzani AR. Maturitas. 2008 Jul-Aug;60(3-4):185-201. Epub 2008 Sep 5. Department of Gynecology and Obstetrics, Université Libre de Bruxelles, Bruxelles, Belgium.

(7) http://www.thorne.com/altmedrev/.fulltext/11/3/208.pdf
A Comprehensive Review of the Safety and Efficacy of Bioidentical Hormones for the Management of Menopause and Related Health Risks Deborah Moskowitz, ND Altern Med Rev 2006;11(3):208-223

(8) http://www.ncbi.nlm.nih.gov/pubmed/17107222
Treat Endocrinol. 2006;5(6):367-374. Is Bio-Identical Hormone Replacement Therapy Safer than Traditional Hormone Replacement Therapy?: A Critical Appraisal of Cardiovascular Risks in Menopausal Women. Curcio JJ, Wollner DA, Schmidt JW, Kim LS. Women's Integrative Medicine Department, Southwest College of Naturopathic Medicine, Tempe, Arizona, USA.

(9) http://www.ncbi.nlm.nih.gov/pmc/articles/PMC2211383/
Breast Cancer Res Treat. 2008 January; 107(1): 103-111. Unequal risks for breast cancer associated with different hormone replacement therapies: results from the E3N cohort study. Agnès Fournier et al.

(10) http://www.solaltech.com/doctors/3/Bioidentical%20Hormone%20Therapy—%20Cirigliano.pdf
Michael Cirigliano MD. J Womens Health (Larchmt). 2007 Jun;16(5):600-31. Bioidentical hormone therapy: a review of the evidence. Cirigliano M. University of Pennsylvania School of Medicine, Philadelphia, Pennsylvania 19104, ACKNOWLEDGMENTS: I received editorial assistance from Eugene R.Tombler, Ph.D., Florencia Schapiro, Ph.D., and Monica Ramchandani, Ph.D., of PharmaWrite,LLC.

(11) http://grassley.senate.gov/about/upload/Senator-Grassley-Report.pdf
Grassley Senate Report

(12) http://graphics8.nytimes.com/2010/06/25/business/SenatorGrassleyReport.pdf
Ghostwriting in Medical Literature Minority Staff Report 111th Congress United States Senate Committee on Finance Sen. Charles E. Grassley, Ranking Member June 24, 2010

(13) http://www.plosmedicine.org/article/info%3Adoi%2F10.1371%2Fjournal.pmed.1000230
Ghostwriting at Elite Academic Medical Centers in the United States," Jeffrey R. Lacasse and Jonathan Leo, "Ghostwriting at Elite Academic Medical Centers in the United States," PLoS Med, 2010; 7(2): 1-4.

(14) http://www.pfizer.com/research/research_clinical_trials/registration_disclosure_authorship.jsp
Authors must also acknowledge individuals who provide editorial support and disclose the funding source. For Pfizer-sponsored studies the fact that the study was funded by Pfizer must be disclosed.

(15) http://www3.interscience.wiley.com/cgi-bin/fulltext/122204938/PDFSTART
Bioethics; 1467-8519 (online) Volume 24 Number 6 2010 pp 267-272 PROFITS AND PLAGIARISM: THE CASE OF MEDICAL GHOSTWRITING TOBENNA D. ANEKWE

(16) http://www3.interscience.wiley.com/cgi-bin/fulltext/122204937/PDFSTART
Bioethics ISSN; 1467-8519 (online) Volume 24 Number 6 2010 pp 273-283 PUBLICATION ETHICS AND THE GHOST MANAGEMENT OF MEDICAL PUBLICATION by SERGIO SISMONDO AND MATHIEU DOUCET

(17) http://publicationethics.org/blogs/ghostauthors-ghost-management-and-manipulation-medical-research
Ghostauthors, ghost management and the manipulation of medical research

(18) http://www.plosmedicine.org/article/info:doi/10.1371/journal.pmed.1000230 Ghostwriting at Elite Academic Medical Centers in the United States. PLoS by Jeffrey R. Lacasse and Jonathan Leo

(19) http://www.nytimes.com/2009/08/19/health/research/19ethics.html?pagewanted=2 One of the authors discussed in DesignWrite documents is Dr. Michelle P. Warren, a professor of obstetrics and gynecology at Columbia. Her article was published in The American Journal of Obstetrics and Gynecology in 2004, when women feared that Wyeth's brand of hormone drugs could be causing particular problems.

(20) http://www.scientificamerican.com/article.cfm?id=ghostwriter-science-industry February 4, 2010 Ghostbusters: Authors of a new study propose a strict ban on medical ghostwriting. A scientist who takes credit as an author on an article secretly written by a pharmaceutical company should face punishment like any other plagiarist. Lacasse and Leo even recommend that scientists who have participated in ghostwriting in the past should confess, and that their ghostwritten papers be reevaluated and even retracted if appropriate.

(21) http://www.thehastingscenter.org/Bioethicsforum/Post.aspx?id=326 How Great Researchers Get By-lines, Get Paid, and Get Medicine in Trouble Medicine and Business Kate Jirik, 12/28/2006

(22) http://www.ama-assn.org/public/peer/7_15_98/jpv80004.htm Prevalence of Articles With Honorary Authors and Ghost Authors in Peer-Reviewed Medical Journals. (JAMA. 1998;280:222-224) Annette Flanagin et al.

(23) http://www.nytimes.com/2008/12/12/business/13wyeth.html?_r=1&scp=2&sq=wyeth&st=cse Drug Maker Said to Pay Ghostwriters for Journal Articles By DUFF WILSON December 12, 2008

(24) http://www.nytimes.com/2009/08/05/health/research/05ghost.html?_r=1&ref=health Medical Papers by Ghostwriters Pushed Therapy August 4, 2009

(25) http://www.nytimes.com/2009/08/19/health/research/19ethics.html?_r=4&hp=&pagewanted=all Senator Moves to Block Medical Ghostwriting By NATASHA SINGER August 18, 2009

(26) http://www.nytimes.com/2009/09/11/business/11ghost.html Ghostwriting Is Called Rife in Medical Journals By DUFF WILSON and NATASHA SINGER Published: September 10, 2009

(27) http://www.ncbi.nlm.nih.gov/pmc/articles/PMC2876906/ Indian J Anaesth. 2010 Jan-Feb; 54(1): 2-4. Transgression in scientific communication. PF KoturEditor, SAARC Journal of Anaesthesia, Former Editor, Indian Journal of Anaesthesia, Sr.Prof. of Anaesthesiology, J.N. Medical College, Belgaum, Karnataka, India.

(28) http://www.cmaj.ca/earlyreleases/9sept09_ghostwriting.dtl Roger Collier, CMAJ September 9, 2009 Prevalence of ghostwriting spurs calls for transparency

(29) http://www.ncbi.nlm.nih.gov/pmc/articles/PMC2219716/?tool=pmcentrez J Gen Intern Med. 2007 July; 22(7): 1030-1034. Published online 2007 March 7. doi: 10.1007/s11606-007-0141-4. PMCID: PMC2219716 Bioidentical Hormones for Menopausal Hormone Therapy: Variation on a Theme Adriane Fugh-Berman, MD and Jenna Bythrow, MS candidate

(30) http://cat.inist.fr/?aModele=afficheN&cpsidt=17214001 Sexuality, Reproduction and Menopause Volume 3, Issue 2, October 2005, Pages 68-71 Elsevier Inc. "Bioidentical" estrogens: Hope or hype? Maida Taylor MD, MPHa, Clinical Director Women's Health, Clinical Research & Medical Affairs—Endocrinology, Novo Nordisk Inc.

(31) http://www.ncbi.nlm.nih.gov/pubmed/12748456 Am J Obstet Gynecol. 2003 May;188(5):1123-31. Progestins and breast cancer. Eden J. Royal Hospital for Women, University of New South Wales, Sydney, NSW, Australia.

(32) http://alethonews.wordpress.com/2010/02/23/pfizers-ghostwritten-journal-articles-are-still-standing-still-bogus/ Pfizer's ghostwritten journal articles are still standing, still bogus By Martha Rosenberg | Online Journal | February 23, 2010

(33) http://www.hrt-legal.com/news/2010/02/09/ghostwritten-medical-journal-articles-about-hrt-should-be-retracted/ Ghostwritten medical journal articles about HRT should be retracted February 9th, 2010 by Jennifer Walker-Journey

(34) http://dida.library.ucsf.edu/documents.jsp The Drug Industry Document Archive (DIDA) contains drug company documents and external resources about drug industry clinical trials, publication of results, pricing, marketing, relations with physicians and involvement in continuing medical education.

CHAPTER 12

Bioidentical Hormones Found Beneficial After Hysterectomy

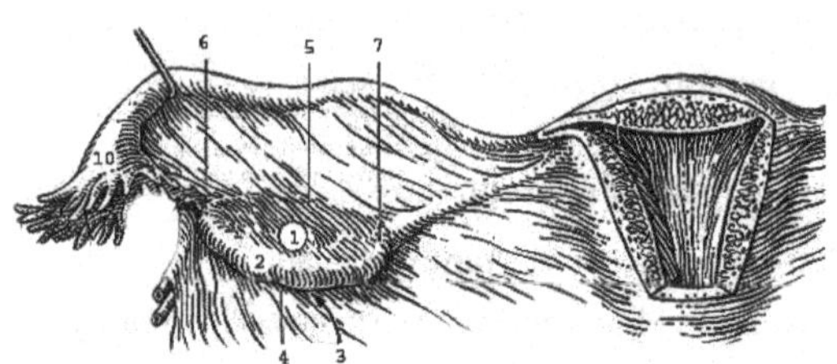

Right Ovary and Fallopian Tube, courtesy of wikimedia commons

Should My Ovaries Be Removed?

Forty Three year old Eva sought medical advice about irregular bleeding from massive uterine fibroids. The continuous bleeding interfered with her lifestyle and caused severe fatigue from the iron deficiency anemia. Uterine artery embolization had been considered and rejected on the grounds the uterine fibroids were much too large for the procedure. The interventional radiologist instead recommended hysterectomy. Eva went home, and after thinking for a few days, finally accepted she would undergo surgery and have the hysterectomy.

What are Uterine Fibroids?

Uterine fibroids are benign growths in the uterus that can grow to large size causing irregular bleeding and pressure on the abdominal organs. They are fairly common and can be detected with pelvic examination, and confirmed with pelvic sonogram and MRI scan. Massive uterine fibroids are most commonly treated with an operation called a hysterectomy operation which removes the uterus along with the fibroid tumors inside the uterus. This form of treatment is usually successful with a good outcome.

Visiting the OB Gyne Surgeon

Next, Eva paid a visit to the Ob-Gyne surgeon to discuss her operation. The surgeon recommended a **COMPLETE** hysterectomy with removal of both ovaries. Sitting in the surgeon's office, Eva timidly protested. "Why remove my ovaries?" asked Eva. The surgeon replied, "Removing the ovaries eliminates the chance of ovarian cancer, and you don't need them anyway."

To Remove or Not to Remove the Ovaries? That is the Question

So now Eva was again in my office asking for my opinion. Should she go against the surgeon's advice and insist on preserving her ovaries, or should she follow the surgeon's advice to have a **COMPLETE** hysterectomy with removal of the ovaries? The ovaries are important because they are the hormone factories that pump out women's hormones on a daily basis. Removing the ovaries removes the source of women's hormones causing all hormone levels to decline to low levels, immediately sending the woman into Menopause.

Studies Show Removing Ovaries Increases Mortality

Luckily, the answer to Eva's question can be found in the medical literature. William Parker MD and Cathleen Rivera MD reported that removing the ovaries is detrimental to overall health and results in increased mortality. (1)(2) Dr. Parker followed 30,000 women for 24 years after their hysterectomy. Half the women had ovaries removed and the other half had their ovaries preserved. The group with ovaries removed did, in fact, have a lower rate of ovarian and breast cancer. However, this was overshadowed by a marked increase in death from heart disease and other cancers. The group with the ovaries removed had a higher all-cause mortality rate, and therefore Dr. Parker recommended that pre-menopausal women preserve the ovaries. Dr Parker also found that postoperative hormone replacement is very beneficial at reducing heart disease risk. (1)

In a second study, Dr Cathleen Rivera followed 1,000 Pre-Menopausal women (under age 45) after hysterectomy, and found that removal of the ovaries resulted in a disturbing 84% increase in death from heart disease. However, if these women were given estrogen replacement after ovarian removal, they were protected with a 35% decrease in mortality from heart disease.(2) I thought this finding was rather impressive.

Bioidentical Hormones After Hysterectomy

These two studies provide convincing evidence of the health benefits of hormone replacement after hysterectomy. Although the patients in these two studies were given Premarin which is a natural hormone (from a pregnant horse), we find that a cocktail of bioidentical hormones including estradiol, estriol, progesterone, DHEA and testosterone works as well or better than the horse hormones. Since all women are humans, it is preferable to prescribe human hormones rather than horse hormones, from pregnant mares, also called Premarin.

Important Point:
Preserving the ovaries during a hysterectomy is beneficial to health, and should be strongly considered in the younger pre-menopausal age group. If the ovaries are removed, bioidentical hormone replacement is then advised as beneficial for health.

What about preventing ovarian cancer and breast cancer in high risk groups?

For women at high risk with familial breast and ovarian cancer, and positive BRCA genetic markers, Dr Parker says it makes sense to go ahead with removing the ovaries for these people in high risk groups.

For references and links, see my web site: www.bioidenticalhormones101.com

References for Chapter 12. Bioidentical Hormones Found Beneficial After Hysterectomy

(1) http://www.ncbi.nlm.nih.gov/pubmed/19384117
Obstet Gynecol. 2009 May;113(5):1027-37. Ovarian conservation at the time of hysterectomy and long-term health outcomes in the nurses' health study. Parker WH et al.

(2) http://www.ncbi.nlm.nih.gov/pmc/articles/PMC2755630/?tool=pubmed
Menopause. 2009 Jan-Feb; 16(1): 15-23. Increased cardiovascular

mortality following early bilateral oophorectomy. Cathleen M. Rivera, MD et al.

(3) http://www.businesswire.com/portal/site/home/permalink/?ndmViewId=news_view&newsId=20090420005411&newsLang=en April 20, 2009 New Study Finds Removing Ovaries During Hysterectomy Increases Risk of Death, Outweighs Benefits

(4) http://www.news-medical.net/news/2009/04/20/48588.aspx Removal of ovaries during hysterectomy increases risk of death, outweighs benefits April 2009

CHAPTER 13

BioIdentical Hormones Relieve Anxiety

56 year old Susan suffered from anxiety and panic attacks, and had been prescribed Valium™, Effexor™ and Wellbutrin™ by her primary care doctor. This cocktail of psychoactive drugs caused Susan adverse side effects, and didn't seem to be helping, so she stopped taking them. A few years ago, after she went through menopause, she started having hot flashes, and this is when she first noticed the anxiety attacks, preceding the hot flashes.

Estrogen Deficiency Causes Anxiety

We sent Susan to the lab for a hormone panel, and sure enough, Susan's estrogen level was low. Susan's symptoms were caused by menopausal estrogen deficiency, a finding commonly seen in the post menopausal age group. Symptoms are promptly relieved with bioidentical estradiol applied as a topical cream twice a day. Additionally, Susan's tests revealed vitamin and mineral deficiencies which were, no doubt, aggravating the anxiety attacks. Susan was started on her bioidentical hormone program which included estradiol and progesterone as a balanced topical cream. She was also started on vitamin B12 and magnesium supplements. Six weeks later, Susan reported that her anxiety and panic attacks had improved and were almost gone. She also noticed better sleep and more clarity of mind, and her night sweats and hot flashes had resolved as well.

Anxiety is Associated with Hot Flashes

A study published in 2005 Menopause reported that anxiety is strongly associated with menopausal hot flashes, and usually precedes the hot flash episode. (13) Hot flashes are caused by estrogen deficiency, and are treated with bioidentical estradiol, which virtually eliminates them. (15)(16)(17)

The Benefits of Bioidentical Estrogen

Previous chapters have discussed the safety and the importance of bioidentical hormones. Uzzi Reiss's book, "Natural SuperWoman", contains an excellent discussion of bioidentical hormones. Chapter 4 covers anxiety, panic attacks and relief with bioidentical estrogen.(1) Numerous articles (see below) summarize the medical literature showing that low estrogen levels cause anxiety and depression in humans and animals. Estrogen treatment relieves anxiety and depression as well as virtually eliminates the hot flashes.

Important Point:
Hot Flashes, anxiety and panic attacks are estrogen deficiency symptoms, relieved with bioidentical estrogen. SSRI anti-depressants do not contain estrogen, and their use for estrogen deficiency is an abuse and victimization of women who suffer from estrogen deficiency. SSRI drugs should not be used to treat estrogen deficiency symptoms.

What is the Mechanism of Action of Estrogen in Eliminating Anxiety and Depression?

Estrogen receptors have been found in the brain, and estrogen increases the expression of an enzyme in the brain called tryptophan hydroxylase-2 (TPH2). This enzyme's job is to convert tryptophan to serotonin, an important neurotransmitter responsible for anti-anxiety and calming effect in the brain. These estrogen receptors have been isolated to specific areas of the brain called the DRN, or the Dorsal Raphe Nuclei (2-6).

Estrogen Effective for Perimenopausal Depression

A study published in the 2001 Archives of General Psychiatry evaluated bioidentical estrogen as treatment for peri-menopausal depression. They evaluated fifty women ages 40-55 years, suffering from a depressive disorder and irregular menstrual periods. These women were treated with bioidentical estrogen or placebo over 12 weeks. Remission of depression was observed in 17 (68%) women treated with bioidentical estradiol compared with only 5 (20%) in the placebo group. The authors concluded, "*Transdermal estradiol is an effective treatment of depression for perimenopausal women.*"(7)

Estrogen Effective for Post-Partum Depression (after child birth)

Postpartum depression is seen in approximately 13% of women who have recently given birth, and often remains untreated. (10) Various treatments have been tried, including antidepressant drug therapy (SSRI's), bioidentical estrogen, individual psychotherapy, and group psychotherapy. (10)

A study published in the 2001 Journal of Clinical Psychiatry showed that bioidentical estrogen is effective for post-partum depression.(8) Twenty-three women suffering from postpartum depression were recruited from a psychiatric emergency unit. The women were treated over 8 weeks with bioidentical estradiol (sublingual form). Baseline serum estradiol levels were very low suggesting ovarian failure. During the first week of estradiol treatment, depressive symptoms resolved rapidly, and serum estradiol levels increased considerably. By the second week of treatment, 83% of patients showed clinical recovery.

A second earlier study published in 1996 Lancet showed that bioidentical estrogen is an effective treatment for post-partum depression. Sixty One women suffering from post partum depression were given transdermal estradiol (0.2 mg daily), and rapid improvement was reported during the first month of treatment.(9)

Many women with post-partum depression are treated with SSRI antidepressants which does not address the underlying estrogen deficiency and ovarian failure. In my opinion, bioidentical hormone treatment is more effective and safer than SSRI antidepressants or other psychoactive drugs, and should be the preferred choice. Bioidentical estrogen has none of the adverse effects associated with SSRI antidepressants which, after all, may end up in mother's milk, and may have adverse effects on the breast feeding baby.

Estradiol for Post Partum Psychosis

While post partum estrogen deficiency causes depression in 13% of patients, a smaller subset go on to develop full blown post partum psychosis. Bioidentical estrogen is also effective for this more severely affected group. A study done in Finland published in the 2001 Journal of Clinical Psychiatry evaluated 10 women suffering from post partum psychosis. All had low serum estradiol (mean of 50 pg/ml) indicating gonadal failure. All were treated with bioidentical estradiol, with serum estradiol levels rising to normal. Remarkably, estradiol treatment reversed psychiatric symptoms in all patients. (11)

Estradiol Improves Cognition for Alzheimer's Dementia

In a study published in 2001 Neurology, twenty postmenopausal women with Alzheimer's dementia were treated with bioidentical estradiol (0.10 mg per day, topical) and compared to placebo. Sophisticated neuropsychological tests showed improvement in attention, and in verbal, visual and semantic memory compared with subjects who received a placebo.(12)

Estradiol Reduces Anxiety in Mouse Model

Alicia A. Walf examined a mouse model in which Estradiol, a bioidentical estrogen, reduces anxiety—and depression-like behavior of aged female mice. Her findings were published in Neuroscience Research in Feb 2010. (14) Matthew N. Hill investigated the mechanism of estradiol as an anxiolytic, and he implicated the enzyme, fatty acid amide hydrolase (FAAH), which degrades the endocannabinoid anandamide. The enzyme, FAAH, is regulated by estrogen.(25) This reveals a biochemical mechanism for how estrogen relieves anxiety. Obviously, this is a fertile area for new research, as the exact mechanism has not yet been elucidated.

For references and links, see my web site: www.bioidenticalhormones101.com

References for 12. BioIdentical Hormones Relieve Anxiety

(5) http://www.uzzireissmd.com/refs/04.html
The Natural SuperWoman, by Uzzi Reiss MD and Yfat Reiss Gendell, Avery Trade, 2008. web site page containing references for the Estrogen chapter.

(6) http://www.ncbi.nlm.nih.gov/pmc/articles/PMC2667128
Neuroscience. 2009 January 23; 158(2): 456-464. Estrogen decreases 5-HT1B autoreceptor mRNA in selective subregion of rat dorsal raphe nucleus: inverse association between gene expression and anxiety behavior in the open field. by Ryoko Hiroiab and John F. Neumaierb

(7) http://endo.endojournals.org/cgi/content/full/endo;146/2/797
Endocrinology Vol. 146, No. 2 797-807, 2005 by The Endocrine Society. Novel Actions of Estrogen Receptor-ß on Anxiety-Related Behaviors by Trent D. Lund, Tomislav Rovis, Wilson C. J. Chung and Robert J. Handa

(8) http://www.ncbi.nlm.nih.gov/pubmed/15820717?dopt=Abstract
Biol Psychiatry. 2005 Apr 15;57(8):938-42. Estrogen receptor-beta regulates tryptophan hydroxylase-1 expression in the murine midbrain raphe. Gundlah C et al.

(9) http://www.ncbi.nlm.nih.gov/pubmed/19559077
Neuroscience. 2009 Oct 6;163(2):705-18. Epub 2009 Jun 23. Estrogen receptor beta regulates the expression of tryptophan-hydroxylase 2 mRNA within serotonergic neurons of the rat dorsal raphe nuclei. Donner N, Handa RJ.

(10) http://www.albany.edu/~cafrye/papers/walfFrye06review.pdf
Neuropsychopharmacology (2006) 31, 1097-1111, 2006 Nature Perspective—A Review and Update of Mechanisms of Estrogen in the Hippocampus and Amygdala for Anxiety and Depression Behavior by Alicia A Walf and Cheryl A Frye

(11) http://www.ncbi.nlm.nih.gov/pubmed/11386980
Arch Gen Psychiatry. 2001 Jun;58(6):529-34. Efficacy of estradiol

for the treatment of depressive disorders in perimenopausal women: a double-blind, randomized, placebo-controlled trial. by Soares CN et al.

(12) http://www.ncbi.nlm.nih.gov/pubmed/11411813
J Clin Psychiatry. 2001 May;62(5):332-6. Estrogen deficiency in severe postpartum depression: successful treatment with sublingual physiologic 17beta-estradiol: a preliminary study.by Ahokas A ET AL.

(13) http://www.ncbi.nlm.nih.gov/pubmed/8598756
Lancet. 1996 Apr 6;347(9006):930-3. Transdermal oestrogen for treatment of severe postnatal depression. by Gregoire AJ ET AL.

(14) http://www.jabfm.com/cgi/reprint/16/5/372.pdf
The Effectiveness of Various Postpartum Depression Treatments and the Impact of Antidepressant Drugs on Nursing Infants Dwenda Gjerdingen, MD, MS (J Am Board Fam Pract 2003;16:372-82.)

(15) http://www.ncbi.nlm.nih.gov/pubmed/10817099
J Clin Psychiatry. 2000 Mar;61(3):166-9. Positive treatment effect of estradiol in postpartum psychosis: a pilot study. Ahokas A et al.

(16) http://www.neurology.org/cgi/content/abstract/57/4/605
Neurology 2001;57:605-612, 2001 American Academy of Neurology High-dose estradiol improves cognition for women with AD Results of a randomized study by S. Asthana, MD et al.

(17) http://www.ncbi.nlm.nih.gov/pubmed/15879914
Menopause. 2005 May-Jun;12(3):258-66. The role of anxiety and hormonal changes in menopausal hot flashes. Freeman EW ET AL.

(18) http://www.ncbi.nlm.nih.gov/pubmed/19804793
Estradiol reduces anxiety—and depression-like behavior of aged female mice by Alicia A. Walf and Cheryl A. Frye Neuroscience Research, The University at Albany-SUNY, United States September 2009

(19) http://www.ncbi.nlm.nih.gov/pubmed/15474758
Maturitas. 2004 Oct 15;49(2):140-7. A short study in the treatment of hot flashes with buccal administration of 17-beta estradiol. Gass MS,

Rebar RW, Cuffie-Jackson C, Cedars MI, Lobo RA, Shoupe D, Judd HL, Buyalos RP, Clisham PR.

(20) http://www.ncbi.nlm.nih.gov/pubmed/11400216
Menopause as a Measure of Population Health—Physiology of hot flashes Robert R. Freedman 1 2 Am. J. Hum. Biol. 13:453-464, 2001

(21) http://jcem.endojournals.org/cgi/content/abstract/61/4/627
Journal of Clinical Endocrinology & Metabolism Vol. 61, No. 4 627-632

(22) http://jcem.endojournals.org/cgi/content/full/82/2/703
Cizza G, Gold PW, Chrousos GP. High-dose transdermal estrogen, corticotropin-releasing hormone, and postnatal depression [letter]. J Clin Endocrinol Metab 1997;82:704.

(23) http://www.ncbi.nlm.nih.gov/pubmed/11411813
Ahokas A, Kaukoranta J, Wahlbeck K, Aito M. Estrogen deficiency in severe postpartum depression: successful treatment with sublingual physiologic 17B-estradiol: a preliminary study. J Clin Psychiatry 2001;62:332-6.

(24) http://www.ncbi.nlm.nih.gov/pubmed/9439497
Ahokas AJ, Turtiainen S, Aito M. Sublingual oestrogen treatment of postnatal depression [letter]. Lancet 1998;351:109.

(25) http://www.ncbi.nlm.nih.gov/pubmed/8598756
Gregoire AJ, Kumar R, Everitt B, Henderson AF, Studd JW. Transdermal oestrogen for treatment of severe postnatal depression. Lancet 1996; 347:930-3.

(26) http://www.ncbi.nlm.nih.gov/pubmed/10591876
Ahokas A, Aito M. Role of estradiol in puerperal psychosis. Psychopharmacology (Berl) 1999;147: 108-10.

(27) http://www.ncbi.nlm.nih.gov/pubmed/10706019
Ahokas A, Aito M, Turiainen S. Association between oestradiol and puerperal psychosis. Acta Psychiatr Scand 2000;101:167-70.

(28) http://www.ncbi.nlm.nih.gov/pubmed/11317610
Granger ACP, Underwood MR. Review of the role of progesterone in the management of postnatal mood disorders. J Psychosom Obstet Gynaecol 2001;22:49-55.

(29) http://science.iowamedicalmarijuana.org/pdfs/psych/Hill%202007.pdf Estrogen recruits the endocannabinoid system to modulate emotionality. Matthew N. Hill, Eda S. Karacabeyli, Boris B. Gorzalka. Psychoneuroendocrinology (2007) 32, 350-357

CHAPTER 14

Menopausal Arthritis and Bioidentical Hormones

Joyce is a 52 years old, post menopausal typist who came to see me in the office because of joint pain in her hands which keeps her up at night with aching, and interferes with her job as a typist. She was fine until about three years ago when her menstrual cycles stopped, and she became post-menopausal. Since then, Joyce has visited a number of doctors with all the usual tests. X-rays of the hands were normal, and blood tests for rheumatoid arthritis were negative. Her doctors told her she had early osteoarthritis and recommended the standard treatments listed here:

Conventional Treatment of Osteoarthritis:

1) NSAID tablets. (Non-Steroidal Anti-Inflammatory Drugs) Such as Aspirin, Acetaminophen (Tylenol™), Ibuprofen™, Naproxen™, Celecoxib™, and Vioxx™. Many of these are over-the counter drugs that do not require a prescription. Some require a prescription.
2) Steroid Injections into the painful joint performed in the Doctor's office.
3) Topical NSAID Creams for pain relief, available over the counter.
4) Physical Therapy.
5) Wait for joint damage, and then offer prosthetic joint replacement.

Menopausal Arthritis

I explained to Joyce that she had fairly classical Menopausal Arthritis caused by an inflammatory response associated with declining estrogen levels. I have noticed this in many of my patients. The inflammatory process is usually relieved by bio-identical estrogen as a topical cream. Joyce's lab panel showed low estrogen levels, and Joyce was started on her bio-identical hormone program. Six weeks later, Joyce reports complete relief of symptoms. Her arthritis pains have gone. In addition, Joyce reports that she went off the bio-identical hormone cream for a week to see what would happen, and sure enough, the arthritis came back, only to be relieved again by resuming the hormone cream. This is a fairly typical story that I have seen over and over again.

Doubts from a Colleague

In casual conversation with a rheumatologist friend of mine, I mentioned Joyce's story and the association of arthritis with declining estrogen levels relieved by bioidentical estrogen. To my surprise, my rheumatologist friend merely laughed and scoffed at the idea, saying he never heard of it. He doubted the association between low estrogen levels and arthritis. As surprising as this might seem, there are many "Denialist Doctors", possibly a result of not keeping up with the medical literature.

Important Point:
Estrogen deficiency can be associated with an arthritis syndrome which is relieved by bioidentical estrogen. This is well established in the medical literature.

Association Well Documented in the Rheumatology Literature

As it turns out, the association of arthritic aches and pains with low estrogen levels is well documented in the mainstream rheumatology literature.(7-10) For example, an article published in Sept 2005 in Arthritis & Rheumatism by Felson and Cummings entitled, "Aromatase Inhibitors and the Syndrome of Arthralgias With Estrogen Deprivation", showed that menopausal women treated with estrogen depleting medications tend to develop aches and pains in their joints. (1) Another report in The Lancet Oncology, September 2008 by Sestak and Cuzick showed the same finding that estrogen depletion is associated with joint aches and pains. (2) The authors state:

"Joint symptoms (eg, arthralgia and arthritis) are a well-known side-effect of certain drugs that reduce estrogen levels. Low estrogen levels and

postmenopausal status are associated with the development of symptoms of arthralgias and arthritis."

Natural Treatments for Osteo-Arthritis

Although bio-identical hormone therapy seems to work for most post-menopausal women for arthritis relief, there are a few women that still have arthritis and arthralgias in spite of the estrogen cream. It just doesn't work for them. Well, here are a few natural therapies that can help.

Anti-Inflammatory Treatments

A Vegetable Juicing Diet is anti-inflammatory and can relieve arthritis: The vegetable juicing diet is an effective lifestyle modification that is very effective for arthritis. I suspect the juicing diet works in part because of the elimination of wheat products, which tend to be pro-inflammatory. In addition, fresh vegetables contain plant compounds which are anti-inflammatory. Credit and thanks goes to Andrew Saul MD for bringing this to my attention in his book, "Doctor Yourself ", Page 36-38 which is devoted to arthritis and the vegetable juicing diet.(3) This is certainly worth a try.

Weight Loss.

Weight loss is anti-inflammatory. Fat in the "spare tire" of the abdomen produces inflammatory chemical mediators. By reducing this fat depot, inflammation is reduced everywhere in the body. This is certainly worth a try.

Anti-inflammatory Remedies

There are a number of anti-inflammatory herbs such as Boswellia, Ginger and Curcumin which can relieve the symptoms. Omega 3 Fish Oil is anti-inflammatory and a number of studies reveal just as effective as NSAID anti-inflammatory medications for rheumatoid arthritis.(5)(12)

Nutritional Supplements to Rebuild Cartilage

Cartilage is an important cushion material in the joints that often wears thin as osteoarthritis progresses. Once cartilage loss is severe enough to show up on an x-ray, this usually indicates irreversible damage to the joint. Cartilage nutrients such as glucosamine, chondroitin, and MSM (methyl sulfonyl methane) have been found to be effective at relieving arthritis. Be patient, it takes about six weeks to get full relief. In addition to cartilage, joints are made of bone material, so taking supplements to build strong bone makes sense. Bone is made of collagen, so supplements that are required for strong collagen formation are ones we want here. Vitamin C is a key vitamin for strong collagen. Bio-available Silica is a supplement that makes strong collagen. Collagen is made from amino acids so, dietary amino acids such as lysine and proline are useful. Collagen strength comes from the sulfur crosslinking, so a dietary source of sulfur such as MSM (Methyl Sulfonyl Methane) is useful as well.

For references and links, see my web site: www.bioidenticalhormones101.com

References for Chapter 14. Menopausal Arthritis and Bioidentical Hormones

(1) http://www.ncbi.nlm.nih.gov/pubmed/16142740
Arthritis Rheum. 2005 Sep;52(9):2594-8. Aromatase inhibitors and the syndrome of arthralgias with estrogen deprivation. Felson DT, Cummings SR.

(2) http://www.ncbi.nlm.nih.gov/pubmed/18703382
Lancet Oncol. 2008 Sep;9(9):866-72. Epub 2008 Aug 12.Risk factors for joint symptoms in patients enrolled in the ATAC trial: a retrospective, exploratory analysis.Sestak I, Cuzick J, Sapunar F, Eastell R, Forbes JF, Bianco AR, Buzdar AU; ATAC Trialists' Group.

(3) http://www.doctoryourself.com/arthritis.html
Doctor Yourself: Natural Healing That Works by Andrew Saul, Basic Health Publications 2003

(4) http://www.doctoryourself.com/JOM1.html
Saul AW. William Kaufman, B-3, and arthritis. J Orthomolecular Med, 2001. Vol. 16, No. 3, Third Quarter, 2001, p 189.

(5) http://www.ncbi.nlm.nih.gov/pubmed/7639807
Arthritis Rheum 1995 Aug;38(8):1107-14. Effects of high-dose fish oil on rheumatoid arthritis after stopping nonsteroidal antiinflammatory drugs. Clinical and immune correlates. Kremer et al.

(6) http://jeffreydach.com/2007/05/22/glucosamine-and-chondroitin-for-arthritis-pain-by-jeffrey-dach-md.aspx Glucosamine and Chondroitin for Arthritis Pain by Jeffrey Dach M.D.

(7) http://cme.medscape.com/viewarticle/512093
"Menopausal Arthritis" May Develop in Women Receiving Estrogen-Depleting Treatments News Author: Laurie Barclay, MD CME Author: Désirée Lie, MD, MSEd

(8) http://www.emaxhealth.com/70/3606.html
Women treated with aromatase inhibitors often experience joint pain and musculoskeletal aching: severe enough, in some cases, to make them stop the treatment.

(9) http://cme.medscape.com/viewarticle/579250
Anastrozole Associated With Joint Symptoms in Patients With Breast Cancer CME News Author: Roxanne Nelson Author: Charles Vega, MD

(10) http://www.ncbi.nlm.nih.gov/pubmed/17368903
Breast. 2007 Jun;16(3):223-34. 2007 Mar 21 Aromatase inhibitor-associated arthralgia syndrome. Burstein HJ.

(11) http://www.jrheum.com/subscribers/06/10/1931.html
Collateral Benefits of Fish Oil Therapy for Rheumatoid Arthritis by CHAK SING LAU, MD, FRCP,Professor of Medicine, Division of Rheumatology & Clinical Immunology, online]

(12) http://www.ncbi.nlm.nih.gov/pubmed/9355207
James MJ, Cleland LG. Dietary n-3 fatty acids and therapy for rheumatoid arthritis. Semin Arthritis Rheum. 1997;27:85-97.

(13) http://www.ncbi.nlm.nih.gov/pubmed/11036827
Volker D, Fitzgerald P, Major G, et al. Efficacy of fish oil concentrate in the treatment of rheumatoid arthritis. J Rheumatol. 2000;27:2343-2346.

(14) http://abcnews.go.com/Health/PainArthritis/story?id=4566412
Are There Any Vitamins Or Herbal Supplements That Can Be Used To Treat Pain Resulting From Osteoarthritis? Tieraona Low Dog, M.D., Director of Education, Program in Integrative Medicine, University of Arizona January 2, 2008

(15) http://www.arthritis.org/media/newsroom/statements/GAIT_Statement_FINAL_2_21_06.pdf Arthritis Foundation Statement on the Glucosamine/chondroitin Arthritis Intervention Trial

(16) http://www.healingdaily.com/conditions/glucosamine.htm
Even JAMA admits glucosamine is effective against osteoarthritic pain. McAlindon TE and others. Glucosamine and chondroitin for treatment of osteoarthritis: A systematic quality assessment and meta-analysis JAMA 283:1469-1475, 2000.

(17) http://www.ncbi.nlm.nih.gov/pubmed/11214126
Reginster JY and others. Long-term effects of glucosamine sulfate on osteoarthritis progression: a randomized, placebo-controlled trial. Lancet 357:251-256, 2001.

CHAPTER 15

Testosterone for Dry Eye Syndrome

Bernice was 58 years old with typical menopausal symptoms of night sweats and hot flashes, and came to see me because of dry itchy, red eyes. The lids sometimes swell because of the irritation. Over the years, Bernice had been to numerous eye doctors who gave her various drops to lubricate the eye, antibiotic drops and steroid drops. She has been given instructions for cleaning and irrigating the eyes. The eye drops seem to help somewhat but the irritation always returns whenever she stops them. Lately, the condition is getting worse and nothing seems to help. A routine hormone panel showed low hormone levels, and the testosterone level was especially low. Bernice listened closely as I explained that her dry eye syndrome was caused by low testosterone levels, and testosterone administered to the eyes would help. Eye drops are available.

Cured With Testosterone, Surely You Must Be Joking, Doctor

A few weeks after starting a bioidentical hormone program including testosterone eye drops, Bernice reported her eyes were much better. Her ophthalmologist was an old friend of mine, and at a social function he informed me that one of his patients with Dry Eye Syndrome was treated by me with testosterone, and surely you must be joking, Doctor. His gesture and facial expression with his eyes rolling back were quite distinctive.

Testosterone for Dry Eyes in the Ophthalmology Medical Literature

Apparently, Bernice's ophthalmologist was unaware of the medical evidence published in the ophthalmology medical journals. We will look at a few of these supportive articles that recommend testosterone for evaporative dry eye syndrome. About 5 million Americans have Dry Eye Syndrome caused by dysfunction of the lubricating glands, the lacrimal and meibomian glands. The small glands at the upper outer eye are the lacrimal glands, while the meibomian glands are located in the edges of the upper and lower lids.

Dr David A Sullivan and Dry Eye Research

Much of the research on testosterone and dry eyes has been done by David A. Sullivan, at Schepens Eye Research Institute at Harvard Medical School.(4) Dr. Sullivan's early work in the 1990's involved Sjogrens syndrome, and the discovery that women with Sjögren's syndrome are androgen-deficient causing meibomian gland dysfunction, tear film instability, and the evaporative dry eye characteristic of Sjögren's, which is an autoimmune disorder. (1) Sullivan published a study in 1991 which showed that testosterone inhibited the progression of autoimmune disease in the lacrimal glands mice with Sjögren's. His mouse model of Sjögren's showed that the testosterone suppressed the magnitude of lymphocyte infiltration in the lacrimal gland 22—to 46-fold.(6)

Lacrimal and Meibomian Glands Regulated by Testosterone

In a 1999 report, Sullivan suggested that androgens (testosterone) regulate both lacrimal and meibomian gland function, and suggest that eye drops containing testosterone may be safe and effective treatment for dry eyes in Sjögren's syndrome.(1)

Men on Testosterone Blockers Get Dry Eyes

In 2000, Dr. Sullivan reported that men taking testosterone blocking drugs have dry eye syndrome. Men on testosterone blocking drug treatment for prostate cancer were found to have poor quality tear fluid. This was demonstrated by analyzing the meibomian gland secretions. The dry eye symptoms included light sensitivity, painful and blurry eyes. Dr. Sullivan said:

"the use of anti-androgen pharmaceuticals was associated with significant changes in the relative amounts of lipids in meibomian gland secretions. Our findings indicate that chronic androgen deficiency is associated with meibomian gland dysfunction and dry eye." (2)

In 2001, Drs. Worda and Nepp from Vienna Austria reported that topically administered androgen can restore the lipid phase of the tear film, and was useful in treatment of "keratoconjunctivitis sicca", the medical term for Dry Eye Syndrome. (3)

Complete Insensitivity to Androgen and Dry Eyes

Next, Dr Sullivan turned his attention to a genetic disorder called Complete Insensitivity to Androgen (CIAS). In this genetic disorder, the androgen receptor is nonfunctional, and subsequently, there is insensitivity to testosterone. Without a functioning receptor, the normal activity of testosterone is completely blocked. Dr Sullivan examined the fluid in tears from Meibomian gland secretions in women with CIAS and compared them to normal controls. The patients with CIAS had alteration in the lipid fractions of tear fluid. This study was published in a 2002 report in Arch Ophthalmology (5).

Trans-Dermal Testosterone For Dry Eye Syndrome

In 2003, Dr. Connor reported transdermal testosterone is safe and effective treatment for dry eye, with the post-menopausal females having the greatest relief of symptoms. (10)

Important Point:
Dry eye syndrome is caused by low testosterone, and is relieved with testosterone delivered to the meibomian glands of the eyelid.

Molecular Biology Mouse Studies of Gene Expression

In 2005, Dr Schirra et al studied the molecular biology of testosterone, and gene expression in the meibomian gland of mice. Dr Schirra reported that testosterone regulates the expression of more than 1500 genes in the mouse meibomian gland which serves to stimulate lipid and fatty acid metabolism in the lubricating eye fluid. (11) The sum total of the above evidence is overwhelming that testosterone plays a key role in production of oil, the lipid component for lubricating the eyes, and that testosterone deficiency is a treatable cause of dry eye syndrome. The treatment is testosterone, a bioidentical hormone.

Conclusion: The evidence is overwhelming that testosterone deficiency plays a role in dry eye syndrome, and testosterone supplementation is curative.

Acknowledgement
Thanks to Carol Peterson, of Women's International Pharmacy, for her pioneering work in formulating eye drops containing testosterone and estradiol for women with dry eye syndrome(14)

For references and links, see my web site: www.bioidenticalhormones101.com

References for Chapter 15. Testosterone for Dry Eyes

(1) http://www.ncbi.nlm.nih.gov/pubmed/10415627 Androgens and dry eye in Sjögren's syndrome. Ann N Y Acad Sci. 1999 Jun 22;876:312-24. Sullivan DA et al.

(2) http://jcem.endojournals.org/cgi/content/abstract/85/12/4874 The Journal of Clinical Endocrinology & Metabolism Vol. 85, No. 12 4874-4882, 2000 Effect of Androgen Deficiency on the Human Meibomian Gland and Ocular Surface Kathleen L. Krenzer, M. Reza Dana, M. David Ullman, Jennifer M. Cermak, Dorothy B. Tolls, James E. Evans and David A. Sullivan

(3) http://www.ncbi.nlm.nih.gov/pubmed/11173183 Maturitas. 2001 Jan 31;37(3):209-12. Treatment of keratoconjunctivitis sicca with topical androgen. by Worda C, Nepp J, Huber JC, Sator MO. Department of Obstetrics and Gynecology, Division of Gynecological Endocrinology and Reproductive Medicine, Vienna University Hospital, Währinger Gürtel 18-20, 1090, Vienna, Austria.

(4) http://www.schepens.harvard.edu/sullivan/research_story.html Sullivan research summary at Schepens Harvard Medical School

(5) http://www.aissg.org/PDFs/BD-Sullivan-CAIS-Meibomian-2002.pdf also see: http://www.ncbi.nlm.nih.gov/pubmed/12470144 Arch Ophthalmol. 2002 Dec;120(12):1689-99. Complete androgen insensitivity syndrome: effect on human meibomian gland secretions. by Sullivan BD, Evans JE, Cermak JM, Krenzer KL, Dana MR, Sullivan DA. Schepens Eye Research Institute,

(6) http://www.iovs.org/cgi/reprint/32/11/3002.pdf http://www.iovs.org/cgi/content/abstract/32/11/3002 Investigative Ophthalmology & Visual Science, Vol 32, 3002-3006.1991 Testosterone-induced suppression of autoimmune disease in lacrimal tissue of a mouse model (NZB/NZW F1) of Sjogren's syndrome AC Vendramini, C Soo and DA Sullivan

(7) http://www3.interscience.wiley.com/journal/120778210/abstract http://www.ncbi.nlm.nih.gov/pubmed/12114274

(8) Sullivan DA et al. Ann N Y Acad Sci. 2002 Jun;966:211-22. Androgen Deficiency, Meibomian Gland Dysfunction, and Evaporative Dry Eye

(9) http://www.aissg.org/INDEX.HTM Androgen Insensitivity Syndrome or AIS (old name Testicular Feminization Syndrome or Testicular Feminisation Syndrome).

(10) http://en.wikipedia.org/wiki/Androgen_insensitivity_syndrome The incidence of complete AIS is about in 1 in 20,000. Androgen Insensitivity Syndrome is a phenotypic female with a chromosomal genotype of 46,XY.The Androgen Insensitivity Syndrome has been linked to mutations in AR, the gene for the human Androgen Receptor, located at Xq11-12 (i.e. on the X chromosome).

(11) http://abstracts.iovs.org/cgi/content/abstract/44/5/2450 Invest Ophthalmol Vis Sci 2003;44: E-Abstract 2450. Treatment of Dry Eye with a Transdermal 3% Testosterone Cream by C.G. Connor Optometry, Southern College of Optometry, Memphis, TN, United States

(12) http://www.iovs.org/cgi/content/full/46/10/3666 Investigative Ophthalmology and Visual Science. 2005;46:3666-3675.) Androgen Control of Gene Expression in the Mouse Meibomian Gland by Frank Schirra,1,2 Tomo Suzuki,1,2 Stephen M. Richards,1 Roderick V. Jensen,3 Meng Liu,1,2 Michael J. Lombardi,3 Patricia Rowley,3 Nathaniel S. Treister,1,4 and David A. Sullivan1,2

(13) http://archopht.ama-assn.org/cgi/content/full/122/2/151 Dry Eye Signs and Symptoms in Women With Premature Ovarian Failure Janine A. Smith, MD; Susan Vitale, PhD, MHS; George F. Reed, PhD; Shirley A. Grieshaber, RN, CRNO; Linda A. Goodman, COT; Vien H. Vanderhoof, RN, CRNP; Karim A. Calis, PharmD, MPH; Lawrence M. Nelson, MBA, MD Arch Ophthalmol. 2004;122:151-156.

(14) http://www.tearfilm.org/dewsreport/pdfs/TOS-0502-DEWS-noAds.pdf Based on data from the largest studies of dry eye to date, the Women's Health Study (WHS), and the Physicians' Health Study (PHS), and other studies,3-14 it has been estimated that about 3.23 million women and 1.68 million men, for a total of 4.91 million Americans 50 years and older have dry eye.

(15) www.womensinternational.com Carol Petersen, R.Ph., C.N.P., Director of Compounding and Dispensing Operations, Women's International Pharmacy, Inc. 2 Marsh Court. Madison, WI 53718. 800. 279. 5708

CHAPTER 16

Newsweek Attacks Oprah and Bioidentical Hormones

An attack article appeared in Newsweek attacking Oprah Winfrey and Bioidentical Hormones. Why should Newsweek attack Oprah Winfrey? (1) Oprah's TV show advocates Natural Medicine and Bioidentical Hormones in direct competition to the interests of the Pharmaceutical Industry and their synthetic hormones. In case you haven't noticed, these are bad times for print media with declining readership caused by competition from the Internet. Newsweek is starving, a magazine described as "an infomercial masquerading as medical news" and "an example of corruption in journalism". Perhaps Newsweek is merely an attack dog for the drug industry, with a typical Newsweek issue representing $2 million in pharmaceutical advertising revenue. (2-5)

Newsweek: a Desperate Mouthpiece for the Pharmaceutical Industry

Five national consumer organizations have complained about Newsweek charging Newsweek with unethical journalism in the promotion of the drug industry's agenda. Specifically, Newsweek ran a special edition, entitled Health for Life, paid for by the drug industry's PhRMA. Newsweek promotes a biased drug agenda, all the while pretending to be impartial and objective. This is truly deceptive. (6-8)

Oprah is Immensely Popular

With a large personal fortune, and 40 million weekly TV viewers, Oprah Winfrey is immensely popular. Her O magazine sells 2 million copies a month. I suggest Oprah's popularity comes directly from championing the interests of the people. In this case, Oprah has championed Natural Medicine and Bioidentical Hormones, topics which are immensely popular with the public. Is Oprah hurt or concerned about the Newsweek article? In this new day of viral marketing, any publicity is good publicity, including this Newsweek hatchet job article. I suspect Oprah is laughing all the way to the bank.

Newsweek is an Infomercial Masquerading as Medical News

For those of you interested in the actual details of the Newsweek errors, distortions and deceptions, I have itemized a few of them for you below:

1) Newsweek says: "bioidentical hormones are unregulated". This is an outright falsehood. Compounded bioidentical hormones are highly regulated at the state levels. Just walk into a pharmacy and ask the pharmacist in charge about the regulations. There are literally hundreds of them. And yes, bio-identical hormones ARE FDA approved. The following table contains a list of FDA-approved bio-identical hormone commercial products available at the drugstore commonly used to treat menopause and andropause:

Hormone Product	Year of FDA Approval	Manufacturer
Alora (estradiol):	FDA approved 1996	Watson Labs
Climara (estradiol):	FDA approved 1994	Bayer
FemPatch: (estradiol)	FDA approved 1997	Parke Davis
Vivelle-Dot (estradiol):	FDA approved 1994	Novartis
Estraderm: (estradiol)	FDA approved 1986	Novartis
Esclim: (estradiol)	FDA approved 1998	Women's First Healthcare
Estrace (estradiol):	FDA approved 1993	Bristol Myers Squibb
Estring: (estradiol)	FDA approved 1996	Pharmacia UpJohn
Prometrium (progesterone):	FDA approved 1998	Solvay Pharmaceuticals
Crinone: (progesterone)	FDA approved 1997	Columbia Labs
AndroGel (testosterone):	FDA approved 1999	Unimed/Abbott
Testim (testosterone):	FDA approved 2002	Auxilium

FDA Approved Bioidentical Hormone Products:
Estradiol products: Estrace, Progynova, Estrofem, Alora, Climara, Vivelle, Vivelle-Dot, Menostar, Estraderm, Estrasorb Topical, Estrogel, Elestrin, Lunelle Estring, Femring.
Progesterone products: Prometrium, Utrogestan, Minagest, Microgest, Crinone, Prochieve, Cyclogest.
Testosterone products: Testoderm, Androderm, AndroGel, Testim.

The Newsweek deception is this: Newsweek says," *there is no FDA approval for Compounded hormones.*" Yes, this is correct. That's because compounded products are not required to be FDA approved. Instead, compounding is regulated by state and local regulatory agencies. For example, every time you receive intravenous antibiotics medications at the hospital, this is a compounded drug which is NON-FDA approved. Compounding is here to stay.

2) Newsweek says: *"Somers is simply repackaging the old, discredited idea that menopause is some kind of hormone-deficiency disease, and that restoring them will bring back youth,"* says Dr. Nanette Santoro, director of reproductive endocrinology at Albert Einstein College of Medicine and head of the Reproductive Medicine Clinic at Montefiore Medical Center." This statement is another outright falsehood. Menopause is characterized by hormone deficiency, and this is the absolute truth proven by lab tests I see every day. This idea has not been discredited. Well, maybe Newsweek wants the public to think so.

3) Newsweek says: "*Hormone therapy can increase a woman's risk of heart attacks, strokes, blood clots and cancer*". Here we see a typical switch tactic by Newsweek. Newsweek is attempting to confuse the public about two very different types of hormones. Yes, Newsweek is correct that synthetic monster hormones (such as Provera) are associated with cancer and heart disease. However, Newsweek has not told the public the truth that bio-identical hormones are safe and are not associated with

increased risk of cancer or heart disease. Obviously that would displease their drug industry masters.

4) Newsweek says: "*And despite Somers' claim that her non-FDA-approved bioidenticals are "natural" and safer, they are actually synthetic, just like conventional hormones and FDA-approved bioidenticals from pharmacies—and there are no conclusive clinical studies showing they are less risky.*" Newsweek is trying to confuse the public into believing that synthetic chemically altered hormones (provera) are the same as bioidentical hormones. They are not. Synthetic means chemically altered, and this creates a monster hormone causing cancer and heart disease. Bio-identical Hormones are not chemically altered. They are identical to the hormones in the human body. The medical literature is replete with studies showing that bioidentical hormones are safe and effective, while, on the other hand, the chemically altered synthetic hormones are monsters and should never have been approved for human use.

5) Newsweek says: "*Unless a woman has significant discomfort from hot flashes—and most women don't—there is little reason to prescribe them.*" Newsweek is wrong again. Hot flashes are only one of many symptoms of estrogen deficiency. Other symptoms include vaginal dryness, sweats, difficulty sleeping, cognitive dysfunction, menopausal arthritis etc. These are all valid symptoms and good reasons for prescribing bioidentical hormones.

6) This Newsweek article also provided misinformation about iodine supplementation, an essential mineral added to table salt since 1924. This means that since 1924, the nation has supplemented with iodine in the form of iodized salt. Supplementation with Iodine is safe and beneficial for health, and highly recommended. For more information, see the chapter on Iodine and Breast Cancer Prevention.

For references and links, see my web site: www.bioidenticalhormones101.com

References for Chapter 16. Newsweek Attacks Oprah and BioIdentical Hormones

(1) http://www.newsweek.com/id/200025 Newsweek. Live Your Best Life Ever! Wish Away Cancer! Get A Lunchtime Face-Lift! Eradicate Autism! Turn Back The Clock! Thin Your Thighs! Cure Menopause! Harness Positive Energy! Erase Wrinkles! Banish Obesity! Live Your Best Life Ever! By Weston Kosova and Pat Wingert, NEWSWEEK, Published May 30, 2009 From the magazine issue dated Jun 8, 2009

(2) http://www.prweb.com/releases/2009/06/prweb2522034.htm Bioidentical Hormone Replacement Is REAL Medical Science, Not Entertainment Medicine by C.W. Randolph, Jr., M.D., Medical Director of the Natural Hormone Institute.

(3) http://www.huffingtonpost.com/deepak-chopra/mainstream-medicine-and-t_b_213132.html Mainstream Medicine and the Oprah Factor by Deepak ChopraAuthor, Sirius radio host, founder of the Alliance for a New Humanity Posted: June 9, 2009

(4) http://www.huffingtonpost.com/claire-shipman-and-katty-kay/did-anyone-else-think-the_b_212819.html Did Anyone Else Think The Newsweek Photo of Oprah Was Misogynistic? And Just Plain Dumb? by Claire Shipman and Katty Kay

(5) http://www.newsweek.com/id/33610 Pat Wingert. Coming to Newsweek after a nine-year journalism career in Chicago, Wingert had worked as a reporter for The Chicago Tribune from 1985 to 1986 and The Chicago Sun-Times from 1977 to 1984.

(6) http://www.ageofautism.com/2009/06/newsweeks-newspeak-pharmas-weapon-against-oprah.html Newsweek's Newspeak: Pharma's Weapon Against Oprah By Jake Crosby Jake Crosby is a history student at Brandeis University

(7) http://www.familiesusa.org/resources/newsroom/statements/2001-statements/press-statement-consumer-groups-criticize-newsweek-for-transgressing-ethical-bounds-by-working-with-the-pharmaceutical-drug-lobby.html Press Statement. CONSUMER GROUPS CRITICIZE NEWSWEEK FOR TRANSGRESSING ETHICAL BOUNDS BY WORKING WITH THE PHARMACEUTICAL DRUG LOBBY. Drug Lobby's Exclusive Sponsorship of Newsweek's Special Health Edition and Other Joint Efforts Improperly Aided Drug Lobby's Agenda, Groups Claim

(8) http://www.nclnet.org/newsweekpr1002.htm Consumer Groups Criticize Newsweek for Transgressing Ethical Bounds by Working with the Pharmaceutical Drug Lobby

(9) http://online.wsj.com/article/SB123717056802137143.html MARCH 16, 2009 The Truth About Hormone Therapy Wall Street Journal By Erika Schwartz, Kent Holtorf, and David Brownstein.

(10) http://newsmax.com/insidecover/newsweek_time_circulation/2009/01/17/172579.html Newsweek May Stop Weekly Circulation January 17 2009

(11) http://www.latimes.com/entertainment/news/la-et-onthemedia20-2009may20,0,7785135.column Can Newsweek relight the readership flame? The newsweekly aims to carve out a perch among its many competitors with a new, deeper focus. But dwindling circulation in the magazine industry points to a tough battle ahead. LA TIMES, James Rainey May 20, 2009.

(12) http://cosmeticmdnation.blogspot.com/2009/06/newsweek-on-oprah-pot-calling-kettle.html Newsweek on Oprah: Pot calling the kettle black when it comes to bioidentical hormones? Dr. Mitchell Matez, D.O. Sanctuary Medical Aesthetic Center, Boca Raton.

(13) http://jeannesmusings.typepad.com/notsogrounded/2009/06/my-entry.html You Go, Oprah! by Jeanne

(14) http://www.suzannesomers.com/Blog/post/Two-Scariest-Women-on-the-Planet.aspx Two Scariest Women on the Planet—Oprah and Suzanne by Suzanne Somers 6/4/2009

(15) http://www.postgradmed.com/index.php?article=1949 Postgraduate Medicine: Volume 121: No.1 Jan 2009. The Bioidentical Hormone Debate:Are Bioidentical Hormones (Estradiol, Estriol, and Progesterone) Safer or More Efficacious than Commonly Used Synthetic Versions in Hormone Replacement Therapy? Kent Holtorf, MD

CHAPTER 17

Bioidentical Hormones Trashed by AP News

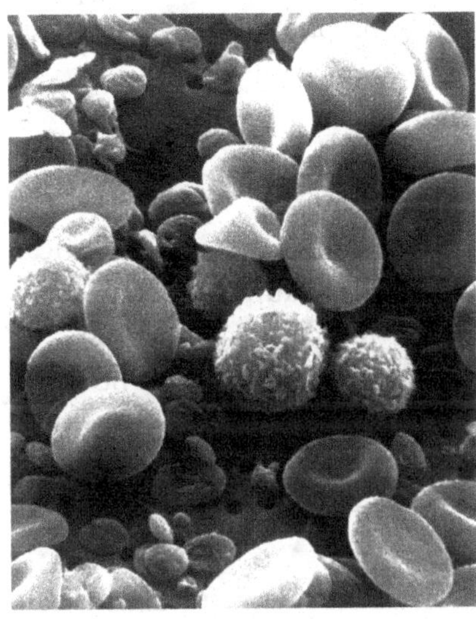

Red Blood Cells Seen with Scanning Electron Microscope, Courtesy of Bruce Wetzel and Harry Schaefer of the National Cancer Institute.

A USA Today article trashing bioidentical hormones caught my attention because it contained almost pure misinformation.(1) Written by an Associated Press AP medical writer, this syndicated article was broadcast over the news media. The writing is a perfect example of trash, or junk journalism. I find it astonishing that the news media feeds this kind of nonsense to the public. The AP article attempts to discredit bioidentical hormones as non-FDA approved, and not proven safe nor effective. Before analyzing the nonsense in the newspaper article, let's take a humorous look at what if the author took her own advice seriously, assuming that naturally occurring human hormones are harmful and dangerous non-approved chemicals. The author, an AP medical writer, might be horrified to know that these non-FDA approved bioidentical hormones, (estradiol, progesterone, estriol and testosterone), are floating around in her blood stream right now, and have been since she was born.

So please don't do anything impulsive and crazy to remove these non-FDA approved chemicals from your body. They are supposed to be there. In fact, these same little non-FDA approved bioidentical hormones have been present in the blood stream of all primates (this includes AP medical news journalists and monkeys) for 40 million years. That's a long time, even for an AP journalist.

Doctors write 65 million prescriptions yearly for non-FDA approved medications, as part of routine medical practice. (8) Two examples are phenobarbital, an anti-convulsant, and chloral-hydrate, a sedative.(8) Another example is intravenous antibiotic treatment at the hospital, a non-FDA approved compounded drug prepared by the hospital compounding pharmacy.

Both FDA Approved and Non-FDA Approved

But Wait! No need to even worry about it, because, Bioidentical Hormones **ARE INDEED** FDA approved. The author even says so in her article. This list of FDA approved bioidentical hormones is presented below. But wait! How can bioidentical hormones be both FDA approved and non-FDA approved? If they are in a bottle at the corner drug store, they are FDA approved, and if they are in my body, they are non-FDA approved. This is really confusing.

The answer can be found in the textbook of biochemistry used by all medical schools, Lehninger's Principles of Biochemistry Chapter 23 on Hormonal Regulation.(16) This authoritative source says the chemical structure of a hormone is independent of where it is. The hormone can be in the human body, in a glass of water, in a bottle at the corner drug store. This doesn't matter; the hormone has the exact same chemical structure. This means that if a bio-identical hormone is FDA approved in a bottle of pills at the drugstore, then the same chemical structure is FDA approved in the human body or anywhere else, it's the same stuff. But for some strange reason, the FDA doesn't work that way and separate paperwork has to be submitted for each one. Welcome to the US government.

Examining the Misinformation Line by Line:

But first, let's take a closer look at the disinformation in the AP article (in bold italic below):

> *"Millions of women have tried custom-compounded hormones . . . . since 2002, when a big federal study found risks from traditional hormone replacement therapy, or HRT."*

The author is correct about the massive switch in 2002, when millions of women abandoned synthetic hormones, and embraced bioidentical hormones after a federal study, the Women's Health Initiative, found that a combination of premarin and provera caused cancer and heart disease. This NIH study used Prempro, a combination of Premarin and Provera, and was terminated early. The culprit was Provera, a synthetic, chemically altered form of progesterone, which has been known for decades to increase risk of cancer and heart disease. The form of estrogen used in the study was Premarin, a horse estrogen from pregnant horse urine. This massive switch to bioidenticals shows that women are smart. Two important things happened after this. Synthetic hormone drug maker Wyeth lost 4 billion dollars in sales, and secondly, breast cancer rates dropped precipitously when masses of women stopped synthetic hormones and started bioidenticals instead. This data was published in 2007 in: "The Decrease in Breast-Cancer Incidence in 2003 in the United States" by Peter M. Ravdin et al. (14) Another study showed a similar decrease in breast cancer rates in Canada after discontinuing synthetic hormones. (15)

> *"However, instead of a safer option, (women) are getting products of unknown risk that still contain the estrogen many of them fear, women's health experts say."*

This is deliberate misinformation. Bioidentical hormones are safer and more effective than the synthetic chemically altered "monster" hormones used in the Women's Health Initiative study. The safety of bioidentical hormones was demonstrated by the French Cohort study, which showed no increased cancer in the bioidentical group. (9) In addition, Dr Holtorf's article cites 196 research studies comparing bio-identical hormones to synthetic patented hormones (like Provera). (10) Dr Holtorf's review of the medical literature concludes:

> *Based on both physiological results and clinical outcomes, current evidence demonstrates that bioidentical hormones are associated with lower risks than their nonbioidentical counterparts. Until there is evidence to the contrary, current evidence dictates that bioidentical hormones are the preferred method of HRT. (10)*

See my article on the safety of bioidentical hormones for more on this topic. The USA Today article continues:

> *"Bioidentical" is a marketing term that has no accepted medical meaning.*

This statement is entirely wrong. The term bioidentical has a definite meaning and is widely used. The term, bioidentical, means a hormone chemical structure which is identical to that found in the human body. Both the Endocrine Society and ACOG (American College of Obstetrics and Gynecology) define the term, "bioidentical", exactly the same, even though the two definitions are worded differently. It is an embarrassment to medical science that the word "bioidentical" has to be used at all. All hormones should have been manufactured as bio-identical hormones. However, because of U.S. patent law which prevents patenting a bioidentical hormone chemical structure, the drug industry created chemically altered hormones which could be patented and sold at higher profit margins. These altered-synthetic hormones are monsters that should never have been approved by the FDA for human consumption.

> *" . . . many prescription drugs contain hormones that chemically match estrogens and progesterones made naturally by the body."*

This is correct. These bioidentical hormones have gone through the FDA approval process showing they are safe and effective. Here a partial list of FDA approved bioidentical hormones available at the corner drug store:

Hormone Product	**Year of FDA Approval**	**Manufacturer**
Alora (estradiol):	FDA approved 1996	Watson Labs
Climara (estradiol):	FDA approved 1994	Bayer
FemPatch: (estradiol)	FDA approved 1997	Parke Davis
Vivelle-Dot (estradiol):	FDA approved 1994	Novartis
Estraderm: (estradiol)	FDA approved 1986	Novartis
Esclim: (estradiol)	FDA approved 1998	Women's First Healthcare
Estrace (estradiol):	FDA approved 1993	Bristol Myers Squibb
Estring: (estradiol)	FDA approved 1996	Pharmacia UpJohn

Prometrium (progesterone):	FDA approved 1998	Solvay Pharmaceuticals
Crinone: (progesterone)	FDA approved 1997	Columbia Labs
AndroGel (testosterone):	FDA approved 1999	Unimed/Abbott
Testim (testosterone):	FDA approved 2002	Auxilium

> *". . . Custom-compounded hormones are not approved by the federal Food and Drug Administration and have not been proved safe or effective."*

This is a misleading and deceptive statement. Custom compounding is regulated at the state level, not by the federal government or the FDA. So, of course compounding is not FDA approved. No FDA approval is required or even desired. Are we going to reject intravenous antibiotic treatment at the hospital because, as a compounded medication, this is also non-FDA approved and not proven safe or effective? Aspirin is FDA approved for over the counter sales. If the compounding pharmacy crushes the aspirin tablet and places the powder into capsules, the aspirin becomes non-FDA approved aspirin, even though it is the same stuff. Starting to make sense now?

The author falsely claims that bioidentical hormones have not been proven safe and effective as required for FDA approval process. Take a look at the list of bioidentical prescription hormones above. These are all FDA approved and proven safe and effective.

> *"They may carry the same cancer and heart risks as traditional treatments and have had even less testing to find out."*

The author is wrong again. The French Cohort study, showed no increased cancer in the bioidentical group. (9) Again, look at Dr Holtorf 's article in Postgraduate Medicine listing 196 research articles showing Bio-identical Hormones are associated with lower risk, and are more efficacious than synthetic counterparts.(10) Two calcium scoring studies showed no increased risk of heart disease associated with bioidentical hormones. A study of CAT calcium scores by Dr. JoAnn E. Manson in the June 2007 JAMA actually showed less heart disease in the women taking unopposed estrogen (they had hysterectomies and were not given the synthetic progestins). (11) These same results had been published 2 years previously in a coronary calcium score study by Dr. Budoff in the 2005 Journal of Women's Health. (12)

> *"Hormone preparations do not need to be customized for each woman; a few standard doses work for almost everyone, medical experts say."*

I don't know who the medical experts were, but I have found dosage varies for bioidentical hormones just as dosage varies for any other drug. Pick up any medical pharmacology text book. What you find is drug dosage varies according to age, body weight, genetics, and hepatic metabolism of the drug.(7) The advice to use standard dosing comes from drug company marketing literature, and is simply wrong.

> *"The saliva tests that some women are given to tailor formulas are of dubious value because hormone levels fluctuate widely throughout the day."*

Again the above statement is an oversimplification that is misleading. For some hormone levels salivary testing is advantageous. For example, saliva testing with four samples throughout the day shows salivary cortisol levels are highest in the morning and lowest in the evening before sleep. Regarding sex hormones, in young cycling females, hormones vary according to a monthly pattern of ovulation called the menstrual cycle. Estrogen and progesterone peaking around day 19-21 of the cycle. Here, salivary hormone testing every two or three days can show this variation and the peaks. In older, post menopausal women who are no longer ovulating, menstrual cycles have stopped and hormone levels typically decline to low levels. As a general rule, wild daily hormone fluctuations simply do not happen for post-menopausal woman. Rather, hormone levels decline to low levels, and since ovulation has stopped, hormone levels don't change much from day to day as revealed by blood testing of hormone levels.

> *"Compounding pharmacists use such different methods that a customized prescription can contain widely varying amounts of hormones depending on who fills it."*

This is a completely wrong and misleading statement. If a prescription for hormone cream is sent to two different compounding pharmacies, and the two creams analyzed, they should have the same amounts of hormones. If they don't, then something is wrong and needs to be fixed. Each compounding pharmacy should make up the exact same formulation when given the same prescription. In other words, there should be reproducibility and consistency from one pharmacy to another. The reality is that there are so many small compounding pharmacies that quality control can be an issue. I have found that this becomes a non-issue when dealing with the larger national compounding pharmacies that specialize in hormones. The quality control is better, and formulations are more consistent.

> *"Many compounders use estriol, a form of estrogen not approved for sale in the United States. The FDA is in a battle with compounding pharmacies over its use."*

Estriol is commonly use in compounding hormone preparations, and like many other natural compounds used for many years, approval was grandfathered in. Formal FDA approval was not required nor was it requested. Medical research shows that of the three estrogens found naturally in humans, estriol is the safest and most protective.

> *The bottom line? "Women need to understand there's no rigorous evidence these preparations are any more effective or any safer than traditional hormone therapy."*

Again, the above statement is false. Dr Holtorf's article published in the medical literature cites 196 references showing safety and efficacy of bioidentical hormones.

> *"For years, medical groups have warned against custom-compounded hormones. The American College of Obstetricians and Gynecologists has denounced claims about their safety. The American Medical Association has urged more FDA oversight. The Federal Trade Commission has filed complaints against online sellers who made health claims for natural progesterone creams without supporting evidence."*

These organizations are all heavily controlled by the drug industry, so of course, they are going to oppose natural substances that cut into profits of the drug industry. Bioidentical hormones compete directly with the synthetic hormone profits of the drug industry. That is what this is all about. This is an information war to protect drug company profits pure and simple.

For references and links, see my web site: www.bioidenticalhormones101.com

References for Chapter 17. BioIdentical Hormones Trashed by AP News

(1) http://www.usatoday.com/news/health/2009-10-29-menopause-herbal_N.htm Bioidenticals: Estrogen without FDA approval for menopause? By Marilynn Marchione,

(2) http://www.thewholechild.us/integrative_/2009/06/alternative-medicine-in-the-news-a-bit-too-much.html Alternative Medicine" in the news

(3) http://blogs.acponline.org/acpinternist/2009/06/throwing-baby-out-with-snake-oil.html Throwing the baby out with the snake oil. Tuesday, June 9, 2009

(4) http://www.usatoday.com/news/health/2008-12-13-breast-cancer-hormone_N.htm New study firmly ties hormone use to breast cancer.

(5) http://content.nejm.org/cgi/content/abstract/360/6/573 NEJM Volume 360:573-587 February 5, 2009 Number 6. Breast Cancer after Use of Estrogen plus Progestin in Postmenopausal Women. Rowan T. Chlebowski, M.D., Ph.D., Lewis H. Kuller, M.D.,et al. for the WHI Investigators.

(6) http://jnci.oxfordjournals.org/cgi/content/full/djm111v1
J Natl Cancer Inst. 2007 Sep 5;99(17):1335-9. Declines in Invasive Breast Cancer and Use of Postmenopausal Hormone Therapy in a Screening Mammography Population. Karla Kerlikowske et al.

(7) http://www.sciencedaily.com/releases/2007/08/070814162852.htm Drop In Breast Cancer Incidence Linked To Hormone Use, Not Mammograms ScienceDaily (Aug. 15, 2007)

(8) http://www.pharmj.com/pdf/cpd/pj_20040626_pharmacokinetics02.pdf Variability in Drug Dosage Requirements, Alison Thompson. Age, Weight, Genetics. Pharmacokinetic variability, hepatic metabolism of drugs, clearance with renal elimination, drug interactions

(9) http://www.cnn.com/2007/HEALTH/conditions/09/26/unapproved.drugs/index.html NEW YORK (CNN)—Every year, doctors write approximately 65 million prescriptions for drugs not yet approved by the U.S. Food and Drug Administration, the federal agency that regulates prescription drugs.

(10) http://www.ncbi.nlm.nih.gov/pubmed/12626212 Climacteric. 2002 Dec;5(4):332-40. Combined hormone replacement therapy and risk of breast cancer in a French cohort study of 3175 women. de Lignières B, de Vathaire F, Fournier S, Urbinelli R, Allaert F, Le MG, Kuttenn F.

(11) http://www.holtorfmed.com/pdf/01-Bioidentical-hormone-debate.pdf also see http://jeffreydach.com/files/80618-70584/The_Bioidentical_Hormone_Debate_Ken_Holtorf_MD.pdf The Bioidentical Hormone Debate: Are Bioidentical Hormones (Estradiol, Estriol, and Progesterone) Safer or More Efficacious than Commonly Used Synthetic Versions in Hormone Replacement Therapy? Kent Holtorf, MD1

(12) http://www.nejm.org/doi/full/10.1056/NEJMoa071513 Estrogen Therapy and Coronary-Artery Calcification JoAnn E. Manson, M.D. et al. N Engl J Med 2007; 356:2591-2602June 21, 2007

(13) http://www.ncbi.nlm.nih.gov/pubmed/15989413 J Womens Health (Larchmt). 2005 Jun;14(5):410-7. Effects of hormone replacement on progression of coronary calcium as measured by electron beam tomography. Budoff MJ et al.

(14) http://jama.ama-assn.org/content/287/17/2215.abstract JAMA. 2002;287(17):2215-2220. Timing of New Black Box Warnings and Withdrawals for Prescription Medications Karen E. Lasser, MD, MPH; et al.

(15) http://www.nejm.org/doi/full/10.1056/NEJMsr070105 The Decrease in Breast-Cancer Incidence in 2003 in the United States. Peter M. Ravdin, Ph.D., M.D., Kathleen A. Cronin, Ph.D et al. N Engl J Med 2007; 356:1670-1674April 19, 2007.

(16) http://jnci.oxfordjournals.org/content/early/2010/09/23/jnci.djq345.abstract Breast Cancer Incidence and Hormone Replacement Therapy in Canada. Prithwish De, C. Ineke Neutel, Ivo Olivotto and Howard Morrison. J Natl Cancer InstVolume102, Issue19Pp. 1489-1495

(17) Lehninger Principles of Biochemistry by Albert Lehninger, David L. Nelson, Michael M. Cox. W. H. Freeman; Fifth Edition edition (June 15, 2008)

CHAPTER 18

Bioidentical Hormones According to the LA Times

An article on bioidentical hormones appeared in the Los Angeles Times.(1) The author was a medical journalist with a master's degree in biology. Sadly, this article contained a number of omissions, errors and falsehoods that require correction:

> The article says: *"Over the decades, millions of women have taken some form of hormone therapy to relieve symptoms of menopause . . . The treatment typically included Premarin, estrogen isolated from the urine of pregnant mares, combined with Provera, a synthetic version of the hormone progesterone."*

The article correctly states that millions of women have taken hormone preparations to relieve symptoms of menopause. However it then presents the biased and narrow viewpoint that all of these women took "synthetic" chemically altered hormones in the form of Provera and Premarin. These are chemically altered hormones sold by the major drug companies. The reality is that millions of women have taken and continue to take human bioidentical hormones, rather than Premarin and Provera for relief of menopausal symptoms.

The Women's Health Initiative Study

The LA Times article then discussed the Women's Health Initiative Study, halted early because the study showed that synthetic, chemically altered hormones (Premarin and Provera) cause cancer and heart disease. In this, they are quite correct.

> *"But when a six-year study of more than 16,600 postmenopausal women that was part of the Women's Health Initiative found that the combination of Premarin and Provera seemed to increase the risk of breast cancer, stroke and heart disease, doctors and patients suddenly had to consider other options."*

Although this is correct, I would remove the word, "seemed" from the text. The synthetic hormones, Premarin and Provera didn't "seem" to cause cancer and heart disease. They DID cause cancer and heart disease in the WHI study. That's why the study was terminated early, a small fact conveniently left out of the story.

> *"Soon after the WHI made headlines, some pharmacies, alternative health clinics and a few outspoken doctors started heavily promoting so-called "bioidentical hormones" for the treatment of menopausal symptoms. Unlike Premarin or Provera, bioidentical hormones—which are produced in laboratories using yam and soy phytoestrogens as a starting point—exactly match the hormone made by human ovaries."*

After the revelations of the WHI study were made public in 2002, millions of smart women abandoned synthetic hormones and switched to bioidentical hormones. This switch was not a product of a massive advertising campaign of the type we see on television for drugs like Lipitor and SSRI antidepressants. As a matter of fact, there was no TV advertising for bioidentical hormones, so I would disagree that bioidentical hormones were "heavily promoted". They weren't. The massive switch was more a product of the rank and file Physicians who stopped writing prescriptions for Medroxyprogesterone (MPA), also called Provera™, the synthetic hormone used in the WHI study. What was conveniently left out of the story is that this sudden drop in the number of synthetic hormone prescriptions in 2003 was accompanied by a nine per cent drop in breast cancer rates as reported in the New England Journal of Medicine by Dr. Ravdin. (22) The author is quite correct in the statement that bioidentical hormones are exactly the same as the hormones made by the ovaries.

FDA Approved Bioidentical Hormones

> *"The Food and Drug Administration has approved several prescription-only drugs that contain bioidentical hormones, including Estrace pills, Estrasorb topical cream and the Alora patch. But many health clinics and pharmacies also sell non-approved creams that contain bioidentical estrogen and/or progesterone. These creams are*

often custom-made—or "compounded"—for each patient, sometimes based on the results of a saliva test that measures a woman's hormone levels."

FDA approved bioidentical hormone preparations are available at the corner drugstore. However, the author omits the fact that compounding pharmacies are regulated at the state level, not by the federal government, so FDA approval is not required or even desired for compounded hormone preparations. Insisting on FDA approval for compounded hormone preparations is similar to insisting that your state driver's license is invalidated because it was not issued by the federal government.

FDA approval is sometimes waved about like a majestic frond, as if it grants magical qualities to a drug. In reality, FDA approval does not automatically mean the drug is effective or desirable. Ten percent of all FDA approved drugs are later recalled or banned and designated as "**Bad Drugs**". Another ten per cent of FDA approved drugs later receive black box warnings. FDA approval means a major drug company has paid a lot of money for studies showing efficacy over placebo. Sometimes, these studies are fudged.

Catch 22 for Natural Substances

Another important omitted fact is that the FDA approval process is so expensive that it makes financial sense only for patented drugs with prospects for large returns. It is unlikely that any drug company will invest the millions for FDA approval studies when the drug in question is a natural substance such as a bioidentical hormone that cannot be protected by a patent. The publicly financed Women's Health Initiative study sponsored by the NIH was done with patented hormones, Premarin and Provera, not the natural non-patentable bioidentical hormones. This no doubt reflects drug company control over NIH research dollars. The NIH should be studying natural substances like bioidentical hormones, but they rarely do.

In One Corner, We Have: Dr Kent Holtorf

> The LA article goes on: *"Dr. Kent Holtorf, a physician and proponent of bioidentical hormones . . . The website for Holtorf's clinic says that women using bioidentical hormones "feel great" without suffering any of the side effects of "synthetic hormones," said to include fatigue, depression and weight gain, along with the increased risk of breast cancer and heart disease. In a phone interview, Holtorf said that bioidentical hormones are more effective and safer than traditional treatments. "Over and over, women have told me that they feel much better" after taking the bioidentical hormones, he says."*

In the Other Corner, We have Dr. Nanette Santoro Representing Mainstream Medicine and Synthetic Hormones

> *"Bioidentical hormones have an obvious appeal to women seeking relief for menopausal symptoms, says Dr. Nanette Santoro, chair of the department of obstetrics and gynecology at the University of Colorado Health Sciences Center in Denver and vice president of clinical science for the Endocrine Society. After all, it just seems to make sense that anything that exactly mimics a woman's own hormones must be better than mare's urine or a man-made compound that doesn't exist in nature."*

> *"But Santoro says there is no proof that bioidentical hormones are any safer or more effective than traditional treatments. "All of the evidence that we have suggests that all of these hormones should be painted with the same brush," she says."*

Dr Santoro represents mainstream medicine and synthetic hormones sold by the major drug companies, and as such uses coded language which requires translation. "*Traditional Treatments*" means synthetic chemically altered hormones sold by the drug companies. *"Painted with the same brush"* is the usual attempt to confuse the difference between chemically altered hormones and bioidentical hormones, claiming they are all the same thing. They are not the same thing. Chemically altered hormones are "**Monster Hormones**" that cause cancer and heart disease. Bioidentical hormones have the same chemical structure as the hormones in the human body and are safe and effective.

Dr Kent Holtorf Review Article Shows Bioidenticals Are Safer and More Effective than Synthetics

Dr Kent Holtorf's review article, "The Bioidentical Hormone Debate", cites 196 medical studies showing bioidentical hormones are safer and more effective than synthetic altered hormones. (2) In my opinion, chemically altered hormones are **MONSTERS** that should never have been approved for human use. Lehninger's textbook of biochemistry uses the word hormone which means a "bioidentical" hormone. Synthetic chemically altered hormones do not exist in the human body. The sole purpose of chemically altering a hormone chemical structure is to obtain a patent to protect profits of the drug industry. These chemically altered monster hormones are a recent invention in the history of medicine and are MONSTERS that should never have been approved for human use. Alternatively, bioidentical hormones and other natural substances by definition cannot be patented and therefore not profitable for the drug industry.

Dr. Nanette Santoro Has Concerns

> *"She has many concerns about bioidentical hormones that don't have FDA approval. For one thing, she says, it's impossible to know if unapproved creams have the promised amounts of hormones. "I've seen patients on these compounds actually losing bone mass because they were getting an insufficient dosage," she says. "Why take that chance?"*

We already discussed the FDA approval issue above. Compounding pharmacies are regulated by the states, not the federal government, so FDA approval is neither required nor desired for compounded preparations. The issue of quality control and proper dosage is a real consideration that applies to ALL TYPES of medications whether FDA approved or not. To get the best quality, I recommend working with a knowledgeable physician familiar with the best compounding pharmacies with the highest reputation for quality and service. Perhaps Dr Santoro's statement is referring here to over-the-counter progesterone creams which are regulated by the cosmetics act. I agree with her point. These are not recommended because the amount of active hormone is not listed on the label, nor is there any assurance of the amount of active hormone inside the product.

"Why take a chance?" says Santoro. This is typical drug company propaganda and fear mongering that is usually seen with drug company television advertising. This plants doubt about compounded preparations. The problem with this logic is that the same doubt can be raised about hospital pharmacies which are all compounding pharmacies. For example, the intravenous medications prepared in the hospital pharmacy are, in fact, compounded medications. The reality is that synthetic hormones are the monsters, and the bioidentical hormones are the safe and effective choice.

Dr. Cynthia Stuenkel, clinical professor of medicine at UC San Diego

> "Dr. Cynthia Stuenkel, clinical professor of medicine at UC San Diego and president of the North American Menopause Society, shares this concern. "*Some progesterone creams may contain little or no progesterone, while others contain so much that they definitely should be available only with a prescription,*" she says. "*Taking hormones without the careful guidance of a doctor is risky business,*" Stuenkel says, "*Among other things, too many hormones can potentially cause blood clots and endometrial hyperplasia, a precursor to uterine cancer.*"

Dr Stuenkel is correct in that progesterone creams are relatively safe, and available OTC (over the counter) without a prescription. These are regulated by the cosmetics act. She is also correct in that the OTC progesterone creams may vary in potency. The highest quality and most reliable progesterone creams are made by prescription at a compounding pharmacy. These are freshly prepared according to the prescribed dosage written by the physician. This is all OK.

Blood Clots and Endometrial Hyperplasia and Uterine Cancer—Omitting History

Dr. Stuenkel is right that certain types of hormones cause blood clots and uterine cancer. However, blood clots are caused by oral estrogen, not progesterone. Uterine cancer is caused by oral estrogen, specifically Premarin. Progesterone is not on this list. Jumping from progesterone to blood clots and endometrial hyperplasia is somewhat misleading and reveals a lack of understanding of the history of medicine. Progesterone does not cause blood clots, endometrial hyperplasia, or uterine cancer. Progesterone is protective. This is taught to first year medical students. Blood clots, endometrial hyperplasia and uterine cancer are all caused by oral estrogen tablets, called Premarin, given without progesterone, which historically was the usual practice from 1950 to 1975. This medical practice was halted with the publication of a NEJM report revealing that Premarin causes uterine cancer. To prevent uterine cancer, a synthetic progesterone called Provera was added to the regimen, hence Prempro (a combo drug of Premarin plus Provera), the drug used in the WHI (women's health initiative) study. This is a little history omitted from the LA Times story.

Also omitted was that oral estrogen tablets cause increased coagulability and increased risk of blood clots. For example, oral estrogen in birth control pills is the cause of blood clots, deep venous thrombosis, pulmonary emboli and stroke in young women. On the other hand, Bioidentical Estrogen in topical cream form is safe, and not associated with increased risk of blood clots.

On the Payroll of Wyeth

Also omitted from the LA Times article was that the two hormone experts, Stuenkel and Santoro both disclosed financial ties to Wyeth and other drug companies that make synthetic chemically altered "Monster'" hormones. These financial ties were publicly disclosed elsewhere as required by medical ethics rules. In addition, The North American Menopause society has financial ties to Wyeth and other synthetic hormone makers. This is publicly disclosed on the NAMS position statement in which many members of the NAMS advisory panel have financial ties to the drug industry.(15-17)

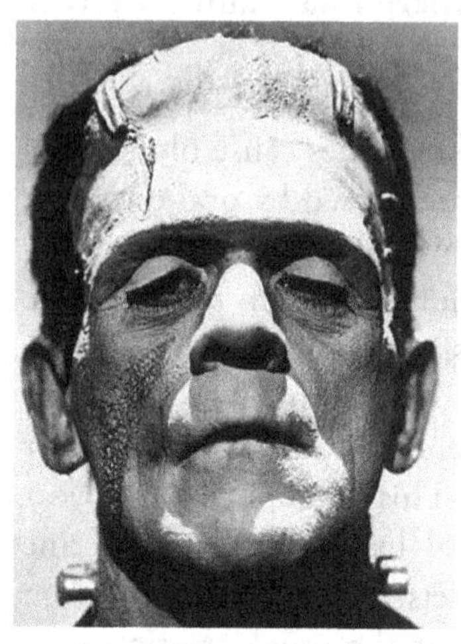

Boris Karloff from The Bride of Frankenstein,1931, courtesy of Universal Studios and Wikimedia Commons

Using Modern Science to Create Frankenstein

The Los Angeles Times also conveniently omits important historical information about the first synthetic hormone invented in 1938, **DES**, Diethylstilbestrol. This monster hormone drug was used from the 1940s until the late 1980s, as an FDA-approved estrogen-replacement therapy. In 1972, the first reports of cervical cancer in the daughters of DES treated women was published in the New England Journal, and the drug was banned in 1975 after millions of women had been exposed. Another early synthetic hormone was Bisphenol A, originally invented in 1936, and now, six billion pounds per year is used for baby bottles, water bottles, and children's toys. These early "monster" hormones gave us a preview of coming attractions with the pharmaceutical industry continuing to sell chemically altered hormones to the public. It's all about money, not health. The take home message is that smart women are avoiding the "monster hormones".

Where to Go For Trusted Information

Rather than rely on newspapers like the LA Times for your medical information, I suggest you go to a more reliable source. Heroic doctors like David Brownstein, Kent Holtorf, Sangeeta Pati, C.W. Randolph, Erika Schwartz, Bruice Kenton, and Jonathan Wright provide their patients with the safer and more effective bioidentical hormones. They also provide the public with trusted and reliable information in their books, web sites and blogs.

For references and links, see my web site: www.bioidenticalhormones101.com

References for Chapter 18. Bioidentical Hormones According to the LA Times

(1) http://articles.latimes.com/2010/jun/07/health/la-he-skeptic-20100607 LA Times, Bioidentical hormones for menopausal symptoms. Proponents boast improvement over older treatments; others say there isn't enough evidence yet. The Healthy Skeptic June 07, 2010,|By Chris Woolston, Special to the Los Angeles Times, Chris Woolston, M.S

(2) http://www.postgradmed.com/index.php?article=1949 Postgraduate Medicine: Volume 121: No.1 by Kent Holtorf, The Bioidentical Hormone Debate: Are Bioidentical Hormones (Estradiol, Estriol, and Progesterone) Safer or More Efficacious than Commonly Used Synthetic Versions in Hormone Replacement Therapy?

(3) http://jeffreydach.com/2009/11/01/bioidentical-hormones-trashed-by-marilynn-marchione-ap-news.aspx BioIdentical Hormone Disinformation From AP Medical Writer, Marilynn Marchione

(4) http://www.usatoday.com/news/health/2009-10-29-menopause-herbal_N.htm Bioidenticals: Estrogen without FDA approval for menopause? By Marilynn Marchione, The Associated Press

(5) http://www.nejm.org/doi/full/10.1056/NEJM197108122850707 Vaginal Cancer after Maternal Treatment with Synthetic Estrogens, Peter Greenwald, M.D., Joseph J. Barlow, M.D., Philip C. Nasca, M.S., and William S. Burnett, M.D. N Engl J Med 1971; 285:390-392August 12, 1971

(6) http://www.cancer.org/docroot/CRI/content/CRI_2_6x_DES_Exposure_Questions_and_Answers.asp DES Exposure: Questions and Answers—What is DES? Amer Cancer Society

(7) http://www.medscape.com/viewarticle/450670_2 Diethylstilbestrol (DES) Update: History of DES

(8) http://www.ourstolenfuture.org/newscience/oncompounds/bisphenola/bpauses.htm Bisphenol A from Our Stolen Future: Are We Threatening

Our Fertility, Intelligence, and Survival?—A Scientific Detective Story, Theo Colborn, Dianne Dumanoski, John Peter Meyers, Plume, 1997.

(9) http://www.environmentcalifornia.org/environmental-health/stop-toxic-toys/bisphenol-a-overview Bisphenol A Overview

(10) http://www.kentonbruicemd.com/blog/Tag/synthetic-hormones Kenton Bruice MD, Why Synthetic Hormones Can Be Dangerous to the Body

(11) http://www.wsu.edu/~delahoyd/frank.comment3.html Frankenstein: The Man and the Monster—Suzanna Storment October 2002—The future of science, if uncontrolled, could be disastrous.

(12) http://www.medpagetoday.com/pdf/IndiciaME03/ Cynthia A. Stuenkel, MD, NCMP Dr. Stuenkel is a consultant for Eli Lilly, Upsher-Smith, and Wyeth.

(13) http://www.clinicianschannel.com/pik/1833/index.cfm Cynthia A. Stuenkel, MD, has received honorarium from Wyeth Pharmaceuticals, Upsher-Smith Laboratories, Inc, and Ally Pharma Options Pvt. Ltd.

(14) http://cme.medscape.com/viewarticle/709447 Cynthia A. Stuenkel, MD, financial relationships

(15) http://www.drugs.com/news/american-association-clinical-endocrinologists-north-american-menopause-society-fail-disclose-7750.html American Association of Clinical Endocrinologists and North American Menopause Society Fail to Disclose Financial Ties to Wyeth Pharmaceuticals—Half of NAMS's Board of Trustees for 2007-2008 receives consulting fees or research support from Wyeth, including Dr. Utian.

(16) http://www.iacprx.org/site/PageServer?pagename=Press_Releases_2007 Wyeth funds research, awards, annual meetings, lectureship funds, educational programs and other activities of NAMS.

(17) http://www.menopause.org/donorlist.pdf
Corporate Supporters of NAMS

(18) http://www.revolutionhealth.com/articles/nanette-santoro-m.d./article.2006-11-27.4097812445 Nanette Santoro, M.D., Grants/Research Support: Ferring Pharmaceuticals Inc., Serono SA. Consultant/Advisory Board: Ferring Pharmaceuticals Inc., Serono SA, Wyeth, Pfizer Inc. Speakers' Bureau: Wyeth, Pfizer Inc., Berlex Inc.

(19) http://www.uchsc.edu/obgyn/ Nanette F. Santoro, M.D.

(20) http://www.clinicianschannel.com/pik/1833/index.cfm
Nanette F. Santoro, MD, has received grants, support, consulting fees honorarium from Wyeth.

(21) http://www.ncbi.nlm.nih.gov/pubmed/171569
N Engl J Med. 1975 Dec 4;293(23):1167-70. Increased risk of endometrial carcinoma among users of conjugated estrogens.Ziel HK, Finkle WD.

(22) http://www.nejm.org/doi/full/10.1056/NEJMsr070105
The Decrease in Breast-Cancer Incidence in 2003 in the United States, Peter M. Ravdin, Ph.D., M.D et al. N Engl J Med 2007; 356:1670-1674April 19, 2007

CHAPTER 19

Ten Bioidentical Hormone Fallacies

A recent article on Huffington Post on the topic of hormones for menopause caught my attention. (1) I was puzzled by the fact that the author had no medical credentials, medical training or even a rudimentary knowledge of biological science. Rather, she is an actress with a theater arts degree from UCLA. She chronicled her menopause experience with a book and blog entitled, "Menopause Makeover". To make up for her lack of medical knowledge, the author joined up with an academic physician who advocates synthetic, chemically altered hormones (progestins), and SSRI antidepressants for menopausal symptoms. The latest article by the two women, "10 Hormone Therapy Facts", is a compilation of nonsense, falsehoods, and half truths, with a hidden agenda promoting the synthetic hormone industry by maligning natural bioidentical hormones.

10 Ten Hormone Facts Should Be Renamed 10 Ten Hormone Fallacies

Firstly, the article attempts to malign bioidentical hormones, claiming they are unregulated, non-FDA approved and not supported by science. These claims against bioidentical hormones are false, and a smokescreen to hide the really frightening fact that synthetic hormones are monsters that cause cancer and heart disease, as shown in the Women's Health Initiative study. Secondly, the article tries to confuse the difference between bioidentical hormones and synthetic, chemically altered hormones made by the pharmaceutical industry. Do not be confused, they are very different. Synthetic hormones are chemically altered monsters that cause cancer and heart disease. Bioidentical hormones are identical to hormones found naturally in the human body, the safe and effective choice. Thirdly, the article contradicts itself, stating that blood testing is not needed, while the author earlier reported that blood testing revealed a high estrogen level. Obviously, blood testing of hormone levels was needed. Fourth, the article quotes the Menopause and Endocrine Societies as authorities without revealing their financial ties to the synthetic hormone makers such as Wyeth. Fifth, the author says that bioidentical hormones did not work for her. Quite to the contrary, millions of women use bioidentical hormones every day for relief of menopausal symptoms and quality of life. Bioidentical hormones work quite well. Sixth, after ranting that bioidentical hormones don't work, the author reports they DO work, and admits she uses estradiol, a bioidentical hormone. Estrogen alone without progesterone causes increased risk of endometrial cancer. This important information is omitted from the article, possibly harming women readers who accept the author as a medical authority, incorrectly concluding that estrogen without progesterone is acceptable. It is not acceptable, and is a disservice to women.

Let's go through the article in detail. Note: the article text is in italics:

Bioidentical hormone treatment made my menopausal symptoms worse.

> *"I splurged for Somers' expensive Beverly Hills doctor recommendation, assuming he must have the answers. He confirmed I was menopausal and gave me tubes of compounded triple estrogen gel and compounded 10 percent micronized progesterone gel, with orders to apply them regularly. After a few months of visiting this overpriced Beverly Hills doctor, my menopause symptoms were exaggerated and my moodiness turned into depression."*

My comment: The above described bioidentical hormone program of topical estrogen and progesterone is the correct one, used by millions of women daily. It is safe and effective. However, close patient monitoring is required, and the patient should be alerted to watch out for signs of hormonal excess.

Blood Test revealed my estrogen levels were 7 times higher than normal

> *"A blood test revealed that my estrogen levels were seven times higher than normal, my increased weight now placed me into the overweight BMI category, and my severe crankiness made it impossible to work.*

> *There is no need for testing of hormone levels, either in saliva or blood. The science has shown that there is no predictable correlation between hormone levels in saliva or in blood and severity of symptoms."*

My comment: The author of this article should have studied Uzzi Reiss's books on bioidentical hormones which explain the symptoms of estrogen excess.(12) These symptoms are fluid retention, bloating, breast enlargement and tenderness. Once these estrogen excess symptoms are identified, the patient should hold off using the estrogen until symptoms dissipate and are relieved. Educating the patient about estrogen excess symptoms, and when to hold hormone dosage is the key to successful treatment program.

Birth Control Pills Can Make Ovarian Function Erratic

Birth control pills complicate the story considerably. Birth control pills are a form of chemical castration, causing artificial cycles without ovulation. Once the pills are stopped, there is usually a delay of months before normal ovarian function and normal cycling resumes, and patients typically experience menopausal symptoms. Upon starting a bioidentical hormone program, the patient will feel better. However, a few months later with resumption of ovarian function, there may be hormonal excess with symptoms of bloating, breast enlargement and mood disorder. This is not a failure of the medication, rather it is a failure of patient monitoring and failure to alert the patient to estrogen excess symptoms. Blood testing is useful here to show elevated estrogen levels. However, in most cases testing is not required since the clinical picture is obvious.

Unregulated Hormones Not Supported by Science

> *"What went wrong? I trusted a resource not supported by science. I was taking unregulated hormones. It was eye-opening to learn that natural compounded bioidentical hormones were unregulated by the FDA. There was no standardization for producing the product, and no tests on the formulations. There are NO real natural hormone products available."*

My comment: The author clearly had a bad experience with this first doctor, and then incorrectly concludes there is something wrong with the bioidentical hormones, saying that bioidentical hormones are not supported by science, unregulated, non-standard, and untested. Of course, this is all nonsense. Bioidentical hormones are heavily regulated, tested and supported by science. The statement, "There are NO real natural hormone products available" is more nonsense. Quite to the contrary, millions of women are using them every day.

Science DOES support the use of bioidentical hormones for menopausal symptoms. Go to Medline and do a search for estrogen or progesterone and 90,000 articles will come up. Dr. Holtorf's review article, "The Bioidentical Hormone Debate", published in PostGraduate Medicine, cites 196 medical studies showing that bioidentical hormones are safer and more effective than synthetic chemically altered hormones. (2)

Bioidentical hormones are heavily regulated as both FDA approved products at the corner drug store and as compounded preparations. Compounding does not fall under the jurisdiction of the FDA, so FDA regulation is not needed or even desired. Instead, Compounding pharmacies have a separate system of regulation at the state and local level which is rigorous and recognized by the AMA. Look for a compounding pharmacy with PCAB accreditation.

1) *"Natural: The word "natural" is a marketing term. There is no scientific evidence that custom-compounded bioidenticals are safer or more effective or more "natural" than standard pharmaceutical bioidentical prescriptions. The only "natural" hormones are the hormones being made by your body."*

My Comment: The word "natural" is not only a marketing term. Natural means anything found in the natural world that cannot be patented. This next comment is a tautology as bioidentical is still bioidentical whether found in FDA approved prescriptions or in compounded preparations. We know from the Women's Health Initiative study JAMA 2002, that synthetic hormones are monsters that cause cancer and heart disease. Bioidentical hormones are safe and do not increase risk of cancer or heart disease as shown in the French Cohort study.

2) *"Bioidenticals: Laboratories create formulations that are either identical (bioidentical) or not (non-bioidentical) to those in your body. There are FDA approved prescription estradiol products that are bioidentical that are not "compounded."*

My Comment: This is correct.

3) *"Compounded hormones: Made in a pharmacy by combining, mixing or altering ingredients to create a customized hormone for an individual patient. Compounding pharmacies must be licensed and regulated by the State Pharmacy boards. However, they do not have to demonstrate the safety, effectiveness and quality control, based on large, scientific studies that the FDA requires of pharmaceutical manufacturers. Compounding pharmacies use chemically synthesized hormones made from plants—the same government-approved ingredients that are used in a manufacturer's laboratory. "Compounded" formulations are neither safer nor more "natural."*

My Comment: Compounded Pharmacies are not under FDA jurisdiction, and that is why they are not regulated by the FDA. Instead, they are regulated by the state and local government. To expect and insist on FDA regulation for compounding pharmacies is like saying your state driver's license is invalid because it was not issued by the federal government. If one rejects compounded medications, then one would also reject intravenous antibiotic treatment at the hospital which is also a compounded medication. Obviously, there is a problem with the logic used here.

What Does FDA Approval Mean? The author creates confusion about the meaning and significance of FDA Approval. Food and Drug Administration approval does not confirm that the drug is the most effective or the safest drug for you. FDA approval means the drug is more effective than placebo for its indicated use and benefits outweigh risks. Drug Manufacturers spend 500 to 800 million doing clinical studies submitted for FDA approval, because of the future prospects for greater profit. The chemical structure of a bioidentical hormone, like other natural substances, cannot be patented, so there is very little financial incentive for a drug company to spend all that money on clinical studies when profits cannot be assured.

Non-FDA Approved Indications

Drugs are FDA approved for certain medical indications. About 20% of the time, doctors prescribe drugs for non-FDA approved indications. For example, the use of SSRI antidepressants as a non-hormonal treatment for hot flashes is a non-FDA approved use of the drug. Mainstream doctors engage in hypocritical reasoning when they criticize others who prescribe compounded bioidentical hormones as non-FDA approved. The problem with this argument is that intravenous medications given at the hospital are also non-FDA approved compounded medications. Get rid of compounding and you must throw out most medications dispensed at the hospital which are, in fact, compounded medications.

Chemically Synthesized Hormones

By using the phrase, "*Compounding pharmacies use chemically synthesized hormones*", the author is again confusing the reader with the difference between synthetic hormones and bioidentical hormones. They are quite different. Synthetic hormones are chemically altered monsters. On the other hand, bioidentical hormones have the same chemical structure as those found in the human body. How the hormone was made or manufactured is not important as long as the chemical structures are identical. A good example is water made by combining an oxygen molecule with two hydrogen molecules. The manufacturing process is irrelevant, since the final chemical structure is H2O, water, a natural substance that cannot be patented.

4) *The North American Menopause Society (NAMS), a non-profit organization of expert scientists and clinicians, "does not recommend custom-compounded products over well-tested, government-approved products for the majority of women." The Endocrine Society has stated that, "Post-market surveys of such (compounded) hormone preparations have uncovered inconsistencies in dose and quality."*

My comment: The author omits that both NAMS and Endocrine Society have publicly acknowledged financial ties to the drug industry. In addition, both organizations advocate the use of synthetic "monster" hormones, and as such, represent the financial interests of the synthetic hormone industry (such as Wyeth and Abbott), rather than the health of the public. Half of the board of trustees of NAMS receives money from Wyeth in the form of consulting fees or research support. Wyeth makes Prempro and Pristiq. These Financial Disclosures are listed page 10 of the NAMS 2007 position statement on Hormones for Menopause. Medical education and research requires authors to publicly disclose financial ties to the drug industry which alerts the reader to a biased pro-industry viewpoint.

5) *To determine whether hormone therapy is appropriate and safe, one's risk factors must be assessed based on personal and family medical history, as well as personal preference. There is no "one size fits all."*

My Comment: Personal and family medical history is always part of any medical evaluation. The above statement refers to risk factors for breast cancer. All women are at risk for breast cancer from environmental carcinogens, and more so if there is an underlying genetic abnormality such as the BRCA gene for breast cancer. The important fact to remember is that Bioidentical Hormone therapy is safe and effective, while synthetic "monster" hormones are the ones that cause cancer and heart disease, and should be avoided.

6) *"Low dose hormone therapy, used judiciously, still remains the most effective way to treat the troubling symptoms of menopause for those who need it and who can use it safely."*

My Comment: Since mainstream physicians know that synthetic "monster" hormones are dangerous, causing cancer and heart disease, they shrug their shoulders and accept "low dose" synthetic hormone therapy as more desirable than the higher dosage used routinely. Less of the harmful monster hormone is given to the patient. Synthetic chemically altered hormones are "Monsters" at any dosage. Stay away.

7) *"There is no need for testing of hormone levels, either in saliva or blood. The science has shown that there is no predictable correlation between hormone levels in saliva or in blood and severity of symptoms. Unless there are unusual complications, it is the standard of care to treat symptoms if needed and adjust medications according to response, not saliva levels."*

My Comment: There are no blood tests for synthetic hormones, so proponents of synthetic hormones pretend that lab testing is not needed. The reality is that very useful blood, urine and saliva testing is available for the entire range of bioidentical hormones. If your doctor doesn't do some sort of testing, you need a new doctor.

8) *"Standard prescription hormone therapy is the safest form available. It has been tested by the FDA and manufactured in a highly regulated manner. Doses are consistent."*

My Comment: "*Standard Prescription hormone therapy*" is coded language for chemically altered synthetic "monster" hormones shown to cause cancer and heart disease in the Women's Health initiative study. That's not so safe. "*Tested by the FDA*" is a misnomer and error. The FDA doesn't do any testing. The drug company pays for testing and then submits the results on paper to the FDA for approval. The testing has to show drug efficacy over placebo. That's all. Sometimes the testing is fudged. Ten percent of FDA approved drugs are later banned, and another ten per cent are given a "black box" warning. (17)

9) *There are also FDA approved non-hormonal therapies available to treat menopause symptoms for those who cannot take hormones.*

My Comment: The above statement a reference to the use of SSRI antidepressants for menopausal symptoms. These drugs were recently shown to be no better than placebo for depression.(16) Regarding efficacy for hot flashes, drug company funded studies showed efficacy over placebo was marginal at best. (14-15) Synthetic altered hormones are bad enough, they cause cancer and heart disease. SSRI antidepressant drugs like Effexor™ and Pristiq™ are even worse; they are chemically addictive with horrendous withdrawal effects.(18-19) The use of SSRI antidepressants for menopausal symptoms should be condemned as a misguided adventure. The practice should be halted.

10) *"Whether hormone therapy is needed depends on severity of symptoms, including hot flashes, night sweats, vaginal dryness and irritability. Hormone therapy should be individualized, which may mean trying different doses and schedules, as well as different routes of administration."*

My Comment: Mainstream medicine will ask patients to "live with it" if the menopausal symptoms are not severe enough to warrant treatment. Millions of smart women have rejected synthetic hormones, and SSRI antidepressants, and are finding success with bioidentical hormone programs.

"Unregulated formulas and inconsistent compounded dosing can be dangerous and has jeopardized the health of many women, including myself. I wished I had known the dangers involved with compounded-hormones. After my menopause symptoms were stabilized with a standard prescription of bioidentical estradiol, I found a new way of eating, lost 30 pounds and updated my beauty regime without cosmetic surgery or alterations. I have never been healthier."

My Comment: The author clearly blames inconsistency in her compounded formula for an episode of hormonal excess. I would disagree, and suggest the hormonal excess may have been due to resumption of hormonal production following cessation of synthetic birth control pills. To avoid hormonal excess, our office staff monitors patients by phone very closely, reminding them of the warning signs of hormonal excess. At the earliest sign of hormonal excess, the patient stops using the estrogen cream. This type of program is very safe. In my experience prescribing compounded hormone preparations and monitoring patients, the formulas have been consistent and standardized, and patients have been happy with the results. For the highest consistency, we use only the large national pharmacies that specialize in bioidentical hormones.

At the end of the article, the author returned to Estradiol, a bioidentical hormone. Yet the author omits the historical information that Estrogen alone (Premarin) causes endometrial hyperplasia and cancer. That is why progesterone must be given with the estrogen to prevent endometrial hyperplasia. Omitting this information is a disservice to women and potentially harmful for readers.

In Conclusion

This "10 Facts" article is a mixture of nonsense, falsehood and half truth. The quality of information reflects the author's credentials, which are none, other than briefly visiting a few doctors for symptoms of hormonal imbalance. The medical information appearing in the article comes from regurgitated drug company propaganda advocating synthetic chemically altered "monster" hormones and SSRI antidepressants for menopause, performing a disservice to women. A safer, more effective alternative is bioidentical hormone therapy. Rather than rely on this type of biased advice, a more balanced viewpoint is available from well known medical experts such as David Brownstein, Kent Holtorf, Bruice Kenton, Sangeeta Pati, C. W. Randolf, Erika Schwartz, and Jonathan Wright. Read their books and articles.

The history of modern medicine is replete with the medical victimization of women. A few discarded examples are: radical mastectomy, excessive hysterectomies, and bone marrow transplant for breast cancer. Synthetic hormones belong on that list. The latest medical hoax is SSRI antidepressants for hot flashes. Take back control of your bodies. Do not allow yourselves to be victims of synthetic hormones and antidepressants for menopausal symptoms. The proper treatment is bioidentical hormone therapy. Bioidentical hormone doctors are available in your area. You can find them with doctor's directories from organizations like ACAM and A4M.

For references and links, see my web site: www.bioidenticalhormones101.com

References for Chapter 19. Ten Bioidentical Hormone Fallacies

(1) http://www.huffingtonpost.com/staness-jonekos/10-hormone-therapy-facts_b_615199.html 10 Hormone Therapy Facts Every Woman Should Know by Staness Jonekos

(2) http://jeffreydach.com/files/80618-70584/TheBioidenticalHormoneDebateKenHoltorfMD.pdf Postgrad Med. 2009 Jan;121(1):73-85. The Bioidentical Hormone Debate: are bioidentical hormones (estradiol, estriol, and progesterone) safer or more efficacious than commonly used synthetic versions in hormone replacement therapy? Holtorf K. Holtorf Medical Group, Inc., Torrance, CA 90505, USA

(3) http://www.ncbi.nlm.nih.gov/pubmed/18928825 Prim Care. 2008 Dec;35(4):669-705.
Hormones in wellness and disease prevention: common practices, current state of the evidence, and questions for the future. Schwartz ET, Holtorf K.

(4) http://www.ncbi.nlm.nih.gov/pubmed/18775609
Could transdermal estradiol + progesterone be a safer postmenopausal HRT? A review.
L'hermite M, Simoncini T, Fuller S, Genazzani AR. Maturitas. 2008 Jul-Aug;60(3-4):185-201. Epub 2008 Sep 5. Department of Gynecology and Obstetrics, Université Libre de Bruxelles, Bruxelles, Belgium.

(5) http://www.jpands.org/vol13no2/hotze.pdf
Point/Counterpoint:The Case for Bioidentical Hormones by Steven F. Hotze, by Steven F. Hotze, M.D. Donald P. Ellsworth, M.D. Journal of American Physicians and Surgeons Volume 13 Number 2 Summer 2008 p43.

(6) http://www.thorne.com/altmedrev/.fulltext/11/3/208.pdf
A Comprehensive Review of the Safety and Efficacy of Bioidentical Hormones for the Management of Menopause and Related

Health Risks by Deborah Moskowitz, ND Altern Med Rev 2006;11(3):208-223

(7) http://www.ncbi.nlm.nih.gov/pubmed/17107222 Treat Endocrinol. 2006;5(6):367-374. Is Bio-Identical Hormone Replacement Therapy Safer than Traditional Hormone Replacement Therapy?: A Critical Appraisal of Cardiovascular Risks in Menopausal Women. Curcio JJ, Wollner DA, Schmidt JW, Kim LS. Women's Integrative Medicine Department, Southwest College of Naturopathic Medicine, Tempe, Arizona, USA.

(8) http://www.ncbi.nlm.nih.gov/pmc/articles/PMC2211383/ Breast Cancer Res Treat. 2008 January; 107(1): 103-111. Unequal risks for breast cancer associated with different hormone replacement therapies: results from the E3N cohort study by Agnès Fournier, 1 Franco Berrino,2 and Françoise Clavel-Chapelon1*

(9) http://bostonreview.net/BR35.3/angell.php Boston Review MAY/ JUNE 2010 Big Pharma, Bad Medicine-How corporate dollars corrupt research and education by Marcia Angell

(10) http://jama.ama-assn.org/content/288/3/321.abstract Risks and Benefits of Estrogen Plus Progestin in Healthy Postmenopausal WomenPrincipal Results From the Women's Health Initiative Randomized Controlled TrialWriting Group for the Women's Health Initiative Investigators JAMA. 2002;288(3):321-333.

(11) http://www.ncbi.nlm.nih.gov/pubmed/171569 N Engl J Med. 1975 Dec 4;293(23):1167-70. Increased risk of endometrial carcinoma among users of conjugated estrogens.Ziel HK, Finkle WD.

(12) http://www.uzzireissmd.com/refs/04.html The Natural SuperWoman, by Uzzi Reiss MD and Yfat Reiss Gendell, Avery Trade, 2008. web site page containing references for Estrogen chapter.

(13) http://www.ncbi.nlm.nih.gov/pubmed/12626212 Climacteric. 2002 Dec;5(4):332-40. Combined hormone replacement therapy and risk of

breast cancer in a French cohort study of 3175 women. de Lignières B, de Vathaire F, Fournier S, Urbinelli R, Allaert F, Le MG, Kuttenn F.

(14) http://www.cnsspectrums.com/aspx/article_pf.aspx?articleid=922 Beyond Remission, Rationale, and Design of the Prevention of Recurrent Episodes of Depression with Venlafaxine for Two Years (PREVENT) Study, Susan G. Kornstein, MD CNS Spectr. 2006;11:12(Suppl 15):28-34 This supplement is sponsored by Wyeth.

(15) http://www.news.vcu.edu/news/Low_Doses_of_AntiDepressant_May_Spell_Relief_for_Some_Women_Suffering Low Doses of Anti-Depressant May Spell Relief for Some Women Suffering from Moderate-to-Severe PMS. Sathya Achia Abraham VCU Communications and Public Relations

(16) http://jama.ama-assn.org/content/303/1/47.short?home Antidepressant Drug Effects and Depression Severity, A Patient-Level Meta-analysis. Jay C. Fournier, MA; Robert J. DeRubeis, PhD; Steven D. Hollon, PhD; Sona Dimidjian, PhD; Jay D. Amsterdam, MD; Richard C. Shelton, MD; Jan Fawcett, MD JAMA. 2010;303(1):47-53

(17) http://www.ncbi.nlm.nih.gov/pubmed/11980521 JAMA. 2002 May 1;287(17):2215-20. Timing of new black box warnings and withdrawals for prescription medications. Lasser KE et al.

(18) http://www.ncbi.nlm.nih.gov/pmc/articles/PMC181155/ Prim Care Companion J Clin Psychiatry. 2001 February; 3(1): 22-27. SSRI Antidepressant Medications: Adverse Effects and Tolerability by James M. Ferguson, M.D.

(19) http://www.psy-world.com/SSRI_problems.pdf
http://www.ncbi.nlm.nih.gov/pubmed/18635702/
J Psychopharmacol. 2009 Nov;23(8):967-74. Epub 2008 Jul 17. Problems associated with long-term treatment with selective serotonin reuptake inhibitors. Moret C, Isaac M, Briley M.

CHAPTER 20

Synthetic Hormones, Pfizer-Wyeth Lose Big Court Case

A jury awarded 112 million dollars in punitive damages for two women who developed breast cancer after taking Prempro, a synthetic hormone pill from Wyeth which contains a synthetic progestin. (1-6) A large jury award is intended to send a message. The jury was outraged at the wanton and reckless conduct of the synthetic hormone maker, Wyeth, for ignoring and suppressing information that Prempro causes breast cancer. In addition, the jury was outraged that Wyeth paid consultants and medical ghostwriters to write medical journal articles playing down the risk of breast cancer. Company profit was placed ahead of patient safety. This jury award is only one of ten thousand cases waiting for their day in court. The jury is still out.

Women's Health Initiative Bombshell

In 2002, a bombshell appeared in the medical literature, and massive numbers of women switched from Prempro to safer bio-identical hormones. This was the 2002 WHI study (Women's Health Initiative) which showed that PremPro™ causes breast cancer. This massive shift away from synthetic Prempro™ reduced breast cancer rates by 10,000 fewer cases per year in the US and Canada.(7-8) This is a reduction of about nine per cent as reported by Ravdin in the New England Journal. (7-8)

The American Public Hoodwinked For 65 Years

This Prempro™ court case teaches us an important lesson. When a "Bad Drug" like Prempro™ gets FDA approval and placed on the market, what happens? The public is hoodwinked, and the drug company profits handsomely. The wheels of justice turn slowly. After 65 years and thousands of victims, our court system has finally ended a bad drug, in this case, a synthetic hormone called Prempro, a combination pill containing Premarin™ and Provera™. The Provera™ component is a progestin, a chemically altered version of bioidentical progesterone. This chemical alteration is done by adding a chemical group to the natural molecule. Why chemically alter a natural hormone? Chemical alteration is required to make the drug patentable, thereby protecting profits of the drug maker. Unfortunately, this chemical alteration of a natural hormone creates a "monster" hormone. The natural bioidentical human hormone is the one that nature made and the one that works best.

Another Important Lesson—Don't Use Synthetic Hormones

Another important lesson from this case is that synthetic hormones like Prempro, which are chemically altered versions of human hormones, are all "Monster Hormones" which should never have been approved by the FDA in the first place. Any alteration in a chemical structure of a hormone creates a Monster, and in the case of Prempro, the result is increased cancer and heart disease.

Changed Chemical Structure Results in Monster Hormones

The drug companies changed the chemical structure of human hormones to obtain patent protection and maximize profits. Human bioidentical hormones cannot be patented because they are found naturally in the human body, therefore they are not profitable for the drug companies.

Just Another Round in the Medical Information War

Drug companies routinely use their influence to control information in the mainstream media and the medical journals. They use medical ghostwriters to downplay adverse side effects of their products in order to maximize profits. They use medical ghostwriters to impugn and cast doubts on the competing product, bioidentical hormones. This is merely part of the Medical Information War played out in the media every day.

For references and links, see my web site: www.bioidenticalhormones101.com

References for Chapter 20. Synthetic Hormones, Pfizer-Wyeth Lose Big Court Case

(1) http://blog.legalbroadcastnetwork.com/the-lbn-blog/2009/11/24/zoe-littlepage-discusses-112-million—wyeth-hrt-verdicts.html Zoe Littlepage Discusses $112 Million Wyeth HRT Verdicts. Tuesday, November 24,

(2) http://menstruationresearch.org/2009/11/23/prempros-losing-streak-continues/ Blog of the Society for Menstrual Cycle Research PremPro's Losing Streak Continues November 23rd, 2009 by Elizabeth Kissling

(3) http://www.nytimes.com/2009/11/24/business/24wyeth.html Another Loss for Pfizer in Drug Suits By DUFF WILSON November 23, 2009 NY Times. Pfizer has been ordered to pay a total of $103 million in punitive damages to two women who were found to have breast cancer after they used hormonal drugs

(4) http://www.philly.com/philly/business/homepage/20091125_Prempro_plaintiffs_lawyers_sold_their_story_to_the_jury.html Posted on Wed, Nov. 25, 2009 Prempro plaintiffs' lawyers sold their story to the jury. By Chris Mondics and Miriam Hill Inquirer Staff Writers The lawyers who won $103 million in two jury verdicts announced Monday against Pfizer Inc. relied as much on their storytelling ability as their knowledge of the law.

(5) http://www.dailymail.com/ap/ApTopStories/200911230561 AP Featured News Monday November 23, 2009 $75M verdict unsealed in Prempro-cancer case PATRICK WALTERS Associated Press Writer

(6) http://www.abajournal.com/news/article/juries_award_103m_in_punitives_in_two_prempro_cases/ Juries Award $103M in Punitives in Two Prempro Cases Posted Nov 24, 2009 By Debra Cassens Weiss Philadelphia juries have awarded two breast-cancer victims $103 million in punitive damages in two separate cases against Pfizer Inc. involving the marketing of the hormone replacement drug Prempro.

(7) http://www.nejm.org/doi/full/10.1056/NEJMsr070105 The Decrease in Breast-Cancer Incidence in 2003 in the United States. Peter M. Ravdin, Ph.D., M.D et al. N Engl J Med 2007; 356:1670-1674 April 19, 2007. A comparison of incidence rates in 2001 with those in 2004 (omitting the years in which the incidence was changing) showed that the decrease in annual age-adjusted incidence was 8.6%.

(8) http://jnci.oxfordjournals.org/content/early/2010/09/23/jnci.djq345.abstract Breast Cancer Incidence and Hormone Replacement Therapy in Canada by Prithwish De, C. Ineke Neutel, Ivo Olivotto and Howard Morrison. JNCI J Natl Cancer Inst (2010). This drop occurred concurrently with a 9.6% decline in the incidence rate of breast cancer.

Section Five: Screening Mammography, and Breast Cancer

This section covers screening mammography for breast cancer, its limitations and failings. Also included is breast cancer prevention with iodine supplementation.

CHAPTER 21

Rethink Pink October Breast Cancer Mammogram

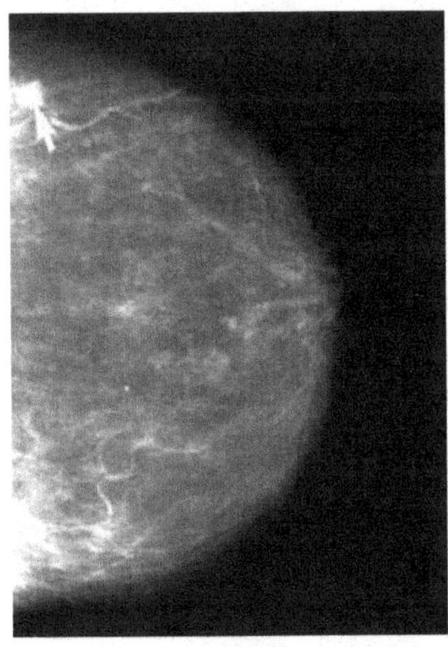

Screening Mammogram showing small cancer (upper left arrow), courtesy of the National Institute of Health and wikimedia commons.

Rethink Pink October Breast Cancer Month—A Closer Look at Screening Mammography

A bombshell article appeared in October 2009 JAMA (the Journal of the American Medical Association) questioning mammography breast cancer screening. (1) Dr. Laura Esserman reviewed 20 years of data and concludes that screening the population for breast cancer has significant drawbacks. The expected survival benefits have not materialized. She says that it is true that early stage breast cancer has decreased due to mammography, however, the data shows **no decrease** in the advanced, "killer" cancers. Overall mortality rates from breast cancer have declined slightly; however, Dr Esserman attributes this to better treatment rather than to screening mammography.

Detected Cases Go Up With Screening Mammography

The combined 20 years of breast cancer data shows essentially no change in the annual cases of breast cancer cases detected, until 1983 when screening mammography was introduced, with an immediate spike and dramatic increase in the number of breast cancer cases detected annually, thanks to this new diagnostic tool, the mammogram.

More Cased Detected, But Only a Modest Decline in Cancer Mortality

Although screening mammography detects dramatically more cases of breast cancer, this increased detection has not translated into decreased mortality in the population. Yes, mortality numbers have decreased slightly. The annual mortality rate for breast cancer from 1930 to 2006 was stable at about 30 cases per 100,000 women, and declined over the last few years to about 25 cases per 100,000. However, this is not due to screening mammography. Dr. Esserman suggests this rather modest decline in mortality is due to improvement in treatment, not increased detection. (1)

Annual Breast Cancer Mortality—Where's the Benefit?

While the incidence of early stage breast cancer has decreased by 2.8 per cent per year since 2001, incidence rates of advanced (distant-stage) disease have remained remarkably stable over this same time period. In 2009, 192,370 women were diagnosed with breast cancer and 40,170 women died of breast cancer. Mammography has increased the detection of very early stage cancer, called DCIS (ductal carcinoma in situ), with 60,000 cases of DCIS detected annually, however, the number of advanced breast cancer cases, the serious fatal type, has not changed by the introduction of mammography screening. This lack of benefit is disappointing.

Dr. Esserman's 2009 Observations Were Made in 2002 by Barnett Kramer

Dr. Barnett Kramer, director of the Office of Disease Prevention at the National Institutes of Health, was interviewed in a 2002 article in the New York Times, in which he said:

"The number of women with breast cancers with the worst prognosis, those that spread to other organs, had been fairly constant in the years before mammography was introduced, and that trend did not change after the introduction of mammography . . . If screening worked perfectly, every cancer found early would correspond to one fewer cancer found later. That did not happen. Mammography, instead has resulted in a huge new population of women with early stage cancer but without a corresponding decline in the numbers of women with advanced cancer." (31)

Important Point: Mammography Has Failed to Live Up To Expectations
Screening Mammography has not lived up to expectations. Although more cases of early breast cancers are found, this has not reduced the number of late stage or killer cancers.

Weighing the Pluses and Minuses of Screening Mammography

Dr Gilbert Welch in his BMJ editorial says the following about mammography screening for breast cancer: (7)(8)(9)

1 in 1,000 women annually screened for 10 years will avoid dying from breast cancer.
2 to 10 women will be over-diagnosed and treated needlessly.
10 to 15 women will be told they have breast cancer earlier than they would otherwise have been told, but this will not affect their prognosis.
100 to 500 women will have at least one "false alarm" (about half of these women will undergo a biopsy)

Mammography—Finding the Reservoir of DCIS

Mammography screening finds the small indolent cancers called DCIS, ductal carcinoma in situ, that represent a reservoir of silent disease in up to 18% of the population, demonstrated by autopsy studies.(18) This leads to over diagnosis and overtreatment. For the invasive cancers which we know are present in one to two per cent of the population, (demonstrated by autopsy series), screening detection is of little help, with little change in the number of advanced cancer cases, and about 40,000 deaths every year. Dr. Gilbert Welch sums it up with the following sage advice: "*doctors who recommend less-aggressive mammography (less frequently, waiting until you are age 50, or stopping it when you are older) or are less quick to biopsy may not be bad doctors but good ones.*"

Important Point:
The reason why mammography has had little impact on breast cancer mortality is that mammography is an X-Ray imaging technique that finds small calcifications indicating DCIS, an indolent, non-aggressive lesion with a good prognosis. (42-50). The data suggests that finding and aggressively treating DCIS does not reduce mortality rates from advanced breast cancer.

Just Stop Calling It Cancer

One glaring problem with screening mammography is the detection of DCIS at a rate of 60,000 cases per year.(17) DCIS is ductal carcinoma in situ, a pathology diagnosis which carries a very good prognosis, a 98 per cent—five year survival. In spite of the rather benign natural history of DCIS, mainstream medicine treats these lesions aggressively with surgery and radiation. Recently, the NIH has called for a change in terminology, asking pathologists to stop calling it "cancer". Here is the NIH consensus statement:

> "*Because of the noninvasive nature of DCIS, coupled with its favorable prognosis, strong consideration should be given to elimination of the use of the anxiety-producing term "carcinoma" from the description of DCIS.*"(2)

Dr Fletcher in the New England Journal Sums IT UP

Dr Suzanne Fletcher summed up the issues with screening mammography detection of DCIS nicely in her 2003 article published in the New England Journal with this quote: (38)

" . . . the risk of death from breast cancer within 10 years after the diagnosis of DCIS (ductal carcinoma in situ) was 1.9 percent. Such an excellent prognosis could be attributable to the detection of lesions before they become invasive cancers, which could save lives. However, if ductal carcinoma in situ were the usual precursor to early invasive cancer, the incidence of early-stage invasive breast cancer should decrease as the incidence of in situ cancer increases, ***but the opposite is happening****. Also, autopsy studies in women who died from causes unrelated to breast cancer have shown a substantial "reservoir" of ductal carcinoma in situ in such women. (Welch) (18) Therefore, detection of ductal carcinoma in situ may be an example of overdiagnosis—finding early neoplasms, many of which will never become invasive breast cancer. Unfortunately, ductal carcinoma in situ can progress to invasive cancer. The eight-year rate of recurrence in one study of treatment with only surgical excision was 27 percent, and half the recurrences were invasive cancers. It is not clear who is at risk for recurrence and whether survival results would be the same if surgery were undertaken only after early invasive cancer had been diagnosed. In sum, women who undergo screening mammography are more likely than other women to be given a diagnosis of ductal carcinoma in situ.* ***Whether finding it (DCIS) saves lives or merely increases the number of women who receive a diagnosis of breast cancer is not yet clear.*** *"endquote Dr Fletcher NEJM.(38)*

We Just Don't Know the Natural Course of Untreated DCIS

A large part of the problem is that we simply do not have a good understanding of the natural course of DCIS. Although we know that some cases of DCIS will progress to invasive cancer, many will not. We have no reliable tools to distinguish the "stable/benign" DCIS cases from the "aggressive" DCIS cases destined to become invasive. Dr. Erbas says, "*The available evidence suggests not all DCIS will progress to invasive cancer in the medium term but precise estimates of progression are not possible given the limitations of the data." (39)* Hopefully, in the near future, new diagnostic tools will be developed to tell us which DCIS cancers need more aggressive treatment and which ones need less aggressive treatment.

Invasive Breast Cancer 15 to 30 years after diagnosis of DCIS!!

Another striking finding is that when following DCIS cases over 30 years, invasive cancers are found fifteen to twenty five years after the initial biopsy. (40-41). This is remarkable. In my opinion, this reflects an underlying nutritional deficiency, biochemical or genetic abnormality which places the patient at increased risk for breast cancer during their lifetime.

DCIS: An Iodine Deficiency Disease?

Breast tissue takes up Iodine by virtue of an active transport called the NIS, Sodium Iodide Symporter. (54-55) In addition, iodine deficiency is a known risk factor for breast cancer, and iodine has been suggested as an adjuvant treatment for breast cancer.(51-53) Are DCIS patients Iodine deficient, and that is why these individuals have a propensity for breast cancer? Unfortunately, most breast cancer studies ignore Iodine, and do not measure urinary Iodine levels, so we don't know the answer. In a few anecdotal cases with a history of treated breast cancer, we have found profoundly low iodine levels. Perhaps new studies sponsored by NIH funding can answer this question. However, in the mean time, it is reasonable to test Iodine levels and provide Iodine supplements to patients at risk for breast cancer or recurrence. Urinary spot iodine testing is widely available at all national labs.

Important Point:
Iodine supplementation is our best tool for breast cancer prevention.

How to Prevent Breast Cancer—Our Program

1) Iodine Supplementation (Iodoral tablets)
2) Natural Progesterone, topical cream
3) Avoid carcinogenic chemicals, xenoestrogens, pesticides, etc.
4) Vitamin D Supplementation. (Vitamin D3 capsules)

For references and links, see my web site: www.bioidenticalhormones101.com

References for Chapter 21. Rethink Pink October Breast Cancer Mammogram

(1) http://jama.highwire.org/cgi/content/abstract/302/15/1685 Rethinking Screening for Breast Cancer and Prostate Cancer. Laura Esserman, MD, MBA; Yiwey Shieh, AB; Ian Thompson, MD JAMA. 2009;302(15):1685-1692.

(2) http://consensus.nih.gov/2009/dcisstatement.htm NIH Consensus statement on DCIS 2009

(3) http://www.medpagetoday.com/HematologyOncology/BreastCancer/16538 Analysis Questions Breast and Prostate Cancer Screening By Peggy Peck, Executive Editor, MedPage Today October 21, 2009

(4) http://movingtotheusa.blogspot.com/2009/10/rethinking-strategies-for-breast-and.html Thursday, 22 October 2009. Rethinking strategies for breast and prostate cancer screening.

(5) http://www.vaoutcomes.org/welch.php H. Gilbert Welch, MD, MPH Professor of Medicine and Community and Family Medicine, Dartmouth Medical School; Co-Director of the White River Junction Outcomes Group

(6) http://www.vaoutcomes.org/papers/NYT_cancer_screening.pdf How Two Studies on Cancer Screening Led to Two Results—New York Times March 13, 2007

(7) http://8.12.42.31/2008/nov/03/opinion/oe-welch3 The excessive focus on mammography. Looking harder to find more may not be the best practice. By H. Gilbert Welch November 03, 2008

(8) http://www.nytimes.com/2008/10/07/health/views/07essa.html Campaign Myth: Prevention as Cure-All By H. GILBERT WELCH, M.D October 6, 2008

(9) http://www.bmj.com/cgi/content/full/339/jul09_1/b1425 9 July 2009, BMJ 2009;339:b1425 Editorials. Gilbert Welch MD. Overdiagnosis and mammography screening.

(10) http://www.huffingtonpost.com/helen-cordes/rethink-pink-now-saner-so_b_329496.html Rethink Pink NOW! Saner Solutions to Breast Cancer, Part 2 Huffington Post, Helen Cordes.

(11) http://archinte.ama-assn.org/cgi/content/abstract/168/21/2311 The Natural History of Invasive Breast Cancers Detected by Screening Mammography by Per-Henrik Zahl, MD, PhD; Jan Mæhlen, MD, PhD; H. Gilbert Welch, MD, MPH Arch Intern Med. 2008;168(21):2311-2316.

(12) http://www.nytimes.com/2008/11/25/health/25breast.html?pagewanted=1&_r=2 Study Suggests Some Cancers May Go Away By GINA KOLATA November 24, 2008. New York Times.

(13) http://jeffreydach.com/2009/10/01/psa-testing-the-failed-medical-experiment-by-jeffrey-dach-md.aspx PSA Screening for Cancer, the Failed Medical Experiment by Jeffrey Dach MD

(14) http://www.greenhealthspot.com/2009/10/rethinking-cancer-screening.html Rethinking Cancer Screening Dr Wang

(15) http://www.dbtechno.com/health/2009/10/21/study-says-screening-for-breast-cancer-is-over-rated/ Study says screening for breast cancer is over rated, dbtechno blog.

(16) http://jeffreydach.com/2009/08/16/the-thyroid-nodule-epidemic-by-jeffrey-dach-md.aspx The Thyroid Nodule Epidemic by Jeffrey Dach MD

(17) http://theoncologist.alphamedpress.org/cgi/content/full/12/11/1276 The Oncologist, Vol. 12, No. 11, 1276-1287, November 2007; Current Treatment and Clinical Trial Developments for Ductal Carcinoma In Situ of the Breast. Judy C. Bougheya, Ricardo J. Gonzalezb, Everett Bonnerc, Henry M. Kuererb

(18) http://www.annals.org/cgi/content/full/127/11/1023 Using Autopsy Series To Estimate the Disease "Reservoir" for Ductal Carcinoma in Situ of the Breast: How Much More Breast Cancer Can We Find? H. Gilbert Welch, MD, MPH, and William C. Black, MD Annals of Internal Med, December 1 1997,| Volume 127, Issue 11, Pages 1023-1028.

(19) http://www.ncbi.nlm.nih.gov/pmc/articles/PMC2002422/?tool=pubmed Br J Cancer. 1987 December; 56(6): 814-819. Breast cancer and atypia among young and middle-aged women: a study of 110 medicolegal autopsies. M. Nielsen et al.

(20) http://www.cancer.org/downloads/STT/F861009_final%209-08-09.pdf Breast Cancer Facts and Figures 2009,2010 American Cancer Society

(21) http://www.cancer.org/docroot/stt/stt_0.asp Breast cancer facts and figures 2009 ACS

(22) http://seer.cancer.gov/statfacts/html/breast.html SEER Cancer Statistics. It is estimated that 192,370 women will be diagnosed with and 40,170 women will die of cancer of the breast in 2009.

(23) http://seer.cancer.gov/csr/1975_2006/results_merged/sect_04_breast.pdf NCI's SEER Cancer Statistics Review, Incidence & Mortality Breast Cancer

(24) http://caonline.amcancersoc.org/cgi/content/full/59/4/225 CA Cancer J Clin 2009; 59:225-249 Cancer Statistics, 2009 Ahmedin Jemal, DVM, PhD1, Rebecca Siegel, MPH2, Elizabeth Ward, PhD3, Yongping Hao, PhD4, Jiaquan Xu, MD5 and Michael J. Thun, MD, MS6

(25) http://seer.cancer.gov/csr/1975_2006/results_single/sect_01_table.01.pdf NCI's SEER Cancer Statistics Review, Incidence & Mortality Breast Cancer

(26) http://www.alternet.org/healthwellness/143195/saving_women_from_breast_cancer%3A_are_mammograms_really_the_answer/ Saving Women From Breast Cancer: Are Mammograms Really the Answer? By Naomi Freundlich, Health Beat. Posted October 21, 2009.

(27) http://www.timesonline.co.uk/tol/comment/letters/article5761650.ece?token=null&offset=0&page=1 February 19, 2009. Breast cancer screening peril. Negative consequences of the breast screening programme.

(28) http://breastcanceradvocate.wordpress.com/2009/10/01/the-truth-about-breast-cancer-is-not-pretty-and-its-not-pink/
The Truth About Breast Cancer is Not Pretty and it's not Pink Posted October 1, 2009

(29) http://ww5.komen.org/contentsimpleleft.aspx?id=6442451356&itc=lefthpban:77 Comments on Mammography Leading to Over-Diagnosis and Over-Treatment (Dr. Eric Winer, October 2009)

(30) http://www.cbcrp.org/publications/papers/Mayer/page_08.php Changes in Breast Cancer Mortality Rates,

(31) http://www.nytimes.com/2002/04/09/ science/confronting-cancer-breast-cancer-mammography-finds-more-tumors-then-debate.html
CONFRONTING CANCER; Breast Cancer: Mammography Finds More Tumors. Then the Debate Begins. By Gina Kolata Published: Tuesday, April 9, 2002. New York Times.

(32) http://nosurrenderbreastcancer.blogspot.com/2009/10/acs-throws-women-under-bus.html Wednesday, October 21, 2009. ACS Throws Women Under the Bus.

(33) http://www.ratical.org/radiation/CNR/XHP/MPDaXrayST.html
Making Personal Decisions about X-ray Screening Tests, Such as Mammography and CT of the Lung, Colon, Heart, or the Entire Body. John W. Gofman, M.D., Ph.D

(34) http://www.noetic.org/research/sr/main.html Database of spontaneous remission.

(35) The Medical Aspects of Carcinoma of the Breast, with a Note on the Spontaneous Disappearance of Secondary Growths OSLER W American Medicine: April 6 1901; 17-19; 63-66 Extracted Summary

(36) http://www.auntminnie.com/index.asp?sec=ser&sub=def&pag=dis&ItemID=87566 'Spontaneous regression' debate erupts anew at ASCO symposium, by Kate Madden Yee AuntMinnie.com staff writer October 12, 2009.

(37) http://www.ncbi.nlm.nih.gov/pmc/articles/PMC164507/ Proc Natl Acad Sci U S A. 2003 May 27; 100(11): 6682-6687. The National Academy of Sciences. Immunology Spontaneous regression of advanced cancer: Identification of a unique genetically determined, age-dependent trait in mice. Zheng Cui et al.

(38) http://www.cwru.edu/CWRU/Med/medicine/newsite/internal/screenbreastcancer.pdf N Engl J Med 2003;348:1672-80. Mammographic Screening for Breast Cancer Suzanne W. Fletcher, M.D., and Joann G. Elmore, M.D., M.P.H. With treatment, the prognosis is excellent.

(39) http://www.springerlink.com/content/pm20211j67150mw4/ Breast Cancer Research and Treatment Volume 97, Number 2, 135-144. The natural history of ductal carcinoma in situ of the breast: a review by Bircan Erbas et al.

(40) http://onlinelibrary.wiley.com/doi/10.1002/1097-0142(19951001)76:7%3C1197::AID-CNCR2820760715%3E3.0.CO;2-0/pdf Cancer Volume 76, Issue 7, pages 1197-1200, 1 October 1995. Continued local recurrence of carcinoma 15-25 years after a diagnosis of low grade ductal carcinoma in situ of the breast treated only by biopsy. David L. Page M.D et al.

(41) http://www.ncbi.nlm.nih.gov/pubmed/6275978 Cancer. 1982 Feb 15;49(4):751-8. Intraductal carcinoma of the breast: follow-up after biopsy only. Page DL, Dupont WD, Rogers LW, Landenberger M.

(42) http://archinte.ama-assn.org/cgi/content/full/160/7/953 Arch Intern Med. 2000 Apr 10;160(7):953-8. Mortality among women with ductal carcinoma in situ of the breast in the population-based surveillance, epidemiology and end results program. Ernster VL, Barclay J, Kerlikowske K, Wilkie H, Ballard-Barbash R.

(43) http://www.ncbi.nlm.nih.gov/pubmed/11350725 Endocr Relat Cancer. 2001 Mar;8(1):33-45. The management of ductal carcinoma in situ of the breast. Skinner KA, Silverstein MJ.

(44) http://www.ncbi.nlm.nih.gov/pmc/articles/PMC1557717/?tool=pubmed Breast Cancer Res. 2006; 8(2): 204. Overdiagnosis and overtreatment of breast cancer: Progression of ductal carcinoma in situ: the pathological perspective. J Louise Jones Tumour Biology Laboratory,

(45) http://www.ncbi.nlm.nih.gov/pubmed/10772968 Cancer Treat Rev. 2000 Apr;26(2):103-25. Ductal carcinoma in situ (DCIS) of the breast: evolving perspectives. Sakorafas GH, Tsiotou AG.

(46) http://www.ncbi.nlm.nih.gov/pubmed/14626378 Int J Fertil Womens Med. 2003 Sep-Oct;48(5):217-25. Treatment of ductal carcinoma in situ of the breast: review of recent advances and future prospects. Mokbel K.

(47) http://www.ncbi.nlm.nih.gov/pubmed/15884091 Cancer. 2005 Jun 15;103(12):2481-4. The natural history of low-grade ductal carcinoma in situ of the breast in women treated by biopsy only revealed over 30 years of long-term follow-up. Sanders ME, Schuyler PA, Dupont WD, Page DL.

(48) http://www.ncbi.nlm.nih.gov/pubmed/17687650 Breast Cancer Res Treat. 2008 Jun;109(3):405-16. 259 Patients with DCIS of the breast applying USC/Van Nuys prognostic index: a retrospective review with long term follow up. Di Saverio S, Catena F, Santini D, Ansaloni L, Fogacci T, Mignani S, Leone A, Gazzotti F, Gagliardi S, De Cataldis A, Taffurelli M.

(49) http://jnci.oxfordjournals.org/content/96/12/906.full Ductal Carcinoma In Situ, Complexities and Challenges JNCI J Natl Cancer Inst (2004) 96 (12): 906-920.

(50) http://annonc.oxfordjournals.org/content/13/8/1236.full Management of women with ductal carcinoma in situ of the breast: a

population-based study. H. M. Verkooijen et al. Ann Oncol (2002) 13 (8): 1236-1245.

(51) http://iodine4health.com/research/cann_2000_iodine_selenium_breast_cancer.pdf Cancer Causes and Control 11: 121±127, 2000. 121. Hypothesis: Iodine, selenium and the development of breast cancer. Stephen A. Cann et al.

(52) http://www.ncbi.nlm.nih.gov/pubmed/16025225 J Mammary Gland Biol Neoplasia. 2005 Apr;10(2):189-96. Is iodine a gatekeeper of the integrity of the mammary gland? Aceves C, Anguiano B, Delgado G.

(53) http://www.ncbi.nlm.nih.gov/pubmed/17956159 Thyroid. 2007 Sep;17(9):851-9. Uptake and gene expression with antitumoral doses of iodine in thyroid and mammary gland: evidence that chronic administration has no harmful effects. Anguiano B, García-Solís P, Delgado G, Aceves Velasco C.

(54) http://www.ncbi.nlm.nih.gov/pubmed/9735978 Clin Nucl Med. 1998 Sep;23(9):585-7. I-131 uptake in the breast for thyroid cancer surveillance with biopsy-proven benign tissue. Allen T, Wiest P, Vela S, Hartshorne M, Crooks LA.

(55) http://www.ncbi.nlm.nih.gov/pubmed/20201784 Curr Cancer Drug Targets. 2010 Mar;10(2):242-67. The biology of the sodium iodide symporter and its potential for targeted gene delivery. Hingorani M et al.

CHAPTER 22

Mammogram Guideline Reversal—What Does It Mean?

In a dramatic break from past guidelines, the US Preventive Task Force now advises beginning screening mammograms at age of 50 instead of age 40, and advises against screening for the 40-50 age group as more harmful than beneficial. Annual frequency of screening mammograms was revised to every other year instead of annually.

Setting Back Evidence-Based-Medicine with Fear Mongering

The mainstream media, government and corporate medicine have come out opposed to these revised guidelines. Using slick marketing, fear mongering, and appealing to emotion, Kathleen Sebelius, appeared on national television and advised women to ignore her own Department's task force panel, and continue with screening mammograms in the 40-50 age group. She avoided discussing the real problem with screening mammography.

Is There a Mortality Benefit, Yes or No?

Surprisingly, this question is still under debate because the 7 or 8 randomized trials of screening mammography found differing mortality benefits. The U.S. Preventive Services Task Force USPSTF reviewed eight randomized controlled trials (RCTs) of mammography screening. The mortality benefit depends on which of the seven or eight randomized trials you regard as valid. Two of the studies had no mortality benefit at all. That is **ZERO** reduction in mortality. One mammography screening study for 40-50 aged women found increased mortality in the screened group (the opposite of what is expected). The most optimistic trials reported mortality reductions of 32 %. The task force did their best to sort out the studies and finally compromised on a 16% mortality reduction as a "best guess".

The 2006 Cochrane report screening for breast cancer with mammography reviewed the same 7 or 8 clinical trials and finally compromised on an estimated 15% reduction in mortality, same as the

USPSTF task force. Considering the harms of screening mammography, over diagnosis, overtreatment and radiation exposure, the Cochrane report concludes. "*It is thus not clear whether screening does more good than harm.*"

Screening Mammography was once thought beneficial in young women with the BRCA gene, which carries a high risk of breast cancer. However, this was abandoned because the excess radiation itself induced breast cancer and offset any benefit. (28-29)

Instead of Mortality—Look at Local, Regional and Distant Disease Numbers

Since mortality benefits of screening mammography vary from zero to 30% depending on the study, let's take a different approach to the numbers by looking at 20 years of data on local vs. advanced breast cancer numbers. This is exactly what Laura Esserman did in JAMA (October 2009). She says:

"*There are several reasons that may help to explain why screening has not led to a more significant reduction in deaths from breast cancer in the United States. First, screening increases the detection of indolent cancers. Second, screening likely misses the most aggressive cancers. In other words, tumor biology dictates and trumps stage, so the basic assumption of these screening programs that finding and treating early stage disease will prevent late stage or metastatic disease may not always be correct.*"

She also says "*Ductal carcinoma in situ, rare prior to widespread screening, now represents 25% to 30% of all breast cancer diagnoses (>60 000 new case-diagnoses annually) . . . Ductal carcinoma in situ is considered to be a precancerous lesion and standard of care is excision and adjuvant treatment. However, after 2 decades of detecting and treating DCIS, there is no convincing evidence of substantial reduction in invasive breast cancer incidence. The 2002 decrease in incidence leveled off in 2005 and is attributed to a reduction in postmenopausal hormone therapy use, not DCIS removal.*"

This point made by Dr Esserman in JAMA is important. Mammography screening is detecting large numbers of DCIS cases which are then treated with surgery and radiation with no real benefit in terms of reducing the numbers of invasive breast cancers.

The Basic Problem With Screening Mammography Not Mentioned by Sebelius

The Reservoir of Silent Disease

The basic underlying problem with screening for breast cancer with mammography is the "reservoir of silent disease". A series of autopsy studies show that indolent breast cancers are common in the population. These early cancers, called DCIS, are silent and rarely cause clinical disease. The most impressive study was from Denmark in 1987.(30-31) The Danish group used specimen radiography on autopsy samples, which most closely approximates screening mammography, searching for small clusters of calcifications. The Danish team found breast cancer in one out of five women, most of which was DCIS (Ductal Carcinoma in Situ). One out of 5 women show breast cancer at autopsy, yet only 2 to 3 women per 10,000 die from breast cancer annually. (20% versus 0.03%) This indicates a paradox, a contradiction between a huge reservoir of silent and clinically insignificant disease, and the much smaller numbers of invasive breast cancers which actually come to medical attention. Something here does not add up.

DCIS in 18% of the Population

Current screening mammography technology detects more than 60,000 cases of DCIS annually, and this is only a small fraction of total DCIS which is present in one out of five women in the population. DCIS is ductal carcinoma in situ, an early form of cancer with good prognosis, a 98% five year survival with no treatment. I expect future refinements in x-ray technology to allow detection of even greater numbers of DCIS cases which have small calcifications. Ultimately the technology will catch up and replicate the Danish autopsy findings. Do we really want this? Do we really want to detect DCIS in one out of every five women, and then submit all these women to surgery for biopsy and lumpectomy? This is exactly what is advocated by the corporate-government-media sponsored mammography screening programs. I question this.

Just Stop Calling It Cancer

Recently, an NIH panel has asked pathologists to stop calling DCIS (ductal carcinoma in situ). Here is the NIH Consensus statement: "*Because of the noninvasive nature of DCIS, coupled with its favorable prognosis, strong consideration should be given to elimination of the use of the anxiety-producing term "carcinoma" from the description of DCIS.*"

Less is Better

I beg to offer a differing opinion more in line with the US Preventive Task Force revisions. The detection of massive numbers of cases of DCIS results in harmful over-treatment of the population with little benefit in terms of reduced mortality from breast cancer. This opinion is echoed by Dr Laura Esserman in a recent JAMA article on the limitations, and disappointing benefits of screening mammography. The discovery of a large reservoir of silent disease is a wake-up call that something is dreadfully wrong. Rather than screen the population for small calcifications, called DCIS, generating massive numbers of lucrative procedures with biopsies and lumpectomies that have little impact on overall mortality, I suggest a better approach.

Breast Cancer Prevention with Iodine Supplementation

The evidence is overwhelming that Iodine deficiency is a major risk factor for breast cancer, and Iodine supplementation prevents and treats breast cancer. Iodine supplementation is less expensive and more effective than corporate-government-media sponsored runaway train called mammogram screening. Iodine tablets are available OTC on the internet without a prescription.

For references and links, see my web site: www.bioidenticalhormones101.com

References for Chapter 22. Mammogram Guideline Reversal

(1) http://www.newsday.com/opinion/oped/opinion-statistics-deny-that-early-screening-for-breast-cancer-saves-lives-1.1625438 Newsday, Opinion: Statistics deny that early screening for breast cancer saves lives November 27, 2009 By Barron H. Lerner, M.D

(2) http://www.latimes.com/news/nationworld/nation/la-na-mammogram17-2009nov17,0,3942708.story By Judith Graham and Thomas H. Maugh II November 17, 2009 Mammogram guidelines spark heated debate. A government panel's recommendation that women under 50 do not need regular mammograms is attacked by oncologists, gynecologists and cancer groups.

(3) http://www.annals.org/content/151/10/716.full Clinical Guidelines. Screening for Breast Cancer: U.S. Preventive Services Task Force Recommendation Statement U.S. Preventive Services Task Force. Annals Int Med. November 17, 2009, vol. 151 no. 10 716-726.

(4) http://www.annals.org/content/151/10/I-44.full Summaries for Patients. Screening for Breast Cancer: U.S. Preventive Services Task Force Recommendations. Annals of Internal Medicine November 17, 2009, vol. 151 no. 10 I-44.

(5) http://www.sfgate.com/cgi-bin/article.cgi?file=/c/a/2009/11/18/MNLT1ALVJA.DTL Anger, shock at new U.S. mammogram guidelines Victoria Colliver, Chronicle Staff Writer San Francisco Chronicle November 18, 2009.

(6) http://www.nature.com/bjc/journal/v93/n5/full/6602683a.html Epidemiology British Journal of Cancer (2005) 93, 590-596. doi:10.1038/sj.bjc.6602683 Published online 31 August 2005. Mammographic screening before age 50 years in the UK: comparison of the radiation risks with the mortality benefits A Berrington de González et al.

(7) http://www.huffingtonpost.com/lauren-cahn/a-mammogram-didnt-save-my_b_362257.html A Mammogram DIDN'T Save My Life, Huffington Post, Lauren Cahn.

(8) http://www.desmoinesregister.com/article/20091119/OPINION03/911190343/-1/debatedem/New-mammogram-guidelines-are-right-approach DesMoines Register, New Mammogram Guidelines.

(9) http://www.msnbc.msn.com/id/33973665/ns/health-womens_health/ MSNBC. New mammogram guidelines raise questions.

(10) http://www.euref.org/ Mammography screening offered every two years to all women aged 50-69 This is in keeping with both International Agency for Research on Cancer (IARC) recommendations and the European Council Recommendation on Cancer.Screening.

(11) http://www.medscape.com/viewarticle/712720 New Breast Cancer Screening Guidelines Opposed by Societies Laurie Barclay, MD

(12) http://www.guardian.co.uk/society/2009/jul/10/breast-cancer-over-diagnosis Breast cancer over-diagnosis results in unnecessary treatment for one in three. Sarah Boseley, health editor guardian.co.uk, Friday 10 July 2009

(13) http://www.huffingtonpost.com/dr-pete-klatsky/when-less-is-more-mammogr_b_367043.html Dr. Peter Klatsky.Physician November 22, 2009 When Less Is More . . . Mammography and Paps

(14) http://www.nytimes.com/2009/11/23/health/23cancer.html?hpw Behind Cancer Guidelines, Quest for Data By GINA KOLATA Published: November 22, 2009

(15) http://www.thehastingscenter.org/Bioethicsforum/Post.aspx?id=4194 Mammography and the Corporate Breast Medicine and Business Adriane Fugh-Berman and Alicia Bell, 11/24/2009

(16) http://www.prospect.org/cs/articles?article=the_mammogram_mess The Mammogram Mess Last week, new guidelines for breast cancer screening inspired a panic. Will we ever be able to discuss effective health care reasonably? by Paul Waldman, November 24, 2009.

(17) http://blog.lib.umn.edu/schwitz/healthnews/2009/11/10-things-that.html 10 things that stand out from the mammography week to remember (forget?) By Gary Schwitzer on November 23, 2009

(18) http://health.blogs.foxnews.com/2009/11/17/ confusion-outrage-over-new-mammogram-recommendations/ Confusion, Outrage Over New Mammogram Recommendations by Dr. Manny Alvarez.

(19) http://www.washingtonpost.com/wp-dyn/content/article/2009/11/19/AR2009111904053.html Sebelius's cave-in on mammograms is a setback for health-care reform By Steven Pearlstein Friday, November 20, 2009, Washington Post.

(20) http://www.latimes.com/news/nation-and-world/la-na-mammogram19-2009nov19,0,6413481.story LA Times, Sebelius distances herself from new mammogram guidelines.

(21) http://www.presstelegram.com/news/ci_13815950?source=rss Health chief says mammograms at 40 right call. by Randolph E. Schmid The Associated Press

(22) http://www.foxnews.com/story/0,2933,575428,00.html Doctors Divided Over New Mammogram Guidelines Tuesday, November 17, 2009. Fox News.

(23) http://www.nytimes.com/2009/11/17/health/17scre.html New Guidelines on Breast Cancer Draw Opposition By RONI CARYN RABIN Published: November 16, 2009, NY Times.

(24) http://www.dotmed.com/news/story/10839
New Mammography Guidelines Could Have Deadly Effects for American Women November 24, 2009 Hologic

(25) http://www.alternet.org/reproductivejustice/144177/47,000 women could die as a result of the new mammogram guidelines 47,000 Women Could Die As a Result of the New Mammogram Guidelines By George Lakoff, AlterNet. Posted November 25, 2009.

(26) http://www.washingtonpost.com/wp-dyn/content/article/2009/11/17/AR2009111704197.html Mammograms and politics: Task force stirs up a tempest. search, recommendations for breast cancer screening have long been debated. Dan Eggen and Rob Stein Washington Post Staff Writer Wednesday, November 18, 2009

(27) http://www.medscape.com/viewarticle/712473 USPSTF Issues New Breast Cancer Screening Guidelines Laurie Barclay, MD Medscape.

(28) http://www.ncbi.nlm.nih.gov/pubmed/11104455 MedGenMed. 2000 Mar 9;2(1):E9. Is mammography indicated for women with defective BRCA genes? Implications of recent scientific advances for the diagnosis, treatment, and prevention of hereditary breast cancer. Friedenson B.

(29) http://www.ncbi.nlm.nih.gov/pubmed/19176458 J Natl Cancer Inst. 2009 Feb 4;101(3):205-9. Estimated risk of radiation-induced breast cancer from mammographic screening for young BRCA mutation carriers. By Berrington de Gonzalez A, Berg CD, Visvanathan K, Robson M.

(30) http://www.ncbi.nlm.nih.gov/pmc/articles/PMC2002422/ Breast cancer and atypia among young and middle-aged women: a study of 110 medicolegal autopsies. M. Nielsen, J. L. Thomsen, S. Primdahl, U. Dyreborg, and J. A. Andersen,tal, Copenhagen, Denmark.

(31) http://www.annals.org/content/127/11/1023.full Using Autopsy Series To Estimate the Disease "Reservoir" for Ductal Carcinoma in Situ of the Breast: How Much More Breast Cancer Can We Find? Ann Intern Med December 1, 1997 127:1023-1028. H. Gilbert Welch, MD, MPH, and William C. Black, MD

CHAPTER 23

Iodine Treats Breast Cancer, Overwhelming Evidence

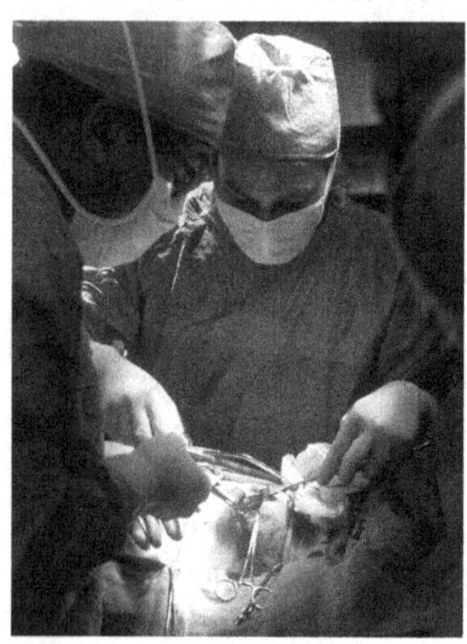

Surgeons performing a breast biopsy courtesy of the NIH, and wikimedia commons

Spontaneous Regression of Breast Cancer after Iodine Supplementation

In his Iodine book, David Brownstein MD reports three cases of spontaneous regression of breast cancer after iodine supplementation.(1) The first patient was a 63 year old English teacher. She was diagnosed with breast cancer in 1989 and after declining conventional treatment, took 50 mg per day of Iodoral, (Iodine). Six weeks later, a PET scan showed "*all of the existing tumors were disintegrating*". The second patient was a 73 year old Delores. She was diagnosed with breast cancer in 2003, declined conventional treatment with radiation and chemotherapy, and instead, Dolores took 50 mg of Iodoral daily. A follow up ultrasound of the breast 18 months later showed," *It appears that these malignancies have diminished in size since the last examination. Interval improvement is definitely seen*". Two years later, a follow up mammogram and ultrasound failed to show any abnormality and were read by the radiologist as normal. The third patient was 52 year old Joyce. She was diagnosed with breast cancer two years prior, and started on Iodoral 50 mg per day. Three years after starting Iodoral, her follow up mammograms and ultrasound exams show decreasing size of the tumor with no progression.(1)

Iodine Deficiency Causes Breast Cancer—The Overwhelming Evidence

Human Studies of Dietary Iodine Intake

Iodine deficiency is associated with a higher rate of goiter and breast cancer. Similarly, higher dietary Iodine intake is associated with less goiter and breast cancer. For example, Japan has the highest dietary intake of iodine (several milligrams per day), and the lowest rates for goiter and breast cancer. However, when Japanese women immigrate and change dietary intake of Iodine to the lower 150 mcg/day in America, breast cancer rates increase.(1) Iceland is another country with high Iodine intake and low rates for goiter and breast cancer. The high dietary iodine came from the fishing industry before World War One. In those days, the fish meal was fed to dairy cows providing milk with high iodine content. After World War One, the fish meal was eliminated from the dairy cows, and breast cancer rates soared ten-fold. (2) Iodine deficient diets in animals induces breast cancer and goiter.(1)

Important Point:
Iodine supplementation is safe, and useful for prevention and treatment of breast cancer.

Iodine Research from Mexico, India and Japan.

The Shrivastava group in India reported molecular iodine induces apoptosis (programmed cell death) in human breast cancer cell cultures. "*Iodine showed cytotoxic effects in the cultured human breast cancer cells*". (3) From Mexico, the Carmen Aceves Velasco Group reported Iodine to be safe, with no harmful effects on thyroid function, and an anti-proliferative effect on human breast cancer cell cultures. (5-7) Their 2009 paper reported the mechanism by which Iodine works as an anti-cancer agent. Iodine binds to membrane lipids called lactones forming iodo-lactones which regulate apoptosis (programmed cell death). Iodine causes apoptosis which makes cancer cells undergo programmed cell death.(4) Dr. Aceves concluded that continuous molecular iodine treatment has a "*potent antineoplastic effect*" on the progression of mammary cancer. (10) From Japan, Dr Funahashi reported a common seaweed food containing high iodine content is more beneficial than chemotherapy on breast cancer. "He found that administration of Lugol's iodine or iodine-rich Wakame seaweed to rats treated with the carcinogen dimethyl benzanthracene suppressed the development of mammary tumors. The same group demonstrated that seaweed induced apoptosis in human breast cancer cells with greater potency than that of fluorouracil, a chemotherapeutic agent used to treat breast cancer."(8)

Mechanism of Action

A 2008 paper by Bernard A. Eskin MD showed that Iodine actually altered gene expression in breast cancer cells, inducing programmed cell death. (9) A 2003 study by Ling Zhang showed that molecular Iodine caused lung cancer cells to undergo programmed cell death (apoptosis). These lung cancer cells had been genetically modified to increase iodine uptake.(12) Interestingly, a 1993 case report describes spontaneous remission of lung cancer in a patient incidentally treated with Amiodorone which contains iodine (about 9 mg per day)(13)

In Conclusion: Current Iodine research calls for use of molecular Iodine for all patients with breast cancer. (10-11) Other cancers such as lung and prostate may also benefit. Further research on Iodine as cancer chemotherapy should receive top priority for NIH funding. Iodine in the form of Iodoral tablets is available OTC, on the internet without a prescription.

Financial Disclosure: The author has no financial interest in the Iodine Book mentioned above, or in any company that manufactures Iodine Supplements.

For references and links, see my web site: www.bioidenticalhormones101.com

References for Chapter 23. Iodine Treats Breast Cancer, Overwhelming Evidence

(1) Iodine, Why You Need It, Why You Can't Live Without It, by David Brownstein MD
Fourth Edition 2009, Medical Alternatives Press.

(2) Breast Cancer and Iodine by David M Derry MD PhD 2001 Trafford.

(3) http://www.jbc.org/content/281/28/19762.abstract July 14, 2006 The Journal of Biological Chemistry, 281, 19762-19771 Molecular Iodine Induces Caspase-independent Apoptosis in Human Breast Carcinoma Cells Involving the Mitochondria-mediated Pathway. Ashutosh Shrivastava et al.

(4) http://www.ncbi.nlm.nih.gov/pmc/articles/PMC2703618/ Mol Cancer. 2009; 8: 33. Published online 2009 June 6. Antineoplastic effect of iodine in mammary cancer: participation of 6-iodolactone (6-IL) and peroxisome proliferator-activated receptors (PPAR). Carmen Aceves et al.

(5) http://iodine4health.com/research/anguiano_2007_uptake_gene_expression.pdf THYROID Volume 17, Number 9, 2007. Uptake and Gene Expression with Antitumoral Doses of Iodine in Thyroid and Mammary Gland: Evidence That Chronic Administration Has No Harmful Effects. Carmen Aceves Velasco et al.

(6) http://erc.endocrinology-journals.org/cgi/content/full/13/4/1147 Endocr Relat Cancer. 2006 Dec; 13 (4): 1147-58. Uptake and antiproliferative effect of molecular iodine in the MCF-7 breast cancer cell line. C Aceves et al. Querétaro, México.

(7) http://erc.endocrinology-journals.org/cgi/content/abstract/15/4/1003 Signaling pathways involved in the antiproliferative effect of molecular iodine in normal and tumoral breast cells: evidence that 6-iodolactone mediates apoptotic effects. C Aceves et al. Querétaro México.

(8) http://iodine4health.com/research/funahashi_2001_seaweed_prevents_breast_cancer.pdf RAPID COMMUNICATION Jpn. J. Cancer Res. 92, 483-487, May 2001 Seaweed Prevents Breast Cancer? Hiroomi Funahashi et al. Japan.

(9) http://www.medsci.org/v05p0189 Int J Med Sci 2008; 5:189-196. Iodine Alters Gene Expression in the MCF7 Breast Cancer Cell Line: Evidence for an Anti-Estrogen Effect of Iodine. Frederick R. Stoddard II1 et al.

(10) http://findarticles.com/p/articles/mi_pwwi/is_200610/ai_n16809836/ Research Calls for Use of Molecular Iodine to Treat Breast Cancer. Market Wire, October, 2006

(11) http://iodine4health.com/research/cann_2000_iodine_selenium_breast_cancer.pdf Cancer Causes and Control 11: 121±127, 2000. Kluwer Academic Publishers. Hypothesis: Iodine, selenium and the development of breast cancer. Stephen A. Cann, Johannes P. van Netten Christiaan van Netten.

(12) http://cancerres.aacrjournals.org/cgi/content/full/63/16/5065 Cancer research 2003;63(16):5065-72. Nonradioactive Iodide Effectively Induces Apoptosis in Genetically Modified Lung Cancer Cells1 Ling Zhang et al.

(13) http://jnci.oxfordjournals.org/cgi/pdf_extract/85/16/1342 J Natl Cancer Inst. 1993 Aug 18;85(16):1342-3. Spontaneous remission of metastatic lung cancer following myxedema coma—an apoptosis-related phenomenon? Hercbergs A, Leith JT.

(14) http://www.fen.bilkent.edu.tr/~tazebay/papers/paper1.pdf 2000 Nature America Inc. The mammary gland iodide transporter is expressed during lactation and in breast cancer. Uygar H. Tazebay et al.

(15) http://web.tiscali.it/iodio/ Dr. Sebastiano Venturi investigator on Iodine Deficiency Disorders and Iodine metabolism

(16) http://web.tiscali.it/iodio/ Is there a role for iodine in breast diseases? S. Venturi

(17) http://osteomed2.com/Documents/Supraphysiological_iodine_and_breastpain.pdf The Effect of Supraphysiologic Levels of Iodine on Patients with Cyclic Mastalgia, Jack H. Kessler, PhD

(18) http://breast-cancer-research.com/content/5/5/235
http://www.biomedcentral.com/content/pdf/bcr638.pdf
The thyroid, iodine and breast cancer by Peter PA Smyth, Breast Cancer Res 2003, 5:235-238

(19) http://www.ncbi.nlm.nih.gov/pubmed/8221402 Can J Surg. 1993 Oct;36(5):453-60. Iodine replacement in fibrocystic disease of the breast. Ghent WR, Eskin BA, Low DA, Hill LP. Department of Surgery, Queen's University, Hotel Dieu Hospital, Kingston, Ont.

(20) http://www.optimox.com/pics/Iodine/opt_Research_I.shtml Guy Abraham Iodine Project Optimox

(21) http://cypress.he.net/~bigmacnc/drflechas/index.htm George Flechas MD

(22) https://www.drbrownstein.com/bookstore_Iodine.php David Brownstein MD Iodine Book

(23) http://www.ei-resource.org/expert-columns/dr.-jacob-teitelbaums-column/iodine-deficiency-%11-an-old-epidemic-is-back/ Jacob Teitelbaum MD on Iodine

(24) http://www.jpands.org/vol11no4/millerd.pdf Extrathyroidal Benefits of Iodine by Donald W. Miller, Jr., M.D. Journal of American Physicians and Surgeons Volume 11 Number 4 Winter 2006.

(25) http://www.breastcancerchoices.org/iodineref2.html Investigating the Relationship Between Iodine and the Breast Part 2: What Are Iodine's Mechanisms of Action? Observations and Theories. Breast Cancer Choices.

(26) http://www.breastcancerchoices.org/iodineref3.html Part 3: What is the Effect of Iodine on Breast Cancer? Breast Cancer Choices. www.breastcancerchoices.org http://www.breastcancerchoices.org/iodine.html

(27) http://iodine4health.com/ http://iodine4health.com/body/breast/breast.htm Iodine and the Breast, Iodine for Health.

(28) http://www.hacres.com/diet/articles/Iodine.pdf Recent Advances in Iodine Nutrition by Michael Donaldson, PhD

(29) http://www.thorne.com/altmedrev/.fulltext/13/2/116.pdf Iodine: Deficiency and Therapeutic Considerations Lyn Patrick, ND Alternative Medicine Review Volume 13, Number 2 2008

(30) http://clincancerres.aacrjournals.org/content/11/4/1483.full In vivo Radioiodide Imaging and Treatment of Breast Cancer Xenografts after MUC1-Driven Expression of the Sodium Iodide Symporter. Roisin M. Dwyer et al. Clin Cancer Res February 15, 2005 11; 1483.

Section Six: Low Testosterone Diagnosis and Treatment

CHAPTER 24

Low Testosterone Could Be Killing You

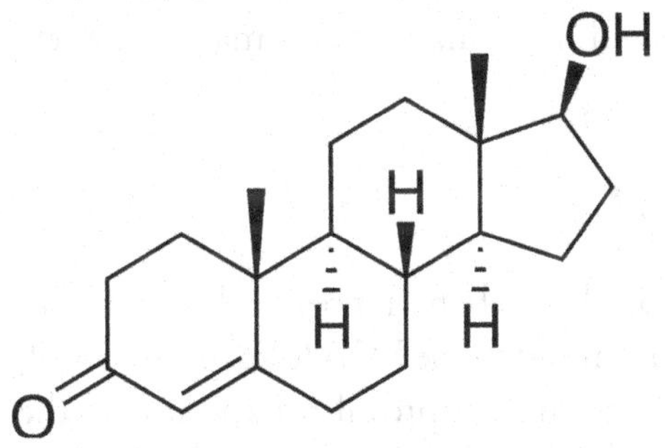

Testosterone chemical structure, courtesy of wikimedia commons

Forty Per Cent More Likely to Die

Therecentmedicalliterature shows that low testosterone is associated with increased mortality.(1-3) One study, published in 2008, tracked 800 California men 50 to 91 years old. Testosterone levels were measured at the beginning of the study, and the men's health was tracked over 20 years. Low testosterone symptoms reported by these men included decreased libido, erectile dysfunction, fatigue, loss of strength, decrease in bone density and decreased muscle mass. The men with low testosterone tended to be overweight, and had increased risk for cardiovascular disease and diabetes. Men with the lowest testosterone, below 241 total serum level, had a **FORTY percent increase in mortality**.(2) I find this astounding.

A Study of EPIC Proportions

The authors of the EPIC Study published in Circulation 2007 said,

> "*In men, endogenous testosterone concentrations are inversely related to mortality due to cardiovascular disease and all causes. Low testosterone may be a predictive marker for those at high risk of cardiovascular disease.*"(9)

Testosterone Blocking Drugs Increase Mortality

A study by Dr. Amy Dosoretz, a radiation oncology resident with the Harvard Radiation Oncology Program in Boston showed that patients treated with the testosterone blocking drugs to "knock out testosterone to shrink the prostate" had a poor outcome. They had a **20% increase in mortality**.(6)(7) A discovery such as this, that a treatment that carries a 20 per cent increased mortality means the treatment is discredited and should be discarded, and should no longer be the "standard of care". Instead it should be considered "substandard care". However, old habits in medicine have a way of lingering on, so it may take a few more years for this to change.

FDA Approval Would Be Denied

FDA approval requires a drug to produce a benefit greater than placebo. Had Amy Doseretz' study been submitted to the FDA for drug approval, the FDA would never have been granted approval for the use of the testosterone blocker, Lupron™, for prostate cancer. A detrimental result of 20 per cent increased mortality would spell disaster, and the FDA approval would be denied.

Other Study Confirms Findings

Dr Amy Dosoretz was not the first to raise doubts about the benefits of testosterone blockade (used as a treatment for prostate cancer). A previous study by Grace L. Lu-Yao was published JAMA 2008 showing that androgen deprivation therapy is not associated with improved survival. (8)

Important Point:
Having a low testosterone level is associated with 40% increased mortality. Blocking testosterone levels with drugs is associated with a 20% increased mortality.

For references and links, see my web site: www.bioidenticalhormones101.com

Chapter 24. Low Testosterone Could Be Killing You

(1) http://jcem.endojournals.org/cgi/content/full/93/1/68 Low Serum Testosterone and Mortality in Male Veterans Arch Intern Med. 2006;166:1660-1665 Molly M. Shores, MD; Alvin M. Matsumoto, MD; Kevin L. Sloan, MD; Daniel R. Kivlahan, PhD.

(2) http://jcem.endojournals.org/cgi/content/full/93/1/68 The Journal of Clinical Endocrinology & Metabolism 2008 Jan;93(1):68-75. Low Serum Testosterone and Mortality in Older Men. Gail A. Laughlin, Elizabeth Barrett-Connor and Jaclyn Bergstrom.

(3) http://abcnews.go.com/Health/ActiveAging/story?id=3247773&page=1&page=1 Low Testosterone Could Kill You. Low Levels of Male Hormone May be More Dangerous Than Previously Thought By SUPINDA BUNYAVANICH, M.D. ABC News Medical Unit June 6, 2007

(4) http://www.medicalnewstoday.com/articles/153822.php Testosterone Replacement For Men With Low Testosterone Improves Liver Function, Metabolic Syndrome. Medical News Today. June 13, 2009.

(5) http://www.news-medical.net/news/2008/03/04/35897.aspx Low testosterone levels linked to depression in older men March 2008. Medical Net News.

(6) http://www.prostatecancerissues.com/ms/news/619639/main.html Hormone Therapy Not Best for Older Prostate Cancer Patients. Study found giving it before radiation raised death risk 20% in this group By Alan Mozes HealthDay Reporter. TUESDAY, Sept. 23

(7) http://www.docguide.com/news/content.nsf/news/852571020057CCF6852574CE006F3F4A Hormone Therapy Before Brachytherapy May Increase Mortality in Prostate Cancer: Presented at ASTRO By Martha Kerr, BSN BOSTON—September 24, 2008—[Presentation title: Mortality in Men Age 70 or More With Localized Prostate Cancer Treated With Brachytherapy With or Without Neoadjuvant Hormonal Therapy. Abstract 84]

(8) http://jama.ama-assn.org/cgi/content/full/300/2/173 Survival Following Primary Androgen Deprivation Therapy Among Men With Localized Prostate Cancer. Grace L. Lu-Yao, MPH, PhD; Peter C. Albertsen, MD; Dirk F. Moore, PhD; Weichung Shih, PhD; Yong Lin, PhD; Robert S. DiPaola, MD; Siu-Long Yao, MD. JAMA. 2008;300(2):173-181.

(9) http://circ.ahajournals.org/cgi/content/short/116/23/2694 Circulation. 2007;116:2694-2701. Endogenous Testosterone and Mortality Due to All Causes, Cardiovascular Disease, and Cancer in Men. European Prospective Investigation Into Cancer in Norfolk (EPIC-Norfolk) Prospective Population Study. Kay-Tee Khaw, MBBChir, FRCP; Mitch Dowsett, PhD; Elizabeth Folkerd, PhD; Sheila Bingham, PhD; Nicholas Wareham, MBBS, PhD; Robert Luben, BSc; Ailsa Welch, PhD; Nicholas Day, PhD

CHAPTER 25

Low Testosterone from Pain Pills

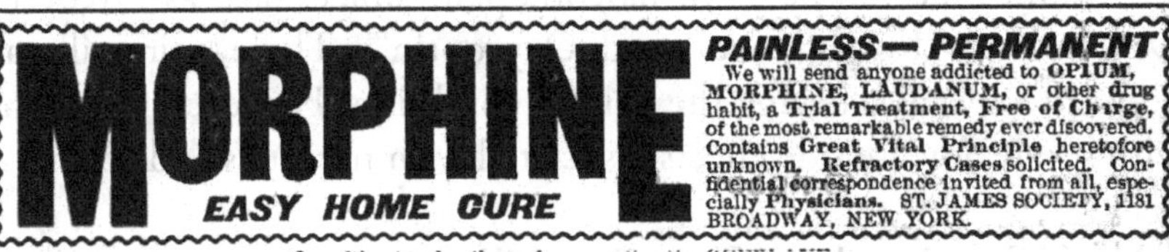

Advertisement for curing morphine addiction from Overland Monthly, January 1900, courtesy of wikimedia commons

Joe has chronic fatigue, loss of muscle strength, and erectile dysfunction. He was doing well until 10 years ago when he started pain pills after a car accident which left him with chronic back pain.

Chronic Pain Treated with Opioid Narcotics

After the car accident, Joe's family doctor prescribed Oxycontin™ pain pills, hoping the chronic back pain would eventually get better. Unfortunately, Joe's back pain did not get better, and he still takes pain pills every day. Even though the pain pills are no longer effective, Joe finds it nearly impossible to get off them because of the severe withdrawal effects.

Low Testosterone Detected on Blood Tests

Joe's lab testing showed very low testosterone levels which explained the fatigue, weakness and low libido. To remedy the low testosterone, Joe was started on bioidentical testosterone program using a topical testosterone gel, and 6 weeks later he reported that the fatigue and weakness are gone, and his wife is much happier with his renewed libido. Joe also reported his chronic pain seemed to decrease in intensity, and he was now interested in pursuing the idea of tapering off the narcotic pain pills.(4)

Doctors Freely Prescribe Narcotic Pain Pills

When patients like Joe seek help from their doctor for a painful condition, they will be given narcotic pain tablets such as Percocet™, Oxycodone™, Roxycodone™ and Oxycontin™. These pain pills are quite effective at relieving the painful condition. However, they come with severe adverse side effects associated with narcotics addiction.

Adverse Effects of Long Term Pain Pills (Opiates)

Narcotic Pain Pills (opioids) are highly addictive with severe adverse effects related to drug withdrawal. Opiate containing narcotic Pain Pills are highly effective for pain, but were never intended for long term use. Over time, these drugs cause profound suppression of the endocrine system, and in men, profound inhibition of testosterone production. This type of testosterone suppression is quite common in our population, and yet, may go unrecognized by the busy primary care doctor. (1)

Another adverse effect of long-term use is opioid-induced hyperalgesia, which means increased sensitivity to pain. This is a form of hypersensitivity to pain in which the original painful condition becomes worsened and magnified. Other adverse effects include impaired cognitive function, and suppression of the immune system, rendering the patient more susceptible to common infections.(6)

Chronic Opioid Pain Pills Lose Effectiveness Long Term

Another problem with long term use of narcotic pain pills is that they lose their effectiveness over time. The brain and nervous system develops a "tolerance" to the drug, and higher doses are required to achieve the same result.(7) The initial pain relief from opioid pain pills may not be sustained long term because of drug tolerance, opioid-induced hyperalgesia, and intermittent drug withdrawal effects. (7) In other words the pills lose their effectiveness, and yet continue to produce dependence and adverse effects.

Low Testosterone Goes Largely Unrecognized

Although quite common, Opioid-induced androgen deficiency has gone largely unrecognized by the medical profession (1). Low testosterone is caused by opioid drug inhibition of LH (Luteinizing Hormone), a pituitary hormone involved in testosterone production, as well direct inhibition of testosterone production, itself. Similarly, there is also inhibition of the entire endocrine system, and adrenal hormone suppression. Symptoms of low testosterone include fatigue, depression, hot flashes, night sweats, diminished libido, erectile dysfunction, and diminished sexual arousal and satisfaction. Men may also develop osteoporosis, anemia, and diminished muscle mass. (2)(3) Women who consume opioid-pain pills will stop having menstrual cycles and will notice greatly diminished libido (sex drive). (5)

Testosterone Treatment Effective and Recommended by Mainstream Medicine

Administration of both topical (transdermal) testosterone and injectable testosterone has been studied and found effective for men with low testosterone on pain pills. (4)

Important Point:
Chronic use of narcotic pain pills causes profound suppression of hormone levels including low testosterone in males, and cessation of menses in females.

Our Approach to Evaluation and Treatment

For men with a chronic pain condition who have been on long-term pain pills, our evaluation includes a complete blood testing panel looking for vitamin, mineral and nutritional deficiencies. We find these deficiencies quite commonly in this group. In addition, evaluation includes a complete hormone panel looking at the entire endocrine system, and adrenal function. If extensive testing shows low hormone levels, then hormone supplementation is offered.

Opiate Detoxification Program is Essential

The reality is that hormone supplementation and nutritional supplementation for the long term opiate pain pill user is only a temporary band aid. To fully restore health, the opiate addiction must be addressed and the patient must ultimately get off the pain pills. Drug withdrawal may be difficult because of severe drug withdrawal symptoms. Therefore, we refer the patient to a center that specializes in narcotics detoxification, and urge the patient to strongly consider this option. (10)

For references and links, see my web site: www.bioidenticalhormones101.com

References for Chapter 25. Low Testosterone From Pain Pills

(1) http://journals.lww.com/co-endocrinology/Abstract/2006/06000/Opioid_induced_androgen_deficiency.6.aspx Current Opinion in Endocrinology and Diabetes: June 2006—Volume 13—Issue 3—p 262-266. Opioid-induced androgen deficiency by Daniell, Harry W.

(2) http://www.amjmed.com/article/S0002-9343(06)00614-0/fulltext American Journal of Medicine, Volume 120, Issue 9, Page 21, September 2007. Opioid-induced Androgen Deficiency Discussion in Opioid Contracts by Harry W. Daniell, MD

(3) http://www.jpain.org/article/S1526-5900(02)00032-9/abstract?refuid=S0002-9343(06)00614-0&refissn=0002-9343 Hypogonadism in men consuming sustained-action oral opioids. Presented in part at the 16th Annual Meeting of the Society for Ambulatory Anesthesia, Palm Springs, CA, May 2-5, 2001. Harry W. Daniell Volume 3, Issue 5, Pages 377-384 (October 2002)

(4) http://www.ncbi.nlm.nih.gov/pubmed/16516826 J Pain. 2006 Mar;7(3):200-10. Open-label pilot study of testosterone patch therapy in men with opioid-induced androgen deficiency. Daniell HW et al.

(5) http://www.ncbi.nlm.nih.gov/pubmed/17936076 J Pain. 2008 Jan;9(1):28-36. Epub 2007 Nov 1. Opioid endocrinopathy in women consuming prescribed sustained-action opioids for control of nonmalignant pain. Daniell HW.

(6) http://www.ncbi.nlm.nih.gov/pubmed/17873598 Curr Opin Anaesthesiol. 2007 Oct;20(5):451-5. An update on the role of opioids in the management of chronic pain of nonmalignant origin. Højsted J, Sjøgren P. Multidisciplinary Pain Center, Rigshospitalet, Blegdamsvej 9, 2100 Copenhagen Ø, Denmark.

(7) http://www.ncbi.nlm.nih.gov/pubmed/18574357 Clin J Pain. 2008 Jul-Aug;24(6):469-78. Efficacy of opioids for chronic pain: a review of the evidence. Ballantyne JC, Shin NS.Division of Pain Medicine, Massachusetts General Hospital, Boston, MA 02114, USA.

(8) http://www.viamedica.pl/gazety/gazetaE/darmowy_pdf.phtml?indeks=33&indeks_art=263 Zbigniew Zylicz, Consultant in Palliative Medicine, Dove House Hospice, Hull, United Kingdom. Opioid-induced hypogonadism: the role of androgens in the well-being and pain thresholds in men and women with advanced disease

(9) http://jcem.endojournals.org/cgi/content/full/85/6/2215 Endocrine Consequences of Long-Term Intrathecal Administration of Opioids, Roger Abs et al., The Journal of Clinical Endocrinology & Metabolism Vol. 85, No. 6 2215-2222

(10) Dr. Marvin "Rick" Sponaugle, Florida Detox and Wellness Institute, 32815 US Highway 19 N, Palm Harbor, FL 34684, Toll-free: 1-888-775-2770 http://floridadetox.com/

CHAPTER 26

Testosterone Found to Cause Heart Attacks?

How Not to Do a Testosterone Clinical Trial

A testosterone study published in the New England Journal was halted early because the testosterone treated group had more heart attacks.(1)(2)(3)(4) Doctors gave topical testosterone to obese, elderly, immobilized men with underlying heart disease. All had limitations in mobility, defined as having difficulty walking two blocks or climbing steps. About half were obese, and 75% were heavy smokers. More than 50% had pre-existing heart disease. Almost all had hypertension. A quarter were diabetics. 60% were on statin drugs like Lipitor. Men younger than 65 were excluded from the study, and the average age was 74.

Starting testosterone levels were low, averaging 250 (ng/dl) for Total and 48 for Free levels. After treatment with 5 to 15 grams/day of topical testosterone gel (Testim™ or Androgel™), levels increased to 574 (ng/dl), after adjustment of the dose, while the placebo group levels remained low at 292 (ng/dl). As you might expect, the Testosterone Group had significant improvements in leg muscle strength.

Sending Old Men Up the Hill

If we recruited a group of immobilized, obese, elderly frail men with heart disease, and then instructed them to run up a mountain hill, these men would be unable to go more than a few steps, and no harm would come from it. However, if we took this same group of men, apply testosterone gel for a few weeks, as they did, and then send them up the hill, this would be a bad thing. The testosterone would give the men the leg muscle strength to run up the hill and many would succumb to heart attacks. In a nutshell, this is what happened in the NEJM study.

Previous Studies Show Opposite Results, Testosterone Benefits the Heart

Low Testosterone Associated with Increased Mortality

Three separate population studies have shown that low testosterone levels in men are associated with increased mortality from cardiovascular disease and all causes. (5-7) A study by Malkin published in 2010 Heart followed 900 men with known coronary artery disease. The men were followed for 8 years, and those with low testosterone had 22% mortality compared to only 12 % for men with normal testosterone levels, almost double the mortality rate for the low testosterone group. (30)

Testosterone Reduces Cardiac Ischemia

In addition, multiple studies have shown testosterone treatment reduces cardiac ischemia in men with known heart disease. For example, an elegant study by English et al.(10) showed less cardiac ischemia in men treated with testosterone. (9-11) Men with known heart disease were given a treadmill test and their Electrocardiogram (EKG) observed while walking up an inclined treadmill. Given enough time on the treadmill, the heart disease shows up as EKG changes and chest pain. The doctors will then stop the test and allow the man to rest. The testosterone group showed longer times on the treadmill before reaching chest pain or critical EKG changes. This indicates improved blood flow with testosterone. However, the men still reach chest pain and critical EKG changes and must be taken off the treadmill. Continuing would bring on a heart attack.

Imagine what would happen if the doctors allowed the men to keep going, to continue up the inclined treadmill in spite of the chest pain? As you might guess, this is an excellent technique for causing heart attacks, and is not advisable. This scenario explains why the men in the NEJM Study had more heart attacks on testosterone. The testosterone gave them the strength to continue up the hill with severe underlying heart disease that caused a heart attack in some of the men.

Dr Morgentaler to the Rescue

A more reasonable approach for testosterone replacement is described by Morgentaler in his 2007 commentary, "Guidelines for Male

Testosterone Therapy: A Clinician's Perspective." Abraham Morgentaler is a Harvard trained Urologist, who says he was taught in medical school that low testosterone was rare and treatment ineffective.(14) Once he started clinical practice in 1988, he was surprised to find that many of his patients had low testosterone associated with erectile dysfunction (ED) which greatly improved with testosterone injections. Patients thanked him for finally "feeling normal again." Nowadays in 2010, testosterone is accepted treatment for diminished libido and erectile dysfunction (ED). Dr. Morgentaler actually prefers to start with transdermal gel testosterone before using the Viagra™ and Cialis™ type drugs, (the phosphodiesterase type-5 inhibitors PDE5i).

Important Point:
Low testosterone is a risk factor for coronary artery disease. In men with known underlying coronary artery disease, lower testosterone levels are associated with higher mortality rate.

Risks of Testosterone Treatment Reviewed by Morgentaler

Dr Morgentaler's 2004 NEJM article is also useful, covering the "*Risks of testosterone-replacement therapy and recommendations for monitoring*". Dr Morgentaler says that 4 million men may be candidates for testosterone treatment, yet only 5 percent are actually treated.(15)(16) Even though there is no large scale, long term clinical studies looking at risks and adverse effects, the number of testosterone prescriptions has increased 500 percent since 1993.

Previous Studies Contradict Bhasin's Conclusions

In his 2004 report, Dr. Morgentaler says that previous studies of men given testosterone-replacement have not shown increased heart disease. There has been no increase rate of heart attacks, myocardial infarction, stroke, or angina (chest pain caused by narrowed coronary arteries). (15) Increased blood count (polycythemia) is an adverse effect noted in about 3% of men after testosterone treatment. This is controlled by reducing dosage or donating blood. Dr Morgentaler also discusses, prostate, PSA, sleep apnea, and other issues. He finds that testosterone treatment is not associated with increased prostate cancer, although he recommends prostate surveillance. Finally he discusses that a small percentage of men may note breast enlargement or tenderness from treatment. For more information, I recommend Dr. Morgentaler's 2009 book, Testosterone for Life. (31)

Conclusion: Testosterone therapy for immobilized elderly men with underlying chronic conditions such as obesity, heart disease, hypertension, and cigarette smoking is not recommended. However, for all other candidates for testosterone therapy, the health benefits clearly outweigh the risks and adverse effects which are quite manageable.

For references and links, see my web site: www.bioidenticalhormones101.com

References for Chapter 26. Testosterone Found to Cause Heart Attacks?

(1) http://www.ncbi.nlm.nih.gov/pubmed/20592293 N Engl J Med. 2010 Jul 8;363(2):109-22. Adverse events associated with testosterone administration. Basaria S, Coviello AD, Travison TG, Storer TW, Farwell WR, Jette AM, Eder R, Tennstedt S, Ulloor J, Zhang A, Choong K, Lakshman KM, Mazer NA, Miciek R, Krasnoff J, Elmi A, Knapp PE, Brooks B, Appleman E, Aggarwal S, Bhasin G, Hede-Brierley L, Bhatia A, Collins L, LeBrasseur N, Fiore LD, Bhasin S.

(2) http://www.nytimes.com/2010/07/06/health/06hormone.html?r=1&ref=health Testosterone Gel Trial Ends After Heart Issue By RONI CARYN RABIN. July 5, 2010

(3) http://www.nejm.org/doi/full/10.1056/NEJMe1006197 Bremner WJ. Testosterone Deficiency and Replacement in Older Men. N Engl J Med;363(2):189-91.

(4) http://www.businessweek.com/news/2010-06-30/auxilium-testosterone-gel-linked-to-heart-problems-in-older-men.html Bloomberg News 07/21/2010—More than one-fifth of patients using a testosterone gel sold by Auxilium Pharmaceuticals Inc. developed heart problems in a study of mobility-impaired men aged 65 and older.

(5) http://www.healther.net/2010/09/testosterone-gel-linked-to-heart-problems/ Testosterone gel linked to heart problems healther 2010/09/26/ 18:04

(6) http://www.nih.gov/news/health/jun2010/nia-30.htm Adverse Cardiovascular Events Reported in Testosterone Trial in Older Men. Treatment Phase of Clinical Trial Halted

(7) http://eurheartj.oxfordjournals.org/content/31/12/1494.abstract Eur Heart J (2010) 31 (12): 1494-1501. Low serum testosterone levels are associated with increased risk of mortality in a population-based cohort of men aged 20-79, Robin Haring et al.

(8) http://circ.ahajournals.org/cgi/content/abstract/116/23/2694 Endogenous Testosterone and Mortality Due to All Causes, Cardiovascular Disease, and Cancer in Men European Prospective Investigation Into Cancer in Norfolk (EPIC-Norfolk) Prospective Population Study (Circulation. 2007;116:2694-2701.)

(9) http://archinte.ama-assn.org/cgi/content/abstract/166/15/1660 Vol. 166 No. 15, Aug 14/28, 2006 Low Serum Testosterone and Mortality in Male Veterans. Molly M. Shores, MD; Alvin M. Matsumoto, MD; Kevin L. Sloan, MD; Daniel R. Kivlahan, PhD Arch Intern Med. 2006;166:1660-1665.

(10) http://circ.ahajournals.org/cgi/content/full/102/16/1906 Low-Dose Transdermal Testosterone Therapy Improves Angina Threshold in Men With Chronic Stable Angina A Randomized, Double-Blind, Placebo-Controlled Study. Katherine M. English et al.

(11) http://circ.ahajournals.org/cgi/content/full/99/13/1666 Rosano GMC, Leonardo F, Pagnotta P, et al. Acute anti-ischemic effect of testosterone in men with coronary artery disease. Circulation. 1999; 99:1666-1670.

(12) http://www.ncbi.nlm.nih.gov/pubmed/10072236 Webb CM, Adamson DL, de Zeigler D, et al. Effect of acute testosterone on myocardial ischemia in men with coronary artery disease. Am J Cardiol. 1999;83:437-439.

(13) http://www.eje-online.org/cgi/content/abstract/161/3/443 CLINICAL STUDY Long-term benefits of testosterone replacement therapy on angina threshold and atheroma in men Atish Mathur, Christopher Malkin et al.

(14) http://jcem.endojournals.org/cgi/content/full/92/2/416 Guideline for Male Testosterone Therapy: A Clinician's Perspective. Abraham Morgentaler Harvard Medical School, Beth Israel Deaconess Medical Center, Boston, Massachusetts The Journal of Clinical Endocrinology & Metabolism Vol. 92, No. 2 416-417, 2007

(15) http://www.ncbi.nlm.nih.gov/pubmed/%2014749457 N Engl J Med. 2004 Jan 29;350(5):482-92. Risks of testosterone-replacement therapy and recommendations for monitoring. Rhoden EL, Morgentaler A.

(16) http://www.ncbi.nlm.nih.gov/pubmed/20104673 J Sex Med. 2010 Jan;7(1 Pt 1):277-83. Symptomatic response rates to testosterone therapy and the likelihood of completing 12 months of therapy in clinical practice. Rhoden EL, Morgentaler A.

(17) http://eurheartj.oxfordjournals.org/content/27/1/57.abstract Testosterone therapy in men with moderate severity heart failure: a double-blind randomized placebo controlled trial Chris J. Malkin et al.

(18) http://content.onlinejacc.org/cgi/content/abstract/56/16/1310 CLINICAL RESEARCH: HEART FAILURE Testosterone Therapy in Women With Chronic Heart Failure A Pilot Double-Blind, Randomized, Placebo-Controlled Study Ferdinando Iellamo, MD et al.

(19) http://circ.ahajournals.org/cgi/content/full/114/17/1829 Circulation. 2006;114:1829-1837. Heart Failure Anabolic Deficiency in Men With Chronic Heart Failure, Prevalence and Detrimental Impact on Survival. Wu FC, Tajar A, Beynon JM, et al.

(20) http://www.ncbi.nlm.nih.gov/pubmed/19929914 J Sex Med. 2010 Apr;7(4 Pt 1):1362-80. Epub 2009 Nov 19. Age-related changes in general and sexual health in middle-aged and older men: results from the European Male Ageing Study (EMAS.

(21) http://www.nejm.org/doi/pdf/10.1056/NEJMoa0911101 Identification of Late-Onset Hypogonadism in Middle-Aged and Elderly Men. Frederick C.W. Wu, M.D., et al for the EMAS Group. N Engl J Med 2010; 363:12 3-135 July 8, 2010

(22) http://www.primaryissues.org/testosterone/ Testosterone Deficiency and Men's Health: A Crucial Connection André T. Guay, MD, and Martin Miner, MD

(23) http://jcem.endojournals.org/cgi/content/abstract/jc.2010-0266v1 Why Is Androgen Replacement in Males Controversial? Glenn R. Cunningham* and Shivani M. Toma Baylor College of Medicine and St. Luke's Episcopal Hospital, Houston, Texas 77030

(24) http://www.slate.com/id/2269042/ The Mel Gibson Excuse Does male menopause actually exist? By Jessica Dweck. Sept. 30, 2010.

(25) http://thestar.com.my/health/story.asp?file=/2010/10/3/health/7143684&sec=health Sunday October 3, 2010 The hormonal male Art of Healing By DR AMIR FARID ISAHAK. The ins and outs of male sex hormones.

(26) http://jcem.endojournals.org/cgi/content/abstract/95/6/2536 Bhasin S, Cunningham GR, Hayes FJ, Matsumoto AM, Snyder PJ, Swerdloff RS, Montori VM, & Task Force, Endocrine Society (2010). Testosterone therapy in men with androgen deficiency syndromes: an Endocrine Society clinical practice guideline. The Journal of clinical endocrinology and metabolism, 95 (6), 2536-59

(27) http://jcem.endojournals.org/cgi/content/abstract/92/11/4241 Araujo, A., Esche, G., Kupelian, V., O'Donnell, A., Travison, T., Williams, R., Clark, R., & McKinlay, J. (2007). Prevalence of Symptomatic Androgen Deficiency in Men Journal of Clinical Endocrinology & Metabolism, 92 (11), 4241-4247 DOI: 10.1210/jc.2007-1245

(28) http://www.myhousecallmd.com/archives/3993 Testosterone: The New Anti-Aging Wonder Drug? by Rebecca Shatsky, MD, 2011

(29) http://media.pituitary.org/pdf/TestTherapyAndDef.pdf Endocrine News June 2006 Article: TESTOSTERONE THERAPY FOR ANDROGEN DEFICIENT MEN New Clinical Guideline from the Endocrine Society By Cathy Kristiansen, Editor

(30) http://heart.bmj.com/content/early/2010/09/28/hrt.2010.195412 Heart 19 October 2010, Low serum testosterone and increased mortality in men with coronary heart disease by Chris J Malkin et al

(31) Testosterone for Life: Recharge Your Vitality, Sex Drive, Muscle Mass, and Overall Health by Abraham Morgentaler McGraw-Hill; 1st edition (October 27, 2008)

Section Seven: Testosterone and PSA Screening for Prostate Cancer

CHAPTER 27

Testosterone, PSA and Prostate Cancer, Myths and Misconceptions

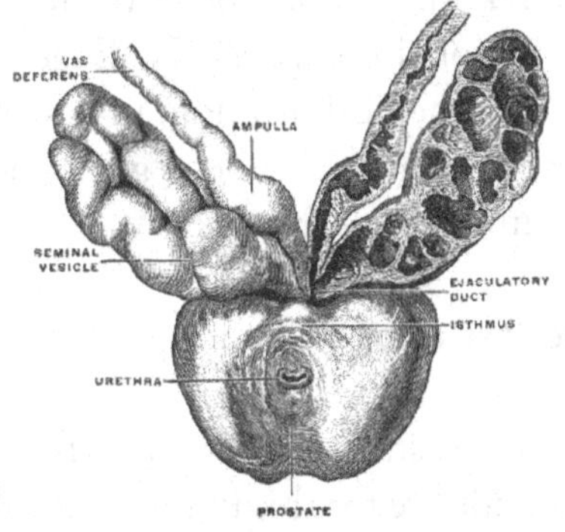

Prostate and seminal vesicals from Gray's Anatomy lithograph, 1918, courtesy of wilimedia commons.

Benefits of Testosterone Therapy

The Nobel Prize in Chemistry was awarded to Butenandt and Ruzicka in 1939 for the synthesis of testosterone.(1) Over the last seventy years, thousands of medical studies have shown that testosterone is beneficial for improving health and prolonging life.(2-27) Testosterone can prevent or reduce the likelihood of osteoporosis, type 2 diabetes, cardiovascular disease, obesity, depression and anxiety and the risk of early mortality(7) Health benefits include positive effects on mood, energy levels, verbal fluency, strength, increased muscle size, decreased body fat and increased bone density.(2-27) Testosterone restores and enhances male libido, and is a treatment for male sexual dysfunction.(33)

Low Testosterone Associated With Increased Mortality

The 2007 EPIC study concluded that testosterone level is inversely related to cardiovascular disease risk and all-cause mortality. Thus, low testosterone may be a marker for increased risk of cardiovascular disease.(35) A low Testosterone level is linked to reduced cognitive performance and onset of Alzheimer's in elderly men.(36)(37)

Testosterone Benefits the Heart

Here are a few studies showing testosterone benefits the heart and circulation. Dr. Dobrzycki studied men with known coronary artery disease and showed they had significantly lower levels of testosterone (J Med Invest 2003).(22) He also showed that lower testosterone levels was associated with reduced pumping ability of the heart. Dr. C.J. Malkin showed that testosterone therapy reduced the risk of death from abnormal heart rhythms (arrhythmias).(23) Dr. Malkin also reported that testosterone improves the pumping action of the heart in patients with Congestive Heart Failure,(24) and acts a protective factor against atherosclerosis and plaque formation in arteries. Dr. Eugene Shippen presented an impressive study at a medical meeting, in which testosterone therapy was used to successfully reverse diabetic gangrene of the lower legs and avoid amputation in many of the cases.

No Evidence of Adverse Effect on the Prostate

Regarding a hypothetical question of prostate cancer risk from testosterone administration, there is no evidence for this in the medical literature. Here are three of many medical studies reporting no adverse effect on the prostate, and no evidence that testosterone is the cause of prostate cancer.

> Dr Morgentaler says: "*It has been part of the conventional medical wisdom for six decades that higher testosterone in some way increases the risk of prostate cancer. This belief is derived largely from the well-documented regression of prostate cancer in the face of surgical or pharmacological castration. However, there is an absence of scientific data supporting the concept that higher testosterone levels are associated with an increased risk of prostate cancer. Specifically, no increased risk of prostate cancer was noted in 1) clinical trials of testosterone supplementation, 2) longitudinal population-based studies, or 3) in a high-risk population of hypogonadal men receiving testosterone treatment. Moreover, hypogonadal men have a substantial rate of biopsy-detectable prostate cancer, suggesting that low testosterone has no protective effect against development of prostate cancer. These results argue against an increased risk of prostate cancer with testosterone*

replacement therapy." Quoted from Testosterone replacement therapy and prostate risks: where's the beef? Morgentaler A. Can J Urol. 2006 Feb;13 Suppl 1:40-3.(28)

Dr Morales says: "*No evidence exists that appropriate androgen administration with knowledgeable monitoring carries significant or potentially serious adverse effects on the prostate gland.*" Quoted from Monitoring androgen replacement therapy: testosterone and prostate safety by Morales A. J Endocrinol Invest. 2005;28 (3 Suppl):122-7(29)

Dr Rhoden says: "*Despite decades of research, there is no compelling evidence that testosterone has a causative role in prostate cancer.*" From Risks of Testosterone-Replacement Therapy and recommendations for Monitoring. N Engl J Med 2004;350:482-92. Rhoden and Morgentaler.(30)

The ADAM Testosterone Questionnaire

This questionnaire is useful for detecting low testosterone levels. ADAM is an acronym for Androgen Deficiency in the Aging Male. (43)(44)

The ADAM Testosterone Questionnaire

1. Do you have a decrease in libido (sex drive)? Yes No
2. Do you have a lack of energy? Yes No
3. Do you have a decrease in strength and/or endurance? Yes No
4. Have you lost height? Yes No
5. Have you noticed a decreased "enjoyment of life" Yes No
6. Are you sad and/or grumpy? Yes No
7. Are your erections less strong? Yes No
8. Have you noticed a recent deterioration in your ability to play sports? Yes No
9. Are you falling asleep after dinner? Yes No
10. Has there been a recent deterioration in your work performance? Yes No

If you answered YES to questions 1 or 7, or any 3 other questions, you may have low testosterone. Next step is a testosterone blood test to determine your level. If low, then testosterone supplementation may be considered. It is important to work closely with a knowledgeable physician who can do a full evaluation, order the appropriate tests, and prescribe treatment.

For references and links, see my web site: www.bioidenticalhormones101.com

References for Chapter 27. Testosterone, PSA and Prostate Cancer Part One

(1) http://nobelprize.org/nobel_prizes/chemistry/laureates/1939/press.html The Nobel Prize in Chemistry 1939 Presentation Speech, Butenandt Discovery of Testosterone.

(2) http://www.hms.harvard.edu/news/pressreleases/mcl/0103testosteronereplace.html Study Suggests Depressed Men May Benefit from Testosterone Replacement Therapy Belmont—January 1, 2003

(3) http://www.revolutionhealth.com/healthy-living/mens-health/hot-topics/mens-health-101/testosterone-therapy-men Testosterone therapy: The answer for aging men? Date updated: April 14, 2006 Mayo Clinic Revolution Health.

(4) http://www.duj.com/Article/Hellstrom2/Hellstrom2.html Digital Urology Journal. Testosterone Replacement Therapy. Wayne J.G. Hellstrom, M.D

(5) http://www.medscape.com/viewarticle/556617_print Testosterone and Ageing: What Have We Learned Since the Institute of Medicine Report and What Lies Ahead? M. M. Miner; A. D. Seftel Int J Clin Pract. 2007;61(4):622-632. 05/21/2007

(6) http://www.aafp.org/afp/20060501/1591.html Testosterone Treatments: Why, When, and How? American Academy of Family Physicians. May 1, 2006 Katherine Margo, M.D.,

(7) http://www.sciencedaily.com/releases/2006/08/060816083120.htm Science News Low Testosterone Levels Associated With Increased Risk Of Death In Men

(8) http://www.sciencedaily.com/releases/2008/01/080109111320.htm Testosterone May Improve Mental Function. ScienceDaily (Jan. 14, 2008

(9) http://www.worldhealth.net/pdf/bookstore/thera6_ch7.pdf Chapter 7 Testosterone, The Male Hormone Connection: Treating Diabetes and Heart Disease. Michael Klentze, M.D., Ph.D.

(10) http://www.hotzehwc.com/attachments/wysiwyg/2/Testosterone101.pdf Testosterone for Men and Women By Steven F. Hotze, M.D., e-book.

(11) https://secure.pharmacytimes.com/lessons/200410-03.asp State-of-the-Art Update on Testosterone Replacement: A Clinical and Pharmacological Approach Narinder Duggal Pharmacy Times

(12) http://www.drmirkin.com/men/M227.html Testosterone Replacement for Older Men?, Gabe Mirkin, M.D.

(13) http://www.endo-society.org/publications/OldContent/testosterone-Feb2004.cfm, Practical Approach to Testosterone Therapy of Elderly Men, Endocrine News Vol 29, N1 Feb 2004.

(14) http://www.hormone.org/Resources/Patient_Guides/upload/patients_guide_low_testosterone.pdf Patient's Guide to Low Testosterone (2003 Edition) Glenn R. Cunningham, MD, Alvin M. Matsumoto, MD, Ronald Swerdloff, MD. From the Family Physicians Inquiries Network.

(15) http://www.healthline.com/sw/hr-nl-a-harvard-expert-shares-his-thoughts-on-testosterone-replacement-therapy An interview with Abraham Morgentaler, M.D.A Harvard expert shares his thoughts on testosterone-replacement

(16) http://www.pubmedcentral.nih.gov/articlerender.fcgi?artid=1502320 Rev Urol. 2003; 5(Suppl 1): S34-S40. New Advances in the Treatment of Hypogonadism in the Aging Male Christopher P Steidle, MD

(17) http://www.ncbi.nlm.nih.gov/pubmed/15799128 Aging Male. 2004 Dec;7(4):319-24. Testosterone therapy—what, when and to whom? Jockenhövel F.

(18) http://www.ncbi.nlm.nih.gov/pubmed/15329035 Drugs. 2004;64(17):1861-91. Androgen replacement therapy: present and future.Gooren LJ, Bunck MC.

(19) http://www.ncbi.nlm.nih.gov/pubmed/16918944 Clin Endocrinol (Oxf). 2006 Sep;65(3):275-81. Testosterone treatment comes of age: new options for hypogonadal men. Nieschlag E.

(20) http://www.med.unc.edu/~mcoward/urology/Harrison's%20Aging-Related%20Changes%20in%20Male%20Reproductive%20Function.pdf Harrison's Internal Medicine. Part 14. Aging-Related Changes in Male Reproductive Function.

(21) http://www.andrologyjournal.org/cgi/content/full/27/2/126 Journal of Andrology, Vol. 27, No. 2, March/April 2006. Review Testosterone Replacement Therapy for Older Men. Moshe Wald et al.

(22) http://www.ncbi.nlm.nih.gov/pubmed/13678385 J Med Invest. 2003 Aug;50(3-4):162-9. An assessment of correlations between endogenous sex hormone levels and the extensiveness of coronary heart disease and the ejection fraction of the left ventricle in males.Dobrzycki S et al.

(23) http://www.ncbi.nlm.nih.gov/pubmed/14609611 Am J Cardiol. 2003 Nov 15;92(10):1241-3. Effect of testosterone therapy on QT dispersion in men with heart failure.Malkin CJ et al.

(24) http://www.ncbi.nlm.nih.gov/pubmed/16093267 Eur Heart J. 2006 Jan;27(1):57-64. Epub 2005 Aug 10. Testosterone therapy in men with moderate severity heart failure: a double-blind randomized placebo controlled trial. Malkin CJ et al.

(25) http://www.drdach.com/wst_page15.html
Testosterone Information Page Jeffrey Dach MD

(26) http://drcranton.com/hrt/testosterone_replacement.htm Testosterone Replacement: The Male Andropause, Taken from a chapter in the book, Resetting the Clock, by Elmer M. Cranton, M.D. and William Fryer.

(27) http://archneur.ama-assn.org/cgi/content/abstract/59/11/1750
Beneficial Effects of Testosterone Replacement for the Nonmotor Symptoms of Parkinson Disease Michael S. Okun, MD et al.

(28) http://www.ncbi.nlm.nih.gov/pubmed/16526980 Can J Urol. 2006 Feb;13 Suppl 1:40-3. Testosterone replacement therapy and prostate risks: where's the beef? Morgentaler A.

(29) http://www.ncbi.nlm.nih.gov/pubmed/16042371
J Endocrinol Invest. 2005;28(3 Suppl):122-7. Monitoring androgen replacement therapy: testosterone and prostate safety. Morales A.

(30) http://www.drdach.com/uploads/testosterone_rhoden.pdf
Risks of Testosterone-Replacement Therapy and Recommendations for Monitoring Ernani Luis Rhoden, M.D., and Abraham Morgentaler, M.D. N Engl J Med 2004;350:482-92.

(31) http://www.ncbi.nlm.nih.gov/pubmed/10415627
Androgens and dry eye in Sjögren's syndrome. Ann N Y Acad Sci. 1999 Jun 22;876:312-24. Sullivan DA et al.

(32) http://www.ncbi.nlm.nih.gov/pubmed/12114274
Androgen deficiency, Meibomian gland dysfunction, and evaporative dry eye. Sullivan DA et al. Ann N Y Acad Sci. 2002 Jun; 966:211-22.

(33) http://www.aace.com/pub/pdf/guidelines/sexdysguid.pdf Male Sexual Dysfunction, Endocr Pract. 2003;9 (No. 1) January/February 2003 77. A Clin Endo Medical Guidelines for clinical practice for evaluation and treatment of male sexual dysfunction: 2003 UPDATE AACE Male Sexual Dysfunction Task Force Andre T. Guay, MD, Richard F. Spark, MD, Sudhir Bansal, MD et al.

(34) http://www.fda.gov/medwatch/SAFETY/2003/03SEP_PI/AndroGel_PI.pdf Androgel FDA approved topical version of testosterone.

(35) http://www.cardiosource.com/cjrpicks/CJRPick.asp?cjrID=3849 Endogenous Testosterone and Mortality due to All Causes, Cardiovascular Disease, and Cancer in Men: European Prospective Investigation Into Cancer in Norfolk (EPIC-Norfolk) Prospective Population Study 2/6/2008 Khaw KT, Dowsett M, Folkerd E, et al. Circulation. 2007;116:2694-2701.

(36) http://www.nih.gov/news/pr/jan2004/nia-26.htm Low Free Testosterone Levels Linked to Alzheimer's Disease in Older Men

(37) http://jcem.endojournals.org/cgi/content/full/87/11/5001 The Journal of Clinical Endocrinology & Metabolism Vol. 87, No. 11 5001-5007. Longitudinal Assessment of Serum Free Testosterone Concentration Predicts Memory Performance and Cognitive Status in Elderly Men Scott D. Moffat et al.

(38) http://www.mbschachter.com/male_andropause.htm The Male Andropause, by Michael B. Schachter M.D., F.A.C.A.M.

(39) http://www.usdoctor.com/Chapter13.html TESTOSTERONE for MEN with DIABETES

(40) http://www.touchbriefings.com/pdf/2782/jones.pdf Testosterone—Clinical Associations with the Metabolic Syndrome and Type 2 Diabetes Mellitus. T Hugh Jones. Consultant Physician and Endocrinologist, Barnsley Hospital NHS Foundation Trust, and Honorary Professor of Andrology, Academic Unit of Diabetes, Endocrinology and Metabolism, University of Sheffield

(41) http://www.svedyn.com/web/revistas/deficit%20androgenos%20adultos.pdf Androgen Deficiency in Men. Daniel S. Tung, MD, Glenn R. Cunningham, MD The Endocrinologist Vol 17, N 2, April 2007.

(42) http://care.diabetesjournals.org/cgi/content/full/30/4/911 Diabetes Care 30:911-917, 2007 Clinical and Biochemical Assessment of Hypogonadism in Men With Type 2 Diabetes, Correlations with bioavailable testosterone and visceral adiposity. Dheeraj Kapoor, MD, et al.

(43) http://jcem.endojournals.org/cgi/content/full/89/12/5920#R4 The Journal of Clinical Endocrinology & Metabolism Vol. 89, No. 12 5920-5926. Prevalence and Incidence of Androgen Deficiency in Middle-Aged and Older Men: Estimates from the Massachusetts Male Aging Study. Andre B. Araujo et al.

(44) http://www.ncbi.nlm.nih.gov/pubmed/11016912
Metabolism. 2000 Sep;49(9):1239-42.Validation of a screening questionnaire for androgen deficiency in aging males. (ADAM) Morley JE, Charlton E et al.

CHAPTER 28

PSA and Testosterone—Part Two—A Medical Myth

A common medical myth is that Testosterone is somehow causative of prostate cancer. This is incorrect, as we will see below. Rather than elevated Testosterone being associated with prostate cancer, it is **LOW testosterone** that is associated with aggressive prostate cancer with poor outcome. Indeed, lower testosterone has been found to be associated with increased all cause mortality in males in the EPIC study.

PSA and Testosterone Observations (see references 1-16)

(1) Lower Testosterone Levels (not higher levels) are associated with increased risk for aggressive prostate cancer. Higher levels within the normal range are associated with less risk for Prostate CA. This is directly opposite to the ingrained urology dogma, and was demonstrated by biopsy studies by Morgentaler and Rhoden. (7)

(2) PSA level will go down when testosterone is withdrawn or given DHT blockade with finasteride.

(3) PSA will rise transiently after starting Testosterone, and then stabilize at new level.(1-19)

(4) Hypogonadal symptomatic patients following treated prostate cancer having undetectable PSA of zero, may be safely treated with testosterone therapy. (9-15)

For references and links, see my web site: www.bioidenticalhormones101.com

References for Chapter 28. PSA and Testosterone, Part Two

(1) http://www.pubmedcentral.nih.gov/articlerender.fcgi?artid=1472885
Rev Urol. 2004; 6 (Suppl 6): S41-S43. Rising PSA during Testosterone Replacement Therapy, John Gore, MD and Jacob Rajfer, MD

(2) http://jcem.endojournals.org/cgi/content/full/92/2/416 The Journal of Clinical Endocrinology & Metabolism Vol. 92, No. 2 416-417. Guideline for Male Testosterone Therapy: A Clinician's Perspective—Abraham Morgentaler Harvard Medical School, Beth Israel Deaconess Medical Center, Boston, Massachusetts.

(3) http://www.urologic.theclinics.com/article/S0302-2838(06)00787-1/abstract Volume 50, Issue 5, Pages 935-939 (November 2006) Urologic Clinics. Testosterone and Prostate Cancer: An Historical Perspective on a Modern Myth? Abraham Morgentaler

(4) http://www.andrologyjournal.org/cgi/content/full/24/3/299 Journal of Andrology, Vol. 24, No. 3, May/June 2003. Managing the Risks of Prostate Disease During Testosterone Replacement Therapy in Older Men: Recommendations for a Standardized Monitoring Plan. Shalender Bhasin et al.

(5) http://www.testosteroneupdate.org/podcasts_d.php Testosterone Update, Presentations held at the 2008 American Urological Association Annual Meeting. May 17-20, 2008, Orlando, Florida.

(6) http://www.ncbi.nlm.nih.gov/pubmed/17113983 J Steroid Biochem Mol Biol. 2006 Dec;102(1-5):261-6. Prostate cancer risk in testosterone-treated men. Raynaud JP.

(7) http://www.ncbi.nlm.nih.gov/pubmed/16434592 Cancer Epidemiol Biomarkers Prev. 2006 Jan;15(1):86-91. Circulating steroid hormones and the risk of prostate cancer. Severi G, Morris HA, MacInnis RJ, English DR,

(8) http://www.ncbi.nlm.nih.gov/pubmed/17169647 Urology. 2006 Dec;68(6):1263-7. Prevalence of prostate cancer among hypogonadal men with prostate-specific antigen levels of 4.0 ng/mL or less. Morgentaler A, Rhoden EL.

(9) http://www.ncbi.nlm.nih.gov/pubmed/17627161 Urol Int. 2007;79(1):13-8. Hormonal predictors of prostate cancer. Sofikerim M, Eskicorapci S, Oruç O, Ozen H.

(10) http://www.ncbi.nlm.nih.gov/pubmed/19154450 BJU Int. 2009 May;103(9):1179-83. Epub 2008 Dec 23. Prostate-specific antigen changes and prostate cancer in hypogonadal men treated with testosterone replacement therapy. Coward RM, Simhan J, Carson CC 3rd.

(11) http://www.ncbi.nlm.nih.gov/pubmed/17105798 JAMA. 2006 Nov 15;296(19):2351-61. Effect of testosterone replacement therapy on prostate tissue in men with late-onset hypogonadism: a randomized controlled trial. Marks LS, Mazer NA,

(12) http://www.ncbi.nlm.nih.gov/pubmed/17183557
Cancer. 2007 Feb 1;109(3):536-41. Testosterone replacement for hypogonadism after treatment of early prostate cancer with brachytherapy. Sarosdy MF.South Texas Urology and Urologic Oncology, San Antonio, Texas 78229, USA.

(13) http://www.ncbi.nlm.nih.gov/pubmed/15643240 J Urol. 2005 Feb;173(2):533-6. Testosterone replacement therapy after primary treatment for prostate cancer. Agarwal PK, Oefelein MG.

(14) http://www.ncbi.nlm.nih.gov/pubmed/12399540 J Androl. 2002 Nov-Dec;23(6):922-6. Prostate-specific antigen changes in hypogonadal men treated with testosterone replacement. Gerstenbluth RE, Maniam PN, Corty EW, Seftel AD.

(15) http://www.ncbi.nlm.nih.gov/pubmed/16904053 Curr Treat Options Oncol. 2006 Sep;7(5):363-9. Testosterone therapy for men at risk for or with history of prostate cancer. Morgentaler A.

(16) http://www.ncbi.nlm.nih.gov/pubmed/19296069 Urologe A. 2009 May;48(5):516-22. Testosterone replacement therapy and prostate cancer. The current position 67 years after the Huggins myth] [Article in German] Rinnab L et al.

(17) http://www.ncbi.nlm.nih.gov/pubmed/17983894 Urol Clin North Am. 2007 Nov;34(4):549-53, vi. The role of testosterone replacement therapy following radical prostatectomy. Khera M et al.

(18) http://www.ncbi.nlm.nih.gov/pubmed/19215619 J Sex Med. 2009 Feb;6(2):574-7 Two years of testosterone therapy associated with decline in prostate-specific antigen in a man with untreated prostate cancer. Morgentaler A. Harvard Medical School, Urology,

(19) http://www.ncbi.nlm.nih.gov/pubmed/19429438 J Steroid Biochem Mol Biol. 2009 Mar;114(1-2):96-105. Epub 2009 Jan 30. Testosterone deficiency syndrome: treatment and cancer risk. Raynaud JP.

CHAPTER 29

PSA Screening for Prostate Cancer, the Failed Medical Experiment

Jim Smith is a 55 year old athlete and outdoors man, who runs marathons and camps outdoors. He was not worried about prostate cancer until he saw the Larry King Show endorsing PSA screening for prostate cancer. Larry King showed celebrity endorsements from Colin Powell, Charlton Heston, Jerry Lewis, Arnold Palmer, Rudy Giuliani, John Kerry, Bob Dole, Norman Schwarzkopf, John McEnroe and Michael Milken all relating personal prostate cancer stories. Watching all these celebrities urging PSA testing on the Larry King show lured Jim into a local Miami hospital offering free screening for prostate cancer. Jim's PSA test showed an elevated PSA of 4.7 (normal is less than 4), so Jim was sent over to a local urologist office all set for a needle biopsy of his prostate.

Pioneering Ultrasound Guided Biopsy

Working as an interventional radiologist in the early days, I actually pioneered ultrasound guided prostate biopsies, and taught many urologists how to do the procedure. This procedure involves placing an ultrasound probe into the patient to image the prostate, and advance a long needle into the prostate gland for the tissue sample. Usually 6 samples are obtained. As uncomfortable as it sounds, it's really not all that bad.

Seeking a Second Opinion

Thinking the rush to biopsy a bit hasty, Jim declined, and instead came to my office seeking a second opinion. After a brief chat, Jim complained of recent urinary symptoms. Sure enough, his urine test indicated a simple infection of the prostate gland which is quite common.

Antibiotics, The Miracle Drug

Inflammation and prostate infection is a common cause of PSA elevation.(27-31) The plan was to treat Jim with antibiotics for his prostate infection and repeat the PSA test. After a few weeks of daily antibiotic called Ciprofloxin™, Jim was smiling ear-to-ear because his repeat PSA was back down to 3.8 and his doctors no longer advised prostate biopsy.

PSA Screening, A 20 Year Failed Medical Experiment

PSA is Prostate Specific Antigen, a protein discovered in 1986, and a marker for prostate cancer and inflammation. This article will show you that PSA screening for prostate cancer is, in fact, a 20 year failed medical experiment which provides little or no benefit in saving lives.

New Studies Oppose PSA Screening

Gina Kolata of the New York Times wrote a scathing indictment of PSA screening citing two studies published from March 2009 New England Journal of Medicine, considered the most important studies in the history of men's health. (1) The large US study, the PLCO, showed no mortality benefit from PSA screening. The European Study, on the other hand, did much better. Their ERSPC study provided a 20% mortality reduction from PSA screening. However, this came at a high cost of significant over-diagnosis. Fifty men were treated for prostate cancer unnecessarily for every life saved. This treatment of surgery, radiation and hormonal castration is associated with erectile dysfunction (ED) and incontinence.(9-12)

One Million Male Victims—Over Diagnosed and Over Treated Since 1986

Dr. Welch reported a very unpleasant finding in the August 2009 issue of the Journal of the National Cancer Institute.(2) Since the invention of the PSA test in 1986, one million men have been treated for a clinically insignificant prostate cancer that did not require treatment.

(3-7) These are 1 million male victims, many suffering from side effects of treatment, such as erectile dysfunction and incontinence.

Sept 2009 BMJ and Archives of Internal Med Papers

Another series of papers just released in the British Medical Journal Sept. 24 2009, again criticizes mass PSA screening, advising against it. (13-16) Another highly critical article from the 2009 Archives of Internal Medicine, by Dr Kirsten Howard from the University of Sydney's School of Public Health, showed that PSA Testing is not a major factor in prostate cancer mortality. Dr Howard says "*men with PSA-detected cancer may often undergo therapies for clinically insignificant cancers*" which does not affect mortality rates from prostate cancer. (115)(116)

Important Point:
PSA testing the population as a screening test for prostate cancer is no longer recommended because it results in unnecessary treatment of many clinically insignificant cancers

Why Doesn't It Work? Where Did We Go Wrong with PSA Screening?

We have known since 1935 with the publication of Arnold Rich's autopsy study that there is a large pool of latent, clinically insignificant prostate cancer in the male population which increases with age.(47) By the age of fifty, 30-40 per cent of males will harbor a clinically insignificant focus of prostate cancer. The vast majority succumb to old age before the prostate cancer bothers them. These prostate cancers are the incidental findings at post mortem exam.

Prostate cancer is a slow growing indolent disease with a 99 per cent 5 year survival after diagnosis. The incidence of latent prostate cancer is estimated to be one half of the male population 65 and over (7 million of the 14 million males), yet there are only 30,000 deaths per year. This means the average male has a 0.5% chance of dying from prostate cancer, (or a 99.5 chance of dying from other causes, not prostate cancer).

PSA screening programs send the screened patients to trans-rectal ultrasound guided biopsy which finds these latent prostate cancers, many of which should not be treated. Mainstream conventional treatment involves radical prostatectomy, radiation therapy, and hormonal castration. The first two are associated with adverse effects of incontinence, and erectile dysfunction. Treatment with androgen blockade, (a form of chemical castration) is associated with increased mortality and osteoporosis.(117)

The Buffalo Hunt Factor—Advanced Prostate Cancer Hunted to Extinction

One impact of wide scale PSA screening for prostate cancer is the eradication of advanced cases of prostate cancer over the past two decades. During my training years in the nuclear medicine department at Rush Medical School in Chicago in the 1970's, the doctors followed dozens of patients with metastatic prostate cancer on serial bone scans. This is rarely seen today. The advanced prostate cancer case is a rare bird driven to extinction, now seen only occasionally.

Stephen Strum, MD, an oncologist from Oregon writes in the comment section of a March 2009 NEJM article, "*The nature of the patient diagnosed with Prostate Cancer has dramatically changed since the introduction of PSA in 1987. Almost gone are men presenting with advanced local or distant Prostate Cancer.*" (20)

Like the vanishing American Buffalo, these advanced metastatic prostate cancer cases have been hunted to the point of near extinction by the PSA Screening Test.

The Vanishing Buffalo—Hunted to Extinction

Stanford's Dr. Thomas Stamey, the first to advocate PSA screening in 1987, has come full circle, and no longer recommends PSA screening. Stamey found the abundance of advanced cases from the early years of PSA Screening are gone, and the PSA test has become useless. Stamey declares, "*The prostate specific antigen era in the United States is over for prostate cancer*". Stamey's data shows there was a substantial decrease in correlation between PSA levels and the amount of prostate cancer—from 43 percent predictive ability in the first five-year group down to 2 percent in the most recent one. "*Our job now is to stop removing every man's prostate who has prostate cancer*," said Stamey. "We originally thought we were doing the right thing, but we are now figuring out how we went wrong." (61)(66)

Organizations Opposed to Routine PSA Screening

In 1997, the American Cancer Society changed its position and no longer recommends screening. Their chief Medical Officer, Otis Brawley MD declined PSA screening for himself. Otis Brawley, MD says in a Jan 2000 interview, "*twenty-three organizations of experts from the Canadian Urology Association to the American College of Physicians to the U.S. Preventive Services Task Force recommend against screening . . . the predominance of professional expert opinion is that (PSA screening) is unproven and should not be done.*" (119)

What is the Clinical Utility of PSA Test?

According Dr Bicker in an article in the August 2009 Anticancer Research, the PSA test is now commonly regarded as an indicator of prostate volume, and is not independently diagnostic or prognostic of prostate cancer. (34) Even though mass screening of asymptomatic men with the PSA test is no longer recommended, the PSA tests remains a very useful tool in the diagnosis and follow up of prostate cancer. For example, the PSA is useful as a cancer marker to follow cancer recurrence, progression or regression after treatment.(45)

Can We Tell Dangerous Prostate Cancers Apart from Insignificant Ones?

What is the Gleason Score? Gleason Score can help separate the aggressive cancers from the non-aggressive cancers. Gleason Score is a histology grading pattern used to grade the biopsy sample. Lower scores (one and two) are associated with better prognosis. Higher scores (4 and 5) are associated with worse prognosis with more aggressive behavior of the tumor.

How to Treat the Aggressive Cancers and Ignore the Others—Watchful Waiting vs. Active Surveillance

One of the major problems with prostate cancer screening with PSA, is the inability of this test to differentiate the clinically insignificant cancers that don't require treatment from the dangerous cancers that do. Various authors have suggested refinements by using parameters such as PSA velocity(23-24)(33)(65-67), Free PSA ratio (21), and of course, the Gleason score (74-76), a form of histology grading, applied to prostate biopsy sample to provide this discrimination. Using these refinements, some doctors such as Laurence Klotz have advocated Active Surveillance based on PSA velocity.(120) Dr Klotz offers treatment for cases having a PSA Doubling Time of 3 years or less (based on a minimum of three determinations over 6 months). Others, such as Mark Soloway MD, feel that Gleason score upgrade or histological evidence of tumor aggression is the most important parameter, and have offered radical treatment if this is found at repeat biopsy. (98-99) The obvious goal is to identify and treat aggressive tumors before they invade the prostatic capsule and beyond. This is not so simple and may require discovery of new biomarkers.

A new bio-marker in prostate cancer cells called Hsp-27 protein indicates an aggressive type of prostate cancer that requires treatment. The absence of the Hsp-27 protein suggests a silent type of cancer that does not require immediate treatment. (35) Do these new protocols and tools work any better than the old ones? We don't know yet. It may take another ten years to find out.

Preventing Prostate Cancer—Diet and LifeStyle Modification

Given the reality that PSA screening for early detection for prostate cancer is a misguided adventure which leads to overdiagnosis and does more harm than good, perhaps another approach to prevention is warranted. Such an approach is suggested by urologist Ronald Wheeler at the Sarosota Prostate Center. (105) Dr Wheeler advocates a nutritional program for prostate cancer prevention with Vitamins C, B6, E, zinc, selenium, Saw palmetto, Pygeum africanum, stinging nettle, pumpkin seed, Echinacea purpurea, garlic, ginkgo biloba, Amino acids-L-glycine, L-alanine, L-glutamic acid and Modified Mediterranean Diet.(105)

Important Point: How to Reduce PSA With Nutritional Supplements
PSA may be reduced by a nutritional program with Vitamins C, B6, E, zinc, selenium, Saw Palmetto, Pygeum africanum, stinging nettle, pumpkin seed, Echinacea purpurea, garlic, ginkgo biloba, Amino acids-L-glycine, L-alanine, L-glutamic acid and Modified Mediterranean Diet.(105)

Results of Diet and Nutrition Program on PSA

In 20 patients with biopsy proven prostate cancer who had declined radical treatment, Dr Wheeler's herbal-nutritional supplement program reduced mean PSA from 6.8 ng/ml to 3.4 ng/ml over three years of follow-up.(105) (121) I would also add digestive enzymes, and optimizing vitamin D level with testing and supplementation, as well as optimizing Iodine levels with Iodoral would also be included in a typical prostate cancer prevention program.

In conclusion, PSA screening for prostate cancer has been a failed medical experiment leaving behind 1 million male victims unnecessarily treated for a type of prostate cancer that was clinically insignificant, providing little or no benefit in terms of lives saved. Leaders in the field are now alerting us to the pitfalls, harms and limitations involved in PSA cancer screening. Recognizing that there are 30,000 prostate cancer deaths per year, the urgent challenge is to identify and treat the aggressive cancers destined to kill the host, and avoid harming the other 7 million men representing a silent reservoir of biologically insignificant disease. Hopefully, this will be the subject of future NIH funded research, so that another one million men in the future will be spared needless over diagnosis and overtreatment.

For references and links, see my web site: www.bioidenticalhormones101.com

References for Chapter 29. PSA Screening for Cancer, the Failed Medical Experiment

(1) http://www.nytimes.com/2009/03/19/health/19cancer.html Prostate Test Found to Save Few Lives By GINA KOLATA NY Times Published: March 18, 2009.

(2) http://jnci.oxfordjournals.org/cgi/content/abstract/djp278v1 Prostate Cancer Diagnosis and Treatment After the Introduction of Prostate-Specific Antigen Screening: 1986-2005. H. Gilbert Welch, Peter C. Albertsen. J Nat Cancer Inst. August 31, 2009

(3) http://www.medicinenet.com/script/main/art.asp?articlekey=105197 PSA Test: More Harm Than Good? Study: 1 Million Men Suffered Needless Treatment After Prostate Cancer Test By Daniel J. DeNoon WebMD Health News Aug. 31, 2009—The PSA prostate cancer screening test does more harm than good, a new study suggests. Medicine.net.

(4) http://www.cnn.com/2009/HEALTH/09/01/prostate.cancer.screening/index.html Study: Prostate cancer test leads to needless diagnoses. CNN News. Tue September 1, 2009 By Denise Mann

(5) http://www.modernmedicine.com/modernmedicine/Enews/Prostate-cancer-overdiagnosis-attributed-to-PSA-te/ArticleStandard/Article/detail/624305?contextCategoryId=40237&ref=25 Prostate cancer overdiagnosis attributed to PSA test—Sep 10, 2009 Urology Times E-News

(6) http://www.webmd.com/prostate-cancer/news/20090831/psa-test-more-harm-than-good PSA Test: More Harm Than Good? Study: 1 Million Men Suffered Needless Treatment After Prostate Cancer Test By Daniel J. DeNoon WebMD Health News—Aug. 31, 2009

(7) http://www.baltimoresun.com/health/bal-md.hs.psa01sep01,0,7710170.story Doubt cast on value of PSA test By Kelly Brewington—Baltimore Sun September 1, 2009.

(8) http://www.foundationforurologicalresearch.com/downloads/PSA%20Best%20Practice%20Statement.pdf Adult Urology Prostate Specific Antigen Best Practice Statement: 2009 Update Kirsten L. Greene.

(9) http://synapse.ucsf.edu/articles/2009/March/26/prostate.html Studies Cast Doubt on Value of Prostate Screenings Synapse Staff Report UCSF.

(10) http://content.nejm.org/cgi/content/full/NEJMoa0810696 Gerald L. Andriole, M.D.,et al. NEJM. Vol 360:1310-1319 March 26, 2009 N 13. Mortality Results from a Randomized Prostate-Cancer Screening Trial.

(11) http://content.nejm.org/cgi/content/full/NEJMoa0810084 NEJM. Volume 360:1320-1328 March 26, 2009 Number 13, Screening and Prostate-Cancer Mortality in a Randomized European Study Fritz H. Schröder, M.D., Jonas Hugosson, M.D.,

(12) http://www.ncbi.nlm.nih.gov/pubmed/19660851 Eur Urol. 2009 Jul 28. Prostate Cancer Mortality Reduction by Prostate-Specific Antigen-Based Screening Adjusted for Nonattendance and Contamination in the European Randomised Study of Screening for Prostate Cancer (ERSPC). Roobol MJ et al.

(13) http://blog.lib.umn.edu/schwitz/healthnews/2009/09/bmj-papers-conc-1.html BMJ papers conclude not enough evidence to support widespread PSA screening—Gary Schwitzer Sept24, 2009.

(14) http://www.bmj.com/cgi/content/abstract/339/sep24_1/b3537 24 September 2009, BMJ 2009;339:b3537. Prostate specific antigen for early detection of prostate cancer: longitudinal study. Benny Holmström et al.

(15) http://www.bmj.com/cgi/content/extract/339/sep24_1/b3601 24 September 2009, BMJ 2009;339:b3601. Analysis Screening for prostate cancer remains controversial. Jennifer R Stark,

(16) http://www.bmj.com/cgi/content/extract/339/sep24_1/b3572 24 September 2009, BMJ 2009;339:b3572. Editorials Prostate specific antigen for detecting early prostate cancer
Evidence is inconclusive, so patient education and shared decision making are essential.

(17) http://health.usnews.com/articles/health/healthday/2009/09/15/watchful-waiting-works-for-older-men-with.html Watchful Waiting Works for Older Men With Prostate Cancer, But experts stress the same does not hold true for patients under 60. Posted September 15, 2009

(18) http://blogs.consumerreports.org/health/2009/09/ whats-wrong-with-free-prostatecancer-screening-yankees-psa-test-bat-for-the-cure-us-open-john-mcenro.html Consumer Reports. Septr 14, 2009. More What's wrong with free prostate-cancer screening?

(19) http://medicalconsumers.org/2009/04/16/just-say-no-to-the-psa-prostate-cancer-test/ Just Say No to the PSA Prostate Cancer Test Posted by medconsumers on April 16, 2009

(20) http://www.nejm.org/perspective-roundtable/screening-for-prostate-cancer/ Comment by Stephen Strum, MD, FACP Ashland, Oregon Physician—Oncologist 03/30/2009. Also see http://www.nejm.org/doi/full/10.1056/NEJMp0901825 See Comments section. Dr Strum's comments to this article. Perspective Perspective Roundtable. Screening for Prostate Cancer. Thomas H. Lee, M.D., Philip W. Kantoff, M.D., and Mary F. McNaughton-Collins, M.D., M.P.H. N Engl J Med 2009; 360:e18March 26, 2009

(21) http://www.psa-rising.com/prostatecancer/fpsa-flowchart.htm The "free" PSA test (PSA-f) and how it may spare you a biopsy. PSA Rising Blog.

(22) http://www.sciencedaily.com/releases/2007/05/070525074607.htm Prostate Cancer: High Pretreatment PSA Velocity Predicts Worse Outcome ScienceDaily (May 25, 2007).

(23) http://www.drcatalona.com/quest/Summer04/quest_summer04_2.asp PSA Velocity: Important New Tool in Fight Against Prostate Cancer—By William J. Catalona, MD

(24) http://content.nejm.org/cgi/content/abstract/351/2/125 Volume 351:125-135 July 8, 2004 Number 2 Preoperative PSA Velocity and the Risk of Death from Prostate Cancer after Radical Prostatectomy Anthony V. D'Amico, M.D., Ph.D., Ming-Hui Chen, Ph.D., Kimberly A. Roehl, M.P.H., and William J. Catalona, M.D.

(25) http://www.ncbi.nlm.nih.gov/pubmed/19682790 Prostate-Specific Antigen Velocity for Early Detection of Prostate Cancer: Result from a Large, Representative, Population-based Cohort. Andrew J. Vickersa et al.

(26) http://www.ncbi.nlm.nih.gov/pubmed/10096388 Urology. 1999 Mar;53(3):581-9 Serum prostate-specific antigen as a predictor of prostate volume in men with benign prostatic hyperplasia. Roehrborn CG et al. Conclusions.

(27) http://www.ncbi.nlm.nih.gov/pubmed/15947609 J Urol. 2005 Jul;174(1):161-4. Treatment of chronic bacterial prostatitis with levofloxacin and ciprofloxacin lowers serum prostate specific antigen. Schaeffer AJ, Wu SC, Tennenberg AM, Kahn JB.

(28) http://www.ncbi.nlm.nih.gov/pubmed/15693428 Arch Ital Urol Androl. 2004 Dec;76(4):154-8. PSA decrease after levofloxacin therapy in patients with histological prostatitis. Guercio S et al.

(29) http://www.ncbi.nlm.nih.gov/pubmed/11912396 J Urol. 2002 Apr;167(4):1723-6 Treatment of chronic prostatitis lowers serum prostate specific antigen. Bozeman CB et al.

(30) http://www.ncbi.nlm.nih.gov/pubmed/17695414 Arch Ital Urol Androl. 2007 Jun;79(2):84-92. Reduction of PSA values by combination pharmacological therapy in patients with chronic prostatitis: implications for prostate cancer detection. Magri V et al,

(31) http://www.ncbi.nlm.nih.gov/pubmed/17637759 Prostate Cancer Prostatic Dis. 2008;11(2):148-52. Epub 2007 Jul 17. PSA reduction (after antibiotics) permits to avoid or postpone prostate biopsy in selected patients. Serretta V et al.

(32) http://psg-mac43.ucsf.edu/ticr/syllabus/courses/26/2004/03/11/Lecture/readings/psa.pdf Surrogate End Point for Prostate Cancer—Specific Mortality After Radical Prostatectomy or Radiation Therapy Anthony V. D'Amico, Judd W. Moul, Peter R. Carroll, Leon Sun, Deborah Lubeck,Ming-Hui Chen

(33) http://www.ncbi.nlm.nih.gov/pubmed/17530618 Cancer. 2007 Jul 1;110(1):56-61. Prostate cancer-specific mortality after radical prostatectomy or external beam radiation therapy in men with 1 or more high-risk factors. D'Amico AV, Chen MH, Catalona WJ, Sun L, Roehl KA, Moul JW.

(34) http://www.ncbi.nlm.nih.gov/pubmed/19661347 Anticancer Res. 2009 Aug;29(8):3289-98. New molecular biomarkers for the prognosis and management of prostate cancer—the post PSA era. Bickers B, Aukim-Hastie C.

(35) http://www.sciencedaily.com/releases/2009/09/090923102335.htm Two-Thirds Of Prostate Cancer Patients Do Not Need Treatment, Study Reveals. ScienceDaily (Sep. 24, 2009)

(36) http://www.ncbi.nlm.nih.gov/pubmed/19707199 Br J Cancer. 2009 Aug 25. [Epub ahead of print] Hsp-27 expression at diagnosis predicts poor clinical outcome in prostate cancer independent of ETS-gene rearrangement. Foster CS et al.

(37) http://www.sciencedaily.com/releases/2008/11/081116142322.htm Men Who Take Aspirin Have Significantly Lower PSA Levels. ScienceDaily (Nov. 17, 2008)

(38) http://www.sciencedaily.com/releases/2008/05/080515072654.htm Low Cholesterol Leads To Lower PSA, Lower Prostate Cancer Risk, Study Suggests. ScienceDaily (May 18, 2008)

(39) http://www.drcatalona.com/quest/Spring04/quest_spring04_1.asp The measurement of PSA, by Dr Catalona.

(40) http://www.themedguru.com/20090926/newsfeature/ studies-highlight-inefficacy-psa-test-86128398.html The Med Guru Blog. Studies highlight inefficacy of PSA test by Jyoti Pal—September 26, 2009

(41) http://www.medpagetoday.com/Urology/ProstateCancer/16142 No Evidence to Support Routine PSA Screening, By Chris Emery, Contributing Writer, MedPage Today, Published: September 25, 2009

(42) http://caonline.amcancersoc.org/cgi/content/full/59/4/220 Editorial—Prostate Cancer: Current Evidence Weighs Against Population Screening. Peter Boyle, PhD, DSc1 and Otis W. Brawley, MD2. Published online before print June 29, 2009 CA Cancer J Clin 2009; 59:220-224

(43) http://jama.ama-assn.org/cgi/content/abstract/296/19/2336 PSA Screening Among Elderly Men With Limited Life Expectancies. Louise C. Walter, MD; Daniel Bertenthal, MPH; Karla Lindquist, MS; Badrinath R. Konety, MD JAMA. 2006;296:2336-2342.

(44) http://www.jurology.com/article/S0022-5347(08)03280-1/abstract Volume 181, Issue 4, Pages 1606-1614 (April 2009) 27 of 126. Prostate Specific Antigen Testing Among the Elderly—When To Stop? Edward M. Schaeffera et al.

(45) http://www.bmj.com/cgi/content/extract/339/sep22_1/b3527 Published 22 September 2009, BMJ 2009;339:b3527. Serum tumour markers: how to order and interpret them, C M Sturgeon.

(46) http://www.ccjm.org/content/76/8/446.full The new data on prostate cancer screening: What should we do now? by Timothy Gilligan, MD, Cleveland Clinic Journal of Medicine August 2009 vol. 76 8 446-448.

(47) http://caonline.amcancersoc.org/cgi/reprint/29/2/115 http://www.ncbi.nlm.nih.gov/pubmed/108001 Classics in oncology.

On the frequency of occurrence of occult carcinoma of the prostate: Arnold Rice Rich, M.D., Journal of Urology 33:3, 1935.

(48) http://www.ncbi.nlm.nih.gov/pubmed/7803731 In Vivo. 1994 May-Jun;8(3):439-43. High grade prostatic intraepithelial neoplasia (HGPIN) and prostatic adenocarcinoma between the ages of 20-69: an autopsy study of 249 cases. Sakr WA et al.

(49) http://www.ncbi.nlm.nih.gov/pubmed/12518329 Prostate. 2003 Feb 15;54(3):238-47. Prevalence of prostate cancer and prostatic intraepithelial neoplasia in Caucasian Mediterranean males: an autopsy study. Sánchez-Chapado M et al.

(50) http://www.ncbi.nlm.nih.gov/pubmed/16203079 Eur Urol. 2005 Nov;48(5):739-44. Epub 2005 Sep 15. The prevalence of prostate carcinoma and its precursor in Hungary: an autopsy study. Soos G, Tsakiris I, Szanto J, Turzo C, Haas PG, Dezso B.

(51) http://www.ncbi.nlm.nih.gov/pubmed/6154966 Scand J Urol Nephrol. 1980;14(1):29-35. Latent prostatic cancer in a consecutive autopsy series. Hølund B.

(52) http://www.ncbi.nlm.nih.gov/pubmed/7107064 Int J Cancer. 1982 Jun 15;29(6):611-6. Geographic pathology of latent prostatic carcinoma. Yatani R et al.

(53) http://www.ncbi.nlm.nih.gov/pubmed/19077395 Urol Int. 2008;81(4):379-82. Epub 2008 Dec 10 Do clinically insignificant tumors of the prostate exist? Stamatiou K et al.

(54) http://ije.oxfordjournals.org/cgi/content/full/36/2/282 Commentary: Implications of the frequent occurrence of occult carcinoma of the prostate, Anthony B Miller, 13 November 2006.

(55) http://prostate-cancer-questions-and-answers.com/2009/09/miami-urology-psa-test/ Miami urology doctors are offering a free PSA Test and DRE exam September 15th, 2009

(56) http://www.nydailynews.com/lifestyle/health/2009/06/08/2009-06-08_free_psa_prostate_screening_locations.html Free PSA Prostate Screening Locations June 8th 2009

(57) http://www.abc15.com/content/living/yourhealth/story/Free-screening-event-to-fight-deadly-cancer-in-men/vfA8Xj-mr0qgyJMbg3-thg.cspx Free screening event to fight deadly cancer in men: Eva Bowen 9/23

(58) http://jnci.oxfordjournals.org/cgi/content/full/djp310 Journal of the National Cancer Institute August 31, 2009. Prostate Cancer Screening; Is This a Teachable Moment? Otis W. Brawley

(59) http://blog.lib.umn.edu/schwitz/healthnews/2009/08/powerful-editor.html The problem with this test is that it tends to create fear and anxiety in many men with no real basis.

(60) http://www.drmcdougall.com/misc/2009nl/aug/king.htm Larry King Live on Prostate Cancer Screening (PSA)—Show Sets a New Standard for Disease Mongering. Dr. MacDougal.

(61) http://www.ncbi.nlm.nih.gov/pubmed/15371827 J Urol. 2004 Oct;172(4 Pt 1):1297-301. The prostate specific antigen era in the United States is over for prostate cancer: what happened in the last 20 years? Stamey TA et al.

(62) http://latimesblogs.latimes.com/booster_shots/2008/08/psa-test-dont-d.html PSA test: Don't do it, say angry men August 4, 2008

(63) http://www.bmj.com/cgi/content/full/324/7332/255/a/DC1 Advocates of PSA testing campaign to silence critics, Annabel Ferriman, BMJ 2002;324:255

(64) http://www.bmj.com/cgi/eletters/324/7332/255/a/DC1#19194 Bertrand M.l Bell, Distinguished University Professor Albert Einstein College of medicine. BMJ.letter.

(65) http://jama.ama-assn.org/cgi/content/abstract/279/19/1542 Use of the Percentage of Free Prostate-Specific Antigen to Enhance Differentiation of Prostate Cancer From Benign Prostatic Disease A Prospective Multicenter Clinical Trial. William J. Catalona, MD et al. JAMA. 1998;279:1542-1547.

(66) http://www.innovations-report.com/html/reports/medicine_health/report-33457.html The PSA era is over in the United States," said Thomas Stamey, MD.

(67) http://www.europeanurology.com/article/S0302-2838(05)00449-5/fulltext The PSA Era is not Over for Prostate Cancer—William J. Catalona, Stacy Loeb. July 2005, pages 541-545. European Urology.

(68) http://www.ncbi.nlm.nih.gov/pubmed/19755699 JAMA. 2009 Sep 16;302(11):1202-9. Outcomes of localized prostate cancer following conservative management. Lu-Yao GL at al.

(69) http://www.ncbi.nlm.nih.gov/pubmed/15870412 20-year outcomes following conservative management of clinically localized prostate cancer. Albertsen PC, Hanley JA, Fine J. JAMA. 2005 May 4;293(17):2095-101.

(70) http://jama.ama-assn.org/cgi/content/abstract/274/8/626 Long-term Survival Among Men With Conservatively Treated Localized Prostate Cancer. Peter C. Albertsen, MD; Dennis G. Fryback, PhD; Barry E. Storer, PhD; Thomas F. Kolon, MD; Judith Fine JAMA. 1995;274(8):626-631.

(71) http://jama.ama-assn.org/cgi/content/abstract/280/11/975 Competing Risk Analysis of Men Aged 55 to 74 Years at Diagnosis Managed Conservatively for Clinically Localized Prostate Cancer. Peter C. Albertsen, MD; James A. Hanley, PhD; Donald F. Gleason, MD, PhD; Michael J. Barry, MD JAMA. 1998;280:975-980.

(72) http://www.ncbi.nlm.nih.gov/pubmed/12604893 Am J Surg Pathol. 2003 Mar;27(3):365-71. Basal cell cocktail (34betaE12 + p63) improves the detection of prostate basal cells. Zhou M et al.

(73) http://www.ncbi.nlm.nih.gov/pubmed/15487448 Am J Clin Pathol. 2004 Oct;122(4):517-23. Usefulness of basal cell cocktail (34betaE12 + p63) in the diagnosis of atypical prostate glandular proliferations. Shah RB et al

(74) http://www.phoenix5.org/Infolink/GleasonGrading.html Understanding Gleason Grading Last Revised May 14, 1997.

(75) http://www.prostate-cancer.org/education/staging/Dowd_GleasonScore.html The Gleason Score: A Significant Biologic Manifestation of Prostate Cancer Aggressiveness On Biopsy By Gerry J. O'Dowd et al. Prostate Cancer Research Institute, Los Angeles, CA Reprinted from PCRI Insights January 2001 v4.1

(76) http://www.yananow.net/Chart-Gleason.htm Gleason Score at Diagnosis

(77) http://jco.ascopubs.org/cgi/content/abstract/23/32/8165 Journal of Clinical Oncology, Vol 23, No 32 (November 10), 2005: pp. 8165-8169. Active Surveillance for Prostate Cancer: For Whom? Laurence Klotz.

(78) http://www.prostatecancerwatchfulwaiting.co.za/ActiveSurveillance.pdf Actuve surveillance: towards a new paradigm in the management of early prostate cancer
Chris Parker.

(79) http://deb.uthscsa.edu/URORiskCalc/Pages/uroriskcalc.jsp The Cancer Risk Calculator for Prostate Cancer

(80) http://caonline.amcancersoc.org/cgi/content/full/56/2/106 Cancer Statistics, 2006 Ahmedin Jemal

(81) http://www.biomedexperts.com/Abstract.bme/18073376/ Interpreting trends in prostate cancer incidence and mortality in the five Nordic countries. Journal of the National Cancer Institute 2007;99(24):1881-7. Kvåle Rune et al.

(82) http://jjco.oxfordjournals.org/cgi/content/abstract/39/6/339 Japanese Journal of Clinical Oncology 2009 39(6):339-351 The Japanese Guideline for Prostate Cancer Screening. Chisato Hamashima et al.

(83) http://theoncologist.alphamedpress.org/cgi/content/full/13/3/306 The Oncologist, Vol. 13, No. 3, 306-308, March 2008; doi:10.1634/theoncologist.2008-0008 Commentary: How Serious Is Getting a Diagnosis of Prostate Cancer? Michael J. Barry et al.

(84) http://www.phac-aspc.gc.ca/publicat/cdic-mcc/16-1sup/c_e.html Trends in Incidence and Mortality of Prostate Cancer in Canada. Isra Levy.

(85) http://jnci.oxfordjournals.org/cgi/content/full/99/24/1881 Interpreting Trends in Prostate Cancer Incidence and Mortality in the Five Nordic Countries. Public Health Rep. 2004 Mar-Apr; 119(2): 174-186.

(86) http://jnci.oxfordjournals.org/cgi/content/full/91/12/1017 Journal of the National Cancer Institute, Vol. 91, No. 12, 1017-1024, June 16, 1999. Cancer Surveillance Series: Interpreting Trends in Prostate Cancer—Part I: Evidence of the Effects of Screening in Recent Prostate Cancer Incidence, Mortality, and Survival Rates. Benjamin F. Hankey et al.

(87) http://jnci.oxfordjournals.org/cgi/content/full/91/12/1025 Journal of the National Cancer Institute, Vol. 91, No. 12, 1025-1032, June 16, 1999. Cancer Surveillance Series: Interpreting Trends in Prostate Cancer—Part II: Cause of Death Misclassification and the Recent Rise and Fall in Prostate Cancer Mortality. Eric J. Feuer, Ray M. Merrill, Benjamin F. Hankey

(88) http://www.eradimaging.com/site/article.cfm?ID=1 Prostate-Specific Antigen Test: Is It a Valid Screening Tool for Prostate Cancer? Pamela C. Cartright.

(89) http://www.renegadeneurologist.com/prostate-treatment-wasted-40-billion-scientist-says/ Prostate Treatment Wasted $40 Billion, Scientist Says From Bloomberg.com:

(90) http://www.usyd.edu.au/news/84.html?newsstoryid=3911 Testing not a major factor in prostate cancer mortality. 29 September 2009. Renegade Neurologist.

(91) http://archinte.ama-assn.org/cgi/content/full/169/17/1554 Weighing the Benefits and Downsides of Prostate-Specific Antigen Screening. Pignone Arch Intern Med.2009; 169: 1554-1556.

(92) http://www.medicalnewstoday.com/articles/143145.php Otis W. Brawley.

(93) http://www.ncbi.nlm.nih.gov/pubmed/16414494 Active surveillance with selective delayed intervention for favorable risk prostate cancer. Klotz L. Division of Urology, University of Toronto,

(94) http://www.europeanurology.com/article/S0302-2838(07)00713-0/pdf Prospective Validation of Active Surveillance in Prostate Cancer: The PRIAS Study RCN van den Bergh, S Roemeling, MJ Roobol European Urology, Volume 52, Issue 6, Pages 1560-1563, December 2007

(95) http://www.prostatecancerwatchfulwaiting.co.za/HardieParker2005.pdf Early outcomes of active surveillance for localized prostate cancer C Hardie, C Parker, A Norman, R Eeles, A. BJU international, 2005.

(96) http://www3.interscience.wiley.com/journal/113385414/abstract PSA doubling time predicts the outcome after active surveillance in screening-detected prostate cancer: Results from the European randomized study of screening for prostate cancer, Sweden section Khatami Ali et al.

(97) http://www3.interscience.wiley.com/cgi-bin/fulltext/118859241/HTMLSTART Cancer. 2008 Jun 15;112(12):2664-70 Active surveillance for the management of prostate cancer in a contemporary cohort. Dall'Era MA et al.

(98) http://www.ncbi.nlm.nih.gov/pubmed/17850361 BJU Int. 2008 Jan;101(2):165-9. Epub 2007 Sep 10. Active surveillance; a reasonable

management alternative for patients with prostate cancer: the Miami experience. Soloway MS, Soloway CT et al.

(99) http://www.ncbi.nlm.nih.gov/pubmed/19233410 J Urol. 2009 Apr;181(4):1635-41;
A multi-institutional evaluation of active surveillance for low risk prostate cancer.
Eggener SE, Mueller A, Berglund RK, Ayyathurai R, Soloway C, Soloway MS et al.

(100) http://www.ncbi.nlm.nih.gov/pubmed/15839912 BJU Int. 2005 May;95(7):956-60. Early outcomes of active surveillance for localized prostate cancer. Hardie C et al.

(101) http://www3.interscience.wiley.com/cgi-bin/fulltext/119142464/HTMLSTART Role of repeated biopsy of the prostate in predicting disease progression in patients with prostate cancer on active surveillance. Mohammed Al Otaibi, MD et al.

(102) http://www.ncbi.nlm.nih.gov/pubmed/16713065 Eur Urol. 2006 Sep;50(3):475-82. Epub 2006 May 3. Management and survival of screen-detected prostate cancer patients who might have been suitable for active surveillance. Roemeling S et al.

(103) http://www.ncbi.nlm.nih.gov/pubmed/18387385 Urology. 2008 Apr;71(4):573-7. Links Staging saturation biopsy in patients with prostate cancer on active surveillance protocol.
Abouassaly R, Lane BR, Jones JS.

(104) http://www3.interscience.wiley.com/cgi-bin/fulltext/114132008/HTMLSTART Prostate-specific antigen velocity and prostate cancer gleason grade and stage Paul F. Pinsky et al.

(105) http://www.ncbi.nlm.nih.gov/pmc/articles/PMC2684075/?tool=pubmed Clin Interv Aging. 2007 March; 2(1): 153-161. Is it necessary to cure prostate cancer when it is possible? (Understanding the role of prostate inflammation resolution to prostate

cancer evolution) Ronald E Wheeler Prostatitis & Prostate Cancer Center, Sarasota, Fl, USA.

(106) http://www3.interscience.wiley.com/cgi-bin/fulltext/116321833/HTMLSTART Prostate-specific antigen velocity and the detection of gleason score 7 to 10 prostate cancer. Rinaa S. Punglia et al.

(107) http://www.ncbi.nlm.nih.gov/pubmed/18762814 Prostate Cancer Prostatic Dis. 2009;12(2):143-7. Biopsy tissue microarray study of Ki-67 expression in untreated, localized prostate cancer managed by active surveillance. Jhavar S, et al

(108) http://jnci.oxfordjournals.org/cgi/content/abstract/97/17/1248 JNCI Journal of the National Cancer Institute 2005 97(17):1248-1253; Prostate Cancer and the Will Rogers Phenomenon Peter C. Albertsen, James A. Hanley, George H. Barrows, David F.

(109) http://www.forbes.com/2009/08/31/ prostate-cancer-screening-business-healthcare-prostate.html Medical Tests—The Dark Side Of Prostate Cancer Screening. Robert Langreth, 8.31.09

(110) http://www.cancer.gov/ncicancerbulletin/090809/page2 Study Questions Value of Prostate Cancer Screening.

(111) http://www.ncbi.nlm.nih.gov/pubmed/19720918
J Clin Oncol. 2009 Aug 31. Prospective Study of Determinants and Outcomes of Deferred Treatment or Watchful Waiting Among Men With Prostate Cancer in a Nationwide Cohort. Shappley WV et al.

(112) http://www.cancer.org/docroot/CRI/ content/CRI_2_4_1X_What_are_the_key_statistics_for_prostate_cancer_36.asp The latest American Cancer Society estimates for prostate cancer in the United States are for 2009: about 192, 280 new cases of prostate cancer will be diagnosed. 27,360 men will die of prostate cancer According to the most recent data, for all men with prostate cancer, the relative 5-year survival rate is nearly100% and the relative 10-year survival rate is 91%.

(113) http://jama.ama-assn.org/cgi/content/short/302/11/1202 Outcomes of Localized Prostate Cancer Following Conservative Management. Grace L. Lu-Yao et al. JAMA. 2009;302(11):1202-1209.

(114) http://www.pubmedcentral.nih.gov/articlerender.fcgi?tool=pubmed&pubmedid=17077805 Br J Cancer. 2006 November 6; 95(9): 1186-1194. Long-term outcome among men with conservatively treated localised prostate cancer J Cuzick et al.

(115) http://www.usyd.edu.au/news/84.html?newsstoryid=3911 "A Model of Prostate-Specific Antigen Screening Outcomes for Low—to High-Risk Men" was published in the Archives on Internal Medicine today. Dr Kirsten Howard from the University of Sydney's School of Public Health was the paper's lead author.

(116) http://www.ncbi.nlm.nih.gov/pubmed/19786680
Arch Intern Med. 2009 Sep 28;169(17):1603-10. A model of prostate-specific antigen screening outcomes for low—to high-risk men: information to support informed choices. Howard K, Barratt A, Mann GJ, Patel MI. Screening and Test Evaluation Program, School of Public Health, University of Sydney, Sydney, Australia.

(117) http://jeffreydach.com/2008/10/26/rethinking-testosterone-suppression-for-prostate-cancer-by-jeffrey-dach-md.aspx Increased Mortality from Androgen Blockade for Prostate Cancer by Jeffrey Dach MD

(118) http://www.medicine.mcgill.ca/mjm/v02n02/psa.html Prostate Specific Antigen (PSA):The Historical Perspective T. Ming Chu, Ph.D. McGill University.

(119) http://www.psa-rising.com/upfront/otisbrawleyfeb00.htm Prostate Cancer Planner Never Takes PSA Test, Compares Prostate Screening to Tuskegee Experiment By Jacqueline Strax. Interview with Otis W. Brawley M.D. January 29 and February 1, 2000

(120) http://jco.ascopubs.org/content/23/32/8165.abstract Journal of Clinical Oncology, Vol 23, No 32 (November 10), 2005: pp. 8165-8169 Active Surveillance for Prostate Cancer: For Whom? Laurence Klotz.

(121) http://www.ronaldwheeler.com/psastats.html PSA stats Dr Ron Wheeler

SECTION EIGHT: SELENIUM, WHY WE NEED IT.

CHAPTER 30

Selenium, from Toxin to Essential Mineral—Part One

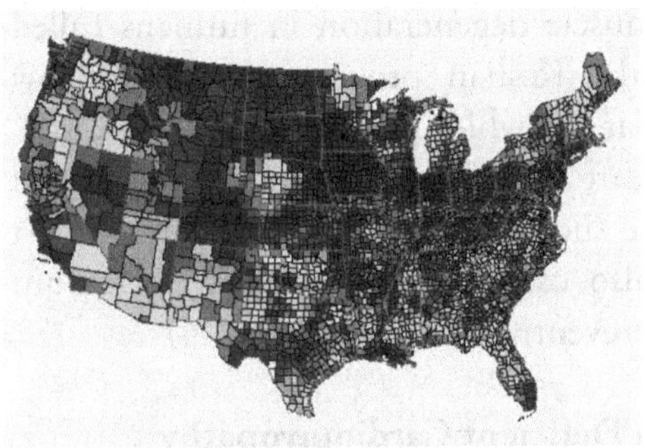

Selenium Soil Content by Counties, with darker counties having higher selenium soil content. Courtesy of the United States Geological Survey (62)

Selenium is an essential trace mineral critical for antioxidant defense, fertility, thyroid hormone metabolism, immune response, and muscle development. First discovered in 1817, selenium was considered a toxic substance best avoided. One hundred and forty years later, in 1957, the status of Selenium dramatically changed with a report of the first selenium deficiency disease. An obscure biochemist at the NIH, Klaus Schwarz, found that giving selenium to Vitamin E deficient mice protected them from liver degeneration.(1)

White Marble Disease in Oregon Cattle

One year later in 1958, scientists at the University of Oregon discovered that selenium deficiency caused "white muscle disease", causing muscle degeneration in cattle foraging grass on selenium depleted soils. They surmised that volcanic soil was low in selenium, and hot volcanic gas caused selenium depletion of the Oregon soil millions of years ago. Selenium supplementation prevented the white muscle disease.(2) A soil selenium map of the United States shows selenium rich areas in the plains states and deficient areas in Oregon, the West coast and the South East.(62-63)

Finland Has Low Selenium Soil

Finland is a country plagued with selenium depleted volcanic soils, and in 1984, was the first to add selenium to crop fertilizer in a mandated program of selenium enrichment.(12-13)

Keshan Disease in China Caused by Selenium Deficiency

In the 1960's and 1970's in China, government sponsored research discovered a form of cardiac muscle degeneration in humans called Keshan disease occurring in the Keshan province noted for low selenium levels in its soil. Similar to "white muscle disease" in cattle, Keshan disease caused the heart muscle to degenerate. Afflicted children of the Keshan province succumbed to cardiac failure with a dilated, nonfunctional heart, also called cardiomyopathy. Selenium supplements were found to be preventive of the disease.(3-4)

Sudden Death From Selenium Deficient Cardiomyopathy

In the early 1980's, selenium deficiency was recognized in the United States when patients on long term artificial feeding died suddenly from cardiomyopathy (a form of heart failure) induced by selenium deficiency. Apparently, the artificial feeding solution had not included selenium, resulting in selenium deficiency and sudden death from heart muscle degeneration. (8-10)

It's Not the Selenium, It's the Seleno-Protein

Selenium is an essential trace mineral because of the selenoproteins critical for antioxidant defense, fertility, thyroid hormone metabolism, immune responses, muscle development and function. Selenoproteins are thought involved in cancer prevention because of inverse correlation between soil selenium, selenium intake, selenium blood levels and cancer incidence. The lower the soil or blood selenium, the higher the incidence of cancer in that geographic area. (5-7)

Seleno-Proteins: When Stop Doesn't Really Mean Stop—What is Selenocysteine?

The amino acid, cysteine, normally contains a sulfur atom. However, when the sulfur atom is replaced by selenium, cysteine becomes seleno-cysteine. Subsequent incorporation of seleno-cysteine into a protein amino acid sequence is called a seleno-protein.

The DNA translation table which maps DNA codons to amino acids was completed in the 1960's. It is quite remarkable that 20 years later, it was discovered that the UGA Stop Codon sometimes is **NOT** a Stop Codon. The UGA stop codon can also translate as seleno-cysteine, the 21st amino acid. This was an unexpected twist which nobody expected, and biochemists were quite surprised by this new information. Notice the translation table below has a code for START and STOP which instructs the cell when to start and stop the amino acid chain under construction. However, there is no code for seleno-cysteine which is incorporated into a seleno-protein. This is because the STOP codon, (UGA) also serves to code for the amino acid, seleno-cysteine, whenever there is a "SECIS" instruction set present in the DNA code.

Inverse Codon Translation Table For Amino Acids			
Amino acid	Codon	Amino Acid	Codon
Ala/A	GCU, GCC, GCA, GCG	**Leu/L**	UUA, UUG, CUU, CUC, CUA, CUG
Arg/R	CGU, CGC, CGA, CGG, AGA, AGG	**Lys/K**	AAA, AAG
Asn/N	AAU, AAC	**Met/M**	AUG
Asp/D	GAU, GAC	**Phe/F**	UUU, UUC
Cys/C	UGU, UGC	**Pro/P**	CCU, CCC, CCA, CCG
Gln/Q	CAA, CAG	**Ser/S**	UCU, UCC, UCA, UCG, AGU, AGC
Glu/E	GAA, GAG	**Thr/T**	ACU, ACC, ACA, ACG

Gly/G	GGU, GGC, GGA, GGG	**Trp/W**	UGG
His/H	CAU, CAC	**Tyr/Y**	UAU, UAC
Ile/I	AUU, AUC, AUA	**Val/V**	GUU, GUC, GUA, GUG
START	AUG	**STOP**	UAA, UGA, UAG

Dr. Vadim Gladyshev and Selenium, Correcting the Human Genome Project

The Genetic Code is a translation table which maps the code in the DNA (called codons) to one of the twenty amino acids, thereby providing the instruction set for the cell machinery to arrange long strings of amino acids into the proper sequence called a protein. The UGA Stop Codon also codes for seleno-cysteine, depending on another instruction set called the SECIS insertion sequence. Thanks to Vadim N. Gladyshev for much of our current knowledge. (Note Vadim N. Gladyshev has since moved from U Nebraska to Harvard). Based on this tricky dual translation of the UGA codon for seleno-cysteine, Gladyshev and his collaborators went about correcting the seleno-cysteine errors in the original DNA database. His new correction software is called Recode2. (14-23)

Selenoproteins—What Do They Do? Here are a Few Selenoproteins and Their Function

1) Glutathione Peroxidase—This is a major antioxidant which works in harmony with vitamin E converting (reducing) hydrogen peroxide to water, and preventing lipid peroxidation and oxidative cellular damage. (24)

2) Iodothyronine De-iodinase Enzyme—This is involved in thyroid function, converts thyroid hormone T4 to T3. (24). See the Iodine Book by David Brownstein MD for an excellent summary of selenium and thyroid function.(64)

3) Thioredoxin reductase—This is an antioxidant responsible for degrading peroxides and hydroperoxides which cause cell death, DNA damage, and tissue atrophy.(24)

4) Sept 15 Selenoprotein—This is a candidate for cancer prevention. (15)

There are about 40 families of selenoproteins. Most still have unknown functions.

Selenium Deficiency and Increased Cancer Risk—The Nutritional Prevention of Cancer Trial (NPC Trial)

The NPC Trial, published in 1996 in JAMA, was the brainchild of Larry C Clark and Gerald Combs, and the first prospective double-blind, placebo-controlled, randomized trial in the Western world to test a selenium supplement on a large population for its effect on cancer prevention. Clark chose selenized yeast containing 200 mcg selenium for residents of the southeastern United States, where soil selenium levels are the lowest in the nation. Between 1983 and 1991, seven dermatology clinics recruited 1,300 patients, with a mean age of 63 years. All had a history of basal and/or squamous cell carcinoma (skin cancer). The NPC Trial showed selenium supplementation significantly decreased the total cancer incidence by 50 percent, and specifically dropped the incidence of lung cancer by 48 percent, prostate cancer by 63 percent, and colorectal cancer by 58 percent. Those who entered the trial with plasma selenium levels less than 106 ng/mL showed both the greatest protection from selenium and the highest rates of subsequent cancer in the control group. (26-27)

The selenized yeast tablet used in the NPC trial was called Seleno-Excell from Cypress Systems which is available at your local vitamin shop or health food store under various brand names. (Note: I have no financial interest in any selenium products mentioned)

The SELECT Study—Selenium and Vitamin E Found Useless at Cancer Prevention

The 1996 NPC trial reigned supreme until it was discredited December 2008, by the disappointing results of the 2009 SELECT study, with Time Magazine and The New York Times proclaiming that selenium and vitamin E useless at prevention of prostate cancer. (32-33) The

SELECT study was a randomized, placebo-controlled trial of Selenium and Vitamin E given to 35,533 men 50 years or older, and PSA of 4.0 ng/mL or less, to determine if the vitamins reduced risk of prostate cancer. The vitamins used were 200 µg L-selenomethionine and 400 IU of synthetic vitamin E. The results showed the vitamins did not prevent prostate cancer in this group. (29)

SELECT—Why Did It Fail?

Hatfield and Gladyshev summarize the reasons why SELECT failed and why the NPC trial and many previous studies succeeded in showing a benefit of selenium supplementation (30). Rayman and Combs also commented on the SELECT study in a JAMA editorial.(31) The major reason for failure is the SELECT patients started with higher serum selenium levels, in the range above 135 mcg/L found not to benefit from selenium supplementation. They already had plenty.

1) SELECT used seleno-methionine whereas the NPC used selenium-enriched yeast.

2) SELECT evaluated prostate cancer. How can selenium be shown to prevent prostate cancer when PSA Screening programs rapidly remove prostate cancers from the population before they progress? The NPC evaluated all cancers in patients with underlying history of skin cancer.

3) The subjects enrolled in SELECT had higher initial plasma levels of selenium than those in the NPC trial (135 ng/ml compared to 113 ng/ml, respectively). The subjects in the NPC trial were selected, in part, on the basis of their having relatively low serum selenium levels it was in this cohort that selenium supplementation was effective in reducing cancer risks.

4) SELECT used synthetic Vitamin E (all racemic), which is clearly inferior to natural vitamin E. Results may have been different for natural vitamin E.

Blood Selenium Levels below 130 ng/ml benefit from supplementation

In agreement with Dr Rayman, a 2008 study published by Bleys in the Archives of internal medicine found an inverse correlation between serum selenium and both cancer mortality, and all cause mortality. They found that selenium supplementation was beneficial up to a serum selenium level of 130 ng/ml. (34) Above 130 ng/ml, they found no further benefit. (34)

Important Point
Low Selenium constitutes a health risk with increased risk for cancer, and immune dysfunction.

Conclusion: The evidence is overwhelming that low selenium blood levels (below 130 ng/ml) constitute a health risk. It is suggested that selenium serum levels be routinely evaluated, and when found low, supplementation is indicated with selenium in the form of selenized yeast or L-seleno-methionine in the amount of 200—300 mcg per day.

References for Chapter 30. Selenium, From Toxin to Essential Mineral, Part One

(1) http://jn.nutrition.org/cgi/content/full/133/11/3331
J. Nutr. 133:3331-3342, November 2003. History of Nutrition. A Short History of Nutritional Science: Part 4 (1945-1985)1 Kenneth J. Carpenter. History of selenium.

(2) http://extension.oregonstate.edu/yamhill/sites/default/files/documents/Selenium.pdf WHAT'S NEW WITH SELENIUM . . . . FERTILIZING OREGON PASTURES By Gene Pirelli, Jim Oldfield, Wayne Mosher and Ron Hathaway—white muscle disease in Oregon

(3) http://www.chiro.org/nutrition/FULL/Selenium_Antioxidant.shtml
Selenium: Antioxidant & Cancer Quencher From The March 1999 Issue of Nutrition Science News By Stephanie Briggs, Ph.D

(4) http://www.ajcn.org/cgi/reprint/57/2/259S.pdf
The epidemiology of selenium deficiency in the etiological study of endemic diseases in China by Kei'ou Ge and Guangqi Yang. Am J Clin Nutr February 1993 vol. 57 no. 2 259S-263S.

(5) http://www.jbc.org/content/284/2/723.full
Selenoproteins by Jun Lu and Arne Holmgren. January 9, 2009 The Journal of Biological Chemistry, 284, 723-727.

(6) http://www.gustrength.com/nutrition:selenium-an-essential-micronutrient Selenium: An Essential Micronutrient Molecules 2009, 14(3), 1263-1278; Review—Selenium as an Essential Micronutrient: Roles in Cell Cycle and Apoptosis. Huawei Zeng

(7) http://physiologyonline.physiology.org/cgi/content/full/21/5/307
Physiology, Vol. 21, No. 5, 307-315, October 2006 Selenoproteins and Their Impact on Human Health Through Diverse Physiological Pathways by Behzad Moghadaszadeh and Alan H. Beggs,

(8) www.ncbi.nlm.nih.gov/pubmed/6807740
Gastroenterology. 1982 Sep;83(3):689-93. Selenium deficiency and fatal cardiomyopathy in a patient on home parenteral nutrition. by Fleming CR ET AL.

(9) http://www.ncbi.nlm.nih.gov/pubmed/6435941
Clin Pharm. 1984 Sep-Oct;3(5):531-5. Selenium deficiency and fatal cardiomyopathy in a patient receiving long-term home parenteral nutrition. Quercia RA, Korn S, O'Neill D, Dougherty JE, Ludwig M, Schweizer R, Sigman R.

(10) http://www.ncbi.nlm.nih.gov/pubmed/11848134
Med Sci Law. 2002 Jan;42(1):10-3. Fulminant heart failure due to selenium deficiency cardiomyopathy (Keshan disease). Burke MP ET AL.

(11) http://www.ncbi.nlm.nih.gov/pubmed/2168125
Am J Clin Nutr. 1990 Sep;52(3):572-7. Cardiomyopathy associated with nonendemic selenium deficiency in a Caucasian adolescent.

Lockitch G, Taylor GP, Wong LT, Davidson AG, Dison PJ, Riddell D, Massing B.

(12) http://www.springerlink.com/content/pt21161703q7hp6v/
The effect of nationwide selenium enrichment of fertilizers on selenium status of healthy Finnish medical students living in south western Finland Journal Biological Trace Element Research Publisher Humana Press Inc. Issue Volume 36, Number 2/February, 1993

(13) http://www.asas.org/Bios/Oldfieldhist.pdf
A brief history of selenium research: From alkali disease to prostate cancer. (from poison to prevention) J. E. Oldfield1 Oregon State University, Corvallis 97331

(14) http://www.ars.usda.gov/pandp/people/people.htm?personid=31990
Gerald Combs.

(15) http://www.nature.com/embor/journal/v5/n2/full/7400080.html
EMBO reports 5, 2, 140-141 (2004) Finding needles in a haystack, In silico identification of eukaryotic selenoprotein genes by Donna M. Driscoll & Laurent Chavatte Department of Cell Biology, Lerner Research Institute

(16) http://digitalcommons.unl.edu/cgi/viewcontent.cgi?article=1035&context=biochemgladyshev Selenoproteins and selenoproteomes Vadim N. Gladyshev, University of Nebraska-Lincoln

(17) http://gladyshevlab.bwh.harvard.edu/research.html
Vadim Gladyshev Lab Selenium and Redox Biology

(18) http://gladyshevlab.bwh.harvard.edu/contact.html
Vadim N. Gladyshev Professor Division of Genetics Department of Medicine Brigham and Women's Hospital Harvard Medical School New Research Building, Room 435 77 Ave. Louis Pasteur Boston, MA 02115

(19) http://scarlet.unl.edu/?p=8 Selenium research lauded Jun 2nd, 2008 BY TROY FEDDERSON,—Vadim Gladyshev, professor of biochemistry

and director of the UNL's Redox Biology Center, received the ORCA award for his research.

(20) http://nar.oxfordjournals.org/cgi/content/abstract/gkp788v1 Nucleic Acids Research Advance Access published online on September 25, 2009. Recode-2: new design, new search tools, and many more genes BY Michaël Bekaert, Vadim N. Gladyshev et al.

(21) http://recode.ucc.ie/about Recode2.

(22) http://www.ncbi.nlm.nih.gov/pmc/articles/PMC372737/?page=1 Universal genetic code late 60s

(23) http://www.ncbi.nlm.nih.gov/pubmed/8744353 Trends Biochem Sci. 1996 Jun;21(6):203-8. Knowing when not to stop: selenocysteine incorporation in eukaryotes.Low SC, Berry MJ.et al.

(24) http://www.thorne.com/altmedrev/.fulltext/9/3/239.pdf Selenium Biochemistry and Cancer: A Review of the Literature Lyn Patrick, ND

(25) http://www.gpmcf.org/JAMA2009.pdf JAMA. 2009;301(18): Margaret P. Rayman; Gerald F. Combs, Jr; David J. Waters Selenium and Vitamin E Supplementation for Cancer Prevention.

(26) http://jama.ama-assn.org/cgi/reprint/276/24/1957.pdf NPC StudyJAMA. 2009;301(18):1876

(27) http://jama.ama-assn.org/cgi/content/abstract/276/24/1957 Effects of Selenium Supplementation for Cancer Prevention in Patients With Carcinoma of the Skin A Randomized Controlled Trial by Larry C. Clark, MPH, PhD et al. JAMA. 1996;276(24):1957-1963.

(28) http://jn.nutrition.org/cgi/reprint/118/2/237.pdf Selenium and Cancer Prevention. CLARK,L. C. and.COMBS,G. F., JR. (1986) Selenium compounds in the prevention of cancer: research needs and public health implications. Nutr. 116: 170-173.

(29) http://jama.ama-assn.org/cgi/content/full/301/1/39
Effect of Selenium and Vitamin E on Risk of Prostate Cancer and Other Cancers. The Selenium and Vitamin E Cancer Prevention Trial (SELECT) BY Scott M. Lippman, MD et al JAMA. 2009;301(1):39-51

(30) http://www.ncbi.nlm.nih.gov/pmc/articles/PMC2718722
http://molinterv.aspetjournals.org/content/9/1/18.full
Mol Interv. 2009 February; 9(1): 18-21. The Outcome of Selenium and Vitamin E Cancer Prevention Trial (SELECT) Reveals the Need for Better Understanding of Selenium Biology Dolph L. Hatfield1 and Vadim N. Gladyshev

(31) http://www.gpmcf.org/JAMA2009.pdf
JAMA. 2009;301(18):1876 Margaret P. Rayman; Gerald F. Combs, Jr; David J. Waters Selenium and Vitamin E Supplementation for Cancer Prevention

(32) http://www.time.com/time/health/article/0,8599,1865464,00.html
Vitamins Do Not Prevent Prostate Cancer, Study Finds By Alice Park Wednesday, Dec. 10, 2008 Time Mag.

(33) http://well.blogs.nytimes.com/2008/10/28/disappointing-news-on-vitamin-e-and-selenium October 28, 2008 Disappointing News on Vitamin E and Selenium By TARA PARKER-POPE NY Times

(34) http://archinte.highwire.org/cgi/content/abstract/168/4/404
Serum Selenium Levels and All-Cause, Cancer, and Cardiovascular Mortality Among US Adults by Joachim Bleys, MD, MPH; Ana Navas-Acien, MD, PhD; Eliseo Guallar, MD, DrPH Arch Intern Med. 2008;168(4):404-410.

(35) http://www.ncbi.nlm.nih.gov/pubmed/12494476
Int J Cancer. 2003 Feb 20;103(5):664-70. Serum selenium and risk of prostate cancer in U.S. blacks and whites. Vogt TM et al.

(36) http://www.ncbi.nlm.nih.gov/pmc/articles/PMC1472449/Proc Natl Acad Sci U S A. 2006 May 23; 103(21): 8179-8184. Selenoprotein

deficiency accelerates prostate carcinogenesis in a transgenic model.Veda Diwadkar-Navsariwala et al.

(37) http://cancerprevention.aacrjournals.org/content/2/5/484.abstract Methyl-Selenium Compounds Inhibit Prostate Carcinogenesis in the Transgenic Adenocarcinoma of Mouse Prostate Model with Survival Benefit. Lei Wang et al Hormel Institute, University of Minnesota, Austin, Minnesota
Cancer Prevention Research May 2009 2; 484

(38) http://www.ncbi.nlm.nih.gov/pmc/articles/PMC2734116 Selenium and Vitamin E: Cell Type—and Intervention-Specific Tissue Effects in Prostate Cancer by Dimitra Tsavachidou et al JNCI Journal of the National Cancer Institute 2009 101(5):306-320

(39) http://www.ncbi.nlm.nih.gov/pubmed/16614422 J Nutr. 2006 May;136(5):1311-7. Both selenoproteins and low molecular weight selenocompounds reduce colon cancer risk in mice with genetically impaired selenoprotein expression. Irons R, Carlson BA, Hatfield DL, Davis CD.

(40) http://www.cypsystems.com/media/anticarcinogenesis.pdf Selenium and anticarcinogenesis: underlying mechanisms by Matthew I. Jackson and Gerald F. Combs Jr Current Opinion in Clinical Nutrition and Metabolic Care 2008, 11:718-726

(41) http://www.ncbi.nlm.nih.gov/pubmed/16313696 Proc Nutr Soc. 2005 Nov;64(4):527-42. Selenium in cancer prevention: a review of the evidence and mechanism of action. Rayman MP.

(42) http://carcin.oxfordjournals.org/cgi/content/full/20/9/1657 Carcinogenesis, Vol. 20, No. 9, 1657-1666, September 1999. Selenium metabolism, selenoproteins and mechanisms of cancer prevention: complexities with thioredoxin reductase Howard E. Ganther

(43) http://archinte.ama-assn.org/cgi/content/abstract/170/3/256 Acute Selenium Toxicity Associated With a Dietary Supplement Jennifer K. MacFarquhar et al Arch Intern Med. 2010;170(3):256-261.

(44) http://www.ajcn.org/cgi/content/abstract/87/2/379
Brazil nuts: an effective way to improve selenium status. Am J Clin Nutr. 2008 Feb. Thomson CD et al.

(45) http://www.mdpi.com/1420-3049/14/10/3975/pdf
Molecules 2009, 14, 3975-3988. Selenium in Oncology: From Chemistry to Clinics, Oliver Micke et al.

(46) http://diss.kib.ki.se/2009/978-91-7409-732-0/thesis.pdf CYTOTOXIC MECHANISMS OF SELENIUM IN CANCERki.se [PDF] E Olm—2009—Karolinska Institutet, Stockholm, Sweden

(47) http://jn.nutrition.org/cgi/reprint/118/2/237.pdf
FOSTER, H. D. (1986) Reducing Cancer Mortality: A Geo graphical Perspective, Western Geographical Series, vol. 23, University of Victoria, Victoria, B.C.

(48) http://www.orthomolecular.org/library/jom/1998/articles/1998-v13n01-p008.shtml The Journal of Orthomolecular Medicine Vol. 13, 1st Quarter 1998 Selenium and Cancer: A Geographical Perspective Harold D. Foster, Ph.D

(49) http://www.ncbi.nlm.nih.gov/pubmed/3924710
Jpn J Cancer Res. 1985 May;76(5):374-7. Selenium in the blood of Japanese and American women with and without breast cancer and fibrocystic disease. Schrauzer GN, Molenaar T, Mead S, Kuehn K, Yamamoto H, Araki E.

(50) http://www.ncbi.nlm.nih.gov/pubmed/2484517
Biol Trace Elem Res. 1988 Jan-Apr;15:205-12. The distribution of selenium in human blood samples of Israeli population—comparison between normal and breast cancer cases. Chaitchik S et al.

(51) http://www.ncbi.nlm.nih.gov/pubmed/20063075
Cancer Causes Control. 2010 Jan 9. Toenail selenium status and DNA repair capacity among female BRCA1 mutation carriers. Kotsopoulos J et al.

(52) http://www.ncbi.nlm.nih.gov/pubmed/19843683
Cancer Epidemiol Biomarkers Prev. 2009 Nov;18(11):2923-8. Selenium supplementation reduced oxidative DNA damage in adnexectomized BRCA1 mutations carriers. by Dziaman T et al.

(53) http://cebp.aacrjournals.org/content/14/5/1302.long
Cancer Epidemiology, Biomarkers & Prevention May 2005 14; 1302. Increased Rates of Chromosome Breakage in BRCA1 Carriers Are Normalized by Oral Selenium Supplementation by Elzbieta Kowalska et al.

(54) http://www.hccpjournal.com/content/4/1/58
A Lowering of Breast and Ovarian Cancer Risk in Women with a BRCA1 Mutation by Selenium Supplementation of Diet. Tomasz Huzarski1, Tomasz Byrski1, Jacek Gronwald1, Elżbieta Kowalska et al.

(55) http://www.cancer-therapy.org/CT1A/HTML/34%20%20Diamond%20et%20al,%20293-29%20c.htm Cancer Therapy Vol 1, 293-298, 2003. Allelic loss at the SEP15 locus in breast cancer by Mohamed A. Nasr et al.

(56) http://cancerres.aacrjournals.org/cgi/content/abstract/51/17/4613
[Cancer Research 51, 4613-4617, September 1, 1991. Inhibition of 7,12-Dimethylbenz(a)anthracene-induced Mammary Tumors and DNA Adducts by Dietary Selenite by Jinzhou Liu et al.

(57) http://www.wjgnet.com/1948-5204/pdf/v1/i1/74.pdf
Selenium as a chemopreventive agent in experimentally induced colon carcinogenesis. World J Gastrointest Oncol 2009 October 15; 1(1): 74-81 by Fereshteh Ezzati Ghadi et al. Panjab University, India

(58) http://www.ncbi.nlm.nih.gov/pubmed/16984549
Int J Urol. 2006 Sep;13(9):1180-4. Selenium is inversely associated with bladder cancer risk: a report from the Belgian case-control study on bladder cancer. Kellen E, Zeegers M, Buntinx F. Belgium.

(59) http://www.ncbi.nlm.nih.gov/pubmed/18953506
Biol Trace Elem Res. 2009 Mar;127(3):200-10. Epub 2008 Oct

25.High-dose sodium selenite can induce apoptosis of lymphoma cells in adult patients with non-Hodgkin's lymphoma. by Asfour IA et al.

(60) http://www.emord.com/media/press-releases/emord-sues-fda.htm Emord Sues FDA: Selenium Claim Suppression Violates First Amendment.

(61) http://jn.nutrition.org/cgi/content/full/135/2/354
2005 The American Society for Nutritional Sciences J. Nutr. 135:354-356, February 2005. The Level of Evidence for Permitting a Qualified Health Claim:
FDA's Review of the Evidence for Selenium and Cancer and Vitamin E and Heart Disease1 Paula R. Trumbo2 Center for Food Safety and Applied Nutrition, Food and Drug Administration, College Park, MD 20740

(62) http://tin.er.usgs.gov/geochem/method.php?element=Se
U.S. Department of the Interior | U.S. Geological Survey. Mineral Resources On-Line Spatial Data. Selenium in Counties of the Conterminous States

(63) http://tin.er.usgs.gov/geochem/doc/averages/se/usa.html
Selenium in Counties of the Conterminous States, U.S. Geological Survey

(64) Iodine, Why You Need It, Why You Can't Live Without It, by David Brownstein MD, Fourth Edition 2009, Medical Alternatives Press.

CHAPTER 31

The Case for Selenium, Part Two

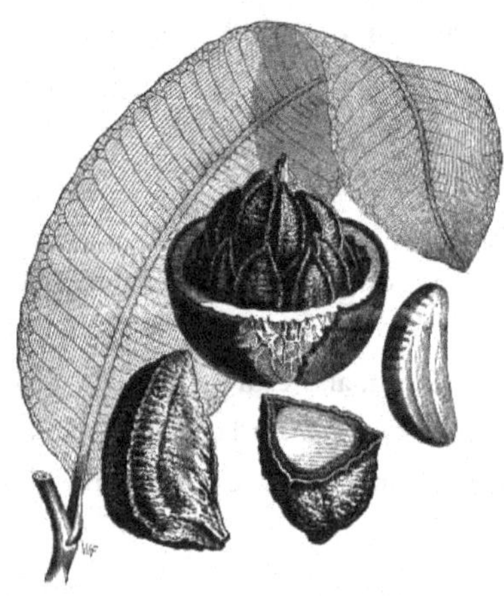

Brazil Nuts are high in selenium, courtesy of Scientific American Supplement, No. 598, June 18, 1887, and Wikimedia Commons

Selenium Toxicity Diagnosed by Dr. House

Selenium Toxicity from overconsumption of Brazil Nuts, called Selenosis, was "reported" on an episode of Dr. House, a medical TV show that often takes artistic liberties to enhance entertainment value. (17-20) In reality, there has never been a reported case of Selenosis from ingesting Brazil nuts. This in merely one example of many egregious errors and biases against natural medicine on the Dr. House series, and is to be expected, considering the massive drug company advertising supporting the show.

Evidence that Selenium Prevents Prostate Cancer

A study published by Vogt in the 2003 International Journal of Cancer evaluated selenium levels in 212 men with prostate cancer, compared with healthy controls. They found "*a moderately reduced risk of prostate cancer at higher serum selenium concentrations*", above 135 ng/ml.(1)

Selenium Prevents Prostate Cancer in Genetic Mice

Another elegant study came from the University of Illinois in the 2006 Proceedings of the National Academy of Science. This study used mice that were genetically manipulated twice. They were genetically modified to have a selenoprotein deficiency as well as an increased risk for prostate cancer. The selenoprotein-deficient mice exhibited accelerated development of prostate cancer in the form of prostate intra-epithelial neoplasia with microinvasion. This study clearly implicated selenoprotein deficiency as a risk factor for prostate cancer, and selenium as a preventive agent. (2) Yet another transgenic mouse prostate cancer study published in May 2009 AACR by Wang showed inhibition of prostate cancer and increased survival in mice treated with selenium compounds.(3)

Selenium Prevents Colon Cancer in Genetic Mice

Irons published a study in the 2006 Journal of Nutrition evaluating colon cancer in genetically altered mice, deficient in selenoproteins. The mice were given dietary selenium, and the colon was studied for cancer formation. The mice supplemented with dietary selenium had reduced colon cancer, with fewer pre-neoplastic lesions of the colon, This was true for both the seleno-protein deficient mice as well as normal mice. (4) A second colon cancer study in mice from India published in the 2009 World Journal of Gastroenterology showed that dietary selenium supplements reduced colon cancer tumors by 40 % in mice chemically treated with carcinogens to produce colon cancer.(5)

Selenium Levels Predict Breast Cancer Risk

A study published in 1985 in Japan Cancer Research looked at serum selenium levels in American and Japanese women with breast cancer. Healthy Japanese women had higher selenium levels of 286 mcg/ml compared to Japanese women with breast cancer who had lower selenium levels of 195 mcg/dl. For healthy American women, serum selenium was higher at 191 compared to American women with breast cancer who had lower selenium of 167 mcg/ml. (6)

Evidence that Selenium Prevents Breast Cancer

A study in Israel published in 1988 evaluated serum selenium levels in 32 breast cancer patients compared to controls. They found significantly lower serum selenium levels in the breast cancer patients (.076 ppm) compared to controls (.119 ppm). (7)

Selenium Prevents Breast Cancer in Mice

In a 1991 publication from Cancer Research, mice with chemically induced breast cancer (using DMBA) were treated with dietary selenite. Tumor incidence correlated inversely with the quantity of selenite consumed, clearly demonstrating inhibition of breast cancer by dietary selenium consumption.(8)

Selenium Beneficial for BRCA Gene Carriers—Reduces Breast Cancer

This may be the most convincing evidence of selenium as a cancer preventive agent. The BRCA gene is a mutation associated with increased risk of breast and ovarian cancer. Women with the BRCA1 gene face an 80 per cent lifetime risk of breast cancer and of 40 per cent lifetime risk of ovarian cancer. The BRCA1 gene manufactures proteins involved in repairing oxidative damage to DNA, with repair of the double-stranded DNA breaks. The BRCA gene test is available from Myriad Genetics, which holds a patent on the human gene sequence. A March 2010 court found the patent invalid, since human gene sequences are part of nature and in the public domain.

Dr. Dziaman from Poland published a study in Nov 2009 looking at DNA damage in BRCA gene carriers. They measured serum and urinary products of DNA oxidation with and without selenium supplementation, finding that damaged DNA products were higher in women with BRCA mutations, and were reduced by selenium supplementation. Their results suggest that BRCA1 deficiency contributes to oxidative damage and breaks in cellular DNA, which may be responsible for cancer development. In addition, selenium supplementation is beneficial, because it protects from oxidative DNA damage.(9)

Strong Evidence for a Selenium as Cancer Preventive Agent

A study of BRCA gene carriers from Kowalska in Poland in 2005 provides strong evidence for selenium as a preventive agent. Fifty five women with the BRCA1 gene mutation were supplemented with

275 μg of sodium selenite, daily for 8 weeks. The amount of DNA damage was assessed from blood lymphocytes showing BRCA gene carriers had twice the DNA damage compared to their normal siblings. However, Selenium supplementation given to BRCA gene carriers reduced the DNA damage to normal levels found in their siblings. (10) A second larger study reported by Kowalska in 2006, verified that selenium supplementation indeed reduces cancer in women with the BRCA1 gene. After two years of selenium supplementation, expected BRCA1-associated cancers were reduced in half.(11)

Sep 15 Selenoprotein genome and breast cancer

Which seleno-protein is the best candidate for breast cancer protection? One of the new selenoproteins discovered is the Sep15 protein, and the gene for this protein is commonly found to be damaged or lost in breast cancer tissue and other solid tumors (12)

Dietary Sources of Selenium

One of the highest dietary sources of selenium is Brazil Nuts, which each provide 12-50 mcg of seleno-methionine. (15) Strunza studied selenium levels in volunteers who ingested 11 Brazil nuts per day for 15 days. Serum selenium rose from 55 mcg/ML to 208 Mcg/mL at the end of the 2 week study. There were no ill effects reported. (16)

A Case of Selenium Toxicity Diagnosed by Dr. House

As mentioned above, Selenium overdose from Brazil nut ingestion (i.e. Selenosis) was "reported" in an episode of Dr House. In reality, there has never been a reported case of Selenosis from ingesting Brazil nuts in the US where selenosis is exceedingly rare, and usually due to exposure to an industrial or chemical plant accident, or dietary supplement manufacturing error.(17-21)

Toxicity of Selenium Excess

A report of selenium toxicity in the US appeared in the 2010 Archives of Internal Medicine. 200 cases of selenosis were caused by an error in manufacturing a liquid dietary supplement, which was subsequently recalled by the FDA. (13-14) The recalled dietary supplement contained 200 times the labeled concentration of selenium, providing 40,000 mcg per day. The recommended dosage for selenium is 200 mcg per day. For the 200 cases of selenosis identified in the report, the average serum selenium level was 751 mcg/ML. Symptoms of selenium toxicity include diarrhea, fatigue, hair loss, joint pain, nail discoloration or brittleness, and nausea. In view of this report, it would appear prudent to avoid liquid selenium preparations, and stick with tablets from known reputable sources. In addition, it is recommended that you work closely with a knowledgeable physician, for monitoring serum selenium levels prior to, and during supplementation.

Warning—Selenium Toxicity
Although exceedingly rare, selenium overdose and toxicity can occur, so it is important to stay within the dosage range recommended by a knowledgeable physician who can monitor selenium blood levels. The usual dosage range for selenium is 200-400 micrograms per day, and the recommended target is a blood level above 135 ng/ml.

Conclusion: The evidence is now overwhelming that dietary selenium is an essential mineral important for health. Selenium deficiency increases risk of cancer, and supplementation is beneficial for those with serum selenium levels below 135 mcg/ML. Since selenium is toxic at high doses, it is recommended that you work closely with a knowledgeable physician who can monitor levels.

References for Chapter 31. Selenium, Part Two, The Case for Selenium as Cancer Preventive

(1) http://www.ncbi.nlm.nih.gov/pubmed/12494476 Int J Cancer. 2003 Feb 20;103(5):664-70.
Serum selenium and risk of prostate cancer in U.S. blacks and whites. Vogt TM et al.

(2) http://www.ncbi.nlm.nih.gov/pmc/articles/PMC1472449/ Proc Natl Acad Sci U S A. 2006 May 23; 103(21): 8179-8184. Selenoprotein

deficiency accelerates prostate carcinogenesis in a transgenic model Veda Diwadkar-Navsariwala et al.

(3) http://cancerprevention.aacrjournals.org/content/2/5/484.abstract Methyl-Selenium Compounds Inhibit Prostate Carcinogenesis in the Transgenic Adenocarcinoma of Mouse Prostate Model with Survival Benefit by Lei Wang et al Hormel Institute, University of Minnesota, Austin, Minnesota Cancer Prevention Research AACR May 2009 2; 484

(4) http://www.ncbi.nlm.nih.gov/pubmed/16614422 J Nutr. 2006 May;136(5):1311-7. Both selenoproteins and low molecular weight selenocompounds reduce colon cancer risk in mice with genetically impaired selenoprotein expression. Irons R, Carlson BA et al.

(5) http://www.wjgnet.com/1948-5204/pdf/v1/i1/74.pdf Selenium as a chemopreventive agent in experimentally induced colon carcinogenesis. World J Gastrointest Oncol 2009 October 15; 1(1): 74-81 by Fereshteh Ezzati Ghadi et al. Panjab University, India

(6) http://www.ncbi.nlm.nih.gov/pubmed/3924710 Jpn J Cancer Res. 1985 May;76(5):374-7. Selenium in the blood of Japanese and American women with and without breast cancer and fibrocystic disease. Schrauzer GN, Molenaar T, Mead S, Kuehn K, Yamamoto H, Araki E.

(7) http://www.ncbi.nlm.nih.gov/pubmed/2484517 Biol Trace Elem Res. 1988 Jan-Apr;15:205-12. The distribution of selenium in human blood samples of Israeli population—comparison between normal and breast cancer cases. Chaitchik S, Shenberg C, Nir-El Y, Mantel M. Elias Sourasky Medical Center Tel-Aviv, Israel.

(8) http://cancerres.aacrjournals.org/cgi/content/abstract/51/17/4613 Cancer Research 51, 4613-4617, September 1, 1991. Inhibition of 7,12-Dimethylbenz(a)anthracene-induced Mammary Tumors and DNA Adducts by Dietary Selenite by Jinzhou Liu et al. University of Illinois

(9) http://www.ncbi.nlm.nih.gov/pubmed/19843683
Cancer Epidemiol Biomarkers Prev. 2009 Nov;18(11):2923-8. Selenium supplementation reduced oxidative DNA damage in adnexectomized BRCA1 mutations carriers. by Dziaman T et al. Poland.

(10) http://cebp.aacrjournals.org/content/14/5/1302.long
Cancer Epidemiology, Biomarkers & Prevention May 2005 14; 1302. Increased Rates of Chromosome Breakage in BRCA1 Carriers Are Normalized by Oral Selenium Supplementation by Elzbieta Kowalska et al.
Although our sample size was small, our results were highly significant; in every case, selenium supplementation resulted in a reduced frequency of chromosome breaks.

(11) http://www.hccpjournal.com/content/4/1/58 A Lowering of Breast and Ovarian Cancer Risk in Women with a BRCA1 Mutation by Selenium Supplementation of Diet by Tomasz Huzarski, Tomasz Byrski1, Jacek Gronwald1, Elżbieta Kowalska et al. Pomeranian Medical University, Szczecin, Poland in Hereditary Cancer in Clinical Practice 2006, 4:58

(12) http://www.cancer-therapy.org/CT1A/HTML/34%20%20Diamond%20et%20al.%20293-29%20c.htm Cancer Therapy Vol 1, 293-298, 2003. Allelic loss at the SEP15 locus in breast cancer by Mohamed A. Nasr, Ya Jun Hu, and Alan M. Diamond Department of Human Nutrition, University of Illinois at Chicago, Chicago, IL

(13) http://archinte.ama-assn.org/cgi/content/abstract/170/3/256 Acute Selenium Toxicity Associated With a Dietary Supplement Jennifer K. MacFarquhar et al Arch Intern Med. 2010;170(3):256-261.

(14) http://www.bt.cdc.gov/agent/selenium/supplements2008.asp Toxic Levels of Selenium in Dietary Supplements The US Food and Drug Administration and Total Body Essential Nutrition, Inc, have recalled approximately 1000 bottles of diet supplements "Total Body Formula" and "Total Body Mega Formula."

(15) http://www.ajcn.org/cgi/content/abstract/87/2/379 Brazil nuts: an effective way to improve selenium status. Am J Clin Nutr. 2008

Feb. Thomson CD, Chisholm A, McLachlan SK, Campbell JM. Department of Human Nutrition, University of Otago, Dunedin, New Zealand.

(16) http://www.vianutricia.com.br/imagens/naMidiaViaNutricia-Nutrition_Research.pdf Brazil nut ingestion increased plasma selenium but had minimal effects on lipids, apolipoproteins, and high-density lipoprotein function in human subjects from Nutrition Research 28 (2008) 151-155 by Célia C. Strunza et al. São Paulo, Brazil

(17) http://www.imdb.com/title/tt1123416/quotes House M.D." Whatever It Takes (2007)

(18) http://en.wikipedia.org/wiki/Whatever_It_Takes_(House) Whatever It Takes" is the sixth episode of the fourth season of House and the seventy-sixth episode overall. It aired on November 6, 2007.

(19) http://www.politedissent.com/archives/1800 November 6th, 2007 House—Episode 6 (Season 4): "Whatever It Takes"

(20) http://hightechsurvivor.blogspot.com/2007/11/brazil-nut-overdose.html Brazil Nut OverDose

(21) http://www.ncbi.nlm.nih.gov/pmc/articles/PMC1002502/pdf/westjmed00108-0050.pdf Fan AM, Kizer KW: Selenium-Nutritional, toxicologic, and clinical aspects. West J Med 1990 Aug; 153:160-167

(22) https://www.myriadpro.com/ Myriad Genetics Web Site.

CHAPTER 32

Selenium Part Three—Mega-Dose Vitamin Therapy in the ICU

Decades ago, when Linus Pauling and Abram Hoffer first proposed Mega-Dose Vitamin Therapy as a serious treatment, mainstream medicine and the news media promptly discredited this idea as quackery. To this day, the media faithfully bombards us with the message that vitamins and minerals are useless, harmful or even killing us.(1-6) When one considers the lowly vitamin pill as an economic rival to pharmaceutical drugs, and the dependence of the media on drug company advertising, the motivation to discredit mega-dose vitamins becomes all too obvious. Seemingly oblivious to this negative message, physicians quietly go about their business using Mega-Dose Vitamin Therapy in the intensive care unit (ICU) with considerable success. Recent reports of this have been appearing in medical journals, finally vindicating Linus Pauling and Abram Hoffer as yes, of course, they were right all along.(7-9)

Septic Shock—a Preterminal Event

Forty years ago, during my training days working in the intensive care unit, the onset of septic shock was a grave sign, and usually a preterminal event. In spite of the best treatment with high powered antibiotics and high dose hydrocortisone, these severely ill patients invariably succumbed. Survival was so rare, it was declared a miracle. While treatments have improved since the old days, septic shock still carries a fifty percent mortality rate.

Intravenous (I.V.) Selenium For Septic Shock in the ICU

In 1999, Dr Angstwurm showed that many critically ill patients have low selenium levels. Selenium is a component of glutathione peroxidase, the key selenoprotein anti-oxidant. In 2007, Dr Angstwurm recruited 249 septic shock patients from eleven intensive care units in Germany, and gave them intravenous (IV) selenium over a 14 day protocol. Results showed mortality reduced to 39% for the selenium treated group, compared to fifty percent mortality otherwise. An impressive result, considering the high mortality rate and futility of most other treatments.(10-11) In 2008, Dr Carlos studied septic shock patients and found that selenium levels could be used to predict clinical course. Those with the highest selenium levels had the best outcome, and the lowest selenium levels had the worst.(12)

A Basket of Mega-Dose Vitamins

If one antioxidant, selenium, was beneficial in the ICU setting, then perhaps a basket of antioxidants would be even more so. In 2008, Dr Giladi of Vanderbilt tested this hypothesis with a shopping cart of antioxidants. Intravenous Vitamin C, E and Selenium was given over a 7 day protocol to 2,200 ICU trauma patients, and compared to placebo. Dr Giladi reported a 28% mortality reduction for the Mega-Dose Vitamin group.(13) A second report on the same patient study group February 2010 showed that the Mega-Dose Vitamin group also benefited from a 53% reduction in abdominal wall infections, and 38% reduction in respiratory failure.(14)

Reducing Infection Rates, and Time on Ventilators

In 2006, Dr Berger reported that a trace mineral infusion with zinc, copper and selenium reduced by half the infection rates for burn patients in the ICU. These infections were nosocomial pneumonia and ventilator associated pneumonia. (15) In 2009, Dr Alison Avenell from Edinburgh, Scotland reported a 10-15% reduction in infection with pneumonia and Clostridia Difficile Enterocolitis in ICU patients treated with a 5 day protocol of IV selenium. (16) In November 2009, Dr El-Attar reported that trace mineral infusions with selenium, zinc and manganese given to patients with chronic lung disease resulted in reducing by half the time on mechanical ventilation.(17)

Animal Model of Inflammatory Hepatic Vasculitis

A 2000 report from China evaluated the effect of selenium and vitamin E on an animal model of experimental hepatic vasculitis (note: vasculitis is inflammation of the arteries). They found the two agents,

Selenium and Vitamin E dramatically reduced hepatic inflammation in the experimental animals down from 100% to 20%. (18)

Why Do We Need Selenium?

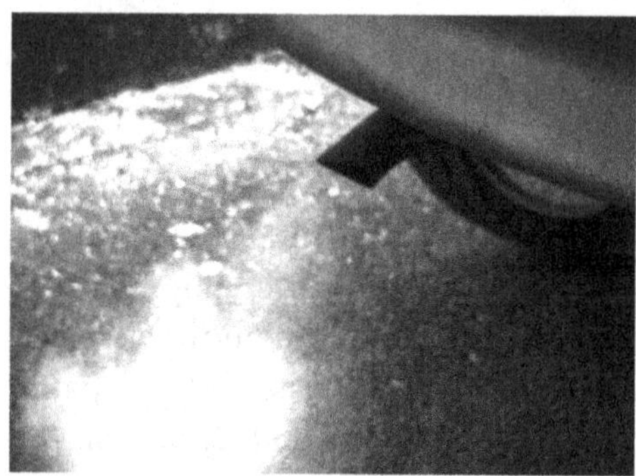

Exhaust from the tailpipe of a car.

To understand the importance of selenium, consider the toxic fumes produced by your automobile. You might be surprised to know your body makes the same foul toxic exhaust called byproducts of oxidation, also known as free radicals. Instead of an exhaust pipe to get rid of the oxidative by-products, our bodies have the selenoprotein anti-oxidant system. The main selenoprotein is glutathione peroxidase which works together with other antioxidants, such as Vitamin C and E, to remove the oxidative by-products of cellular energy production. Severe illness leads to depletion of selenoproteins and build up of oxidative by products which may overwhelm the body's defenses leading to catastrophic outcomes. Replenishing selenium and other anti-oxidants in this setting makes sense, and is in fact extremely beneficial.

Mega-Dose Vitamins outside the ICU

Dr Lamm reported Mega-Dose vitamins useful in prevention of cancer recurrence. Published in the 1994 Journal of Urology, Dr Lamm gave megadose vitamins A, B6, C, E and Zinc 65 to patients with biopsy proven bladder cancer. The patients were followed, and cancer recurrence was reduced in half for patients on the mega-dose vitamin therapy. (19)

For references: see web site www.bioidenticalhormones101.com

References for Chapter 32. Selenium Reduces Mortality in the ICU

(1) http://well.blogs.nytimes.com/2008/11/20/news-keeps-getting-worse-for-vitamins/ New York Times—November 20, 2008, News Keeps Getting Worse for Vitamins By TARA PARKER-POPE

(2) http://cbs5.com/health/vitamins.study.damaging.2.679134.html CBS News—Mar 17, 2008 Doctor: Vitamins Don't Work, Could Be Harmful (CBS 5)

(3) http://www.necn.com/Boston/Health/2009/02/09/Study-Multivitamins-not-that/1234208748.html Study: Multi-vitamins not that effective-

(4) http://articles.latimes.com/2008/dec/21/science/sci-vitamins21 LA Times—Vitamins aren't a cure-all, In fact, taking them does nothing to fight cancer, studies find. December 21, 2008 by Karen Kaplan—

(5) http://www.dailytelegraph.com.au/lifestyle/vitamins-could-be-killing-you/story-e6frf00i-1111113075043 Daily Telegraph—Vitamins could be killing you, By Tamara McLean From: The Daily Telegraph March 01, 2007

(6) http://www.throng.co.nz/inside-new-zealand/inside-new-zealand-series-premiere-are-vitamins-killing-you Inside New Zealand: Are Vitamins Killing You?

(7) http://journal.ics.ac.uk/pdf/1001038.pdf Review articles—Selenium in critically ill patients by S Strachan, D Wyncoll. The Intensive Care Society 2009 Volume 10, Number 1, January 2009 JICS

(8) http://www.pulmonaryreviews.com/09may/C1.html How Can Pharmaconutrition Benefit Patients in the ICU? Pulmonary Reviews Vol. 14, No. 5 May 2009.

(9) http://www.ncbi.nlm.nih.gov/pubmed/15605227
Intensive Care Med. 2005 Mar;31(3):327-37. Epub 2004 Dec 17. Antioxidant nutrients: a systematic review of trace elements and vitamins in the critically ill patient. by Heyland DK, Dhaliwal R, Suchner U, Berger MM. Department of Medicine, Queen's University, Kingston, ONT, Canada.

(10) http://www.ncbi.nlm.nih.gov/pubmed/17095947
Selenium in Intensive Care (SIC): Results of a prospective randomized, placebo-controlled, multiple-center study in patients with severe systemic inflammatory response syndrome, sepsis, and septic shock by Matthias W. A. Angstwurm, MD et al. Crit Care Med 2007 Vol. 35, No. 1

(11) http://www.ncbi.nlm.nih.gov/pubmed/10507602
Crit Care Med. 1999 Sep;27(9):1807-13. Selenium replacement in patients with severe systemic inflammatory response syndrome improves clinical outcome. Angstwurm MW, Schottdorf J, Schopohl J, Gaertner R.

(12) http://www.advancesinsepsis.com/pdfs/4407.pdf
Selenium in Early Sepsis: A Marker for Change? by W Graham Carlos, MD, Curtis Ramsey MS, and Joseph Fraiz, MD St Vincent Hospital and Health Systems, Indianapolis, IN, USA Adv Sepsis 2008;6(3):99-102.

(13) http://www.ncbi.nlm.nih.gov/pubmed/18596309
Impact of High-Dose Antioxidants on Outcomes in Acutely Injured Patients JPEN J Parenter Enteral Nutr. 2008 Jul-Aug;32(4):384-8. Bryan R. Collier, Aviram Giladi et al

(14) http://www.ncbi.nlm.nih.gov/pubmed/20149369
Injury. 2010 Feb 9. High-dose antioxidant administration is associated with a reduction in post-injury complications in critically ill trauma patients. by Giladi AM et al

(15) http://www.ncbi.nlm.nih.gov/pmc/articles/PMC1794452
Crit Care. 2006; 10(6): R153. Reduction of nosocomial pneumonia

after major burns by trace element supplementation: aggregation of two randomised trials. Mette M Berger,1 Philippe Eggimann,1 Daren K Heyland,2 René L Chioléro,1 Jean-Pierre Revelly,1 Andrew Day,2 Wassim Raffoul,3 and Alan Shenkin4

(16) http://www.bapen.org.uk/res_press_signet_results.html
Issued: 15 October 2009 RESULTS OF 'SIGNET' TRIAL REVEALED EXCLUSIVELY AT BAPEN CONFERENCE 2009 by Dr Alison Avenell, Health Services Research Unit, University of Aberdeen AB25 2ZD 2Professor P J Andrews, Dept of Anaesthesia, Critical Care and Pain Medicine, University of Edinburgh, Western General Hospital, Edinburgh Scotland.

(17) http://www.ncbi.nlm.nih.gov/pubmed/19761535
Respirology. 2009 Nov;14(8):1180-7. Epub 2009 Sep 16. Serum trace element levels in COPD patient: the relation between trace element supplementation and period of mechanical ventilation in a randomized controlled trial. El-Attar M, Said M, El-Assal G, Sabry NA, Omar E, Ashour L.Chest Department, Faculty of Medicine, Ain Shams University, Cairo, Egypt.

(18) http://www.ncbi.nlm.nih.gov/pubmed/11866925
Zhonghua Bing Li Xue Za Zhi. 2000 Aug;29(4):279-83. [Study on the modulation of the inflammatory response in mouse hepatic vasculitis with sodium selenite and vitamin E antioxidants] [Article in Chinese] by Xu M, Hou J, Wu Y, Ling Y. Institute of Basic Medical Sciences, Peking Union Medical College and Chinese Academy of Medical Sciences, Beijing 100005, China.

(19) http://www.ncbi.nlm.nih.gov/pubmed/8254816
J Urol. 1994 Jan;151(1):21-6. Megadose vitamins in bladder cancer: a double-blind clinical trial. Lamm DL, Riggs DR, Shriver JS, vanGilder PF, Rach JF, DeHaven JI. Department of Urology, West Virginia University School of Medicine, Morgantown.

(20) http://www.ncbi.nlm.nih.gov/pubmed/20424130
Cancer Prev Res (Phila Pa). 2010 Apr 27. [Epub ahead of print] A Large Prospective Study of SEP15 Genetic Variation, Interaction with Plasma

Selenium Levels, and Prostate Cancer Risk and Survival. Penney KL, Schumacher FR, Li H, Kraft P, Morris JS, Kurth T, Mucci LA, Hunter DJ, Kantoff PW, Stampfer MJ, Ma J.

(21) http://www.ncbi.nlm.nih.gov/pubmed/20413070
J Trace Elem Med Biol. 2010 Apr;24(2):119-23. Epub 2009 Oct 23. Supplementation of selenium reduces chemical hepatocarcinogenesis in male Sprague-Dawley rats. Alwahaibi N, Mohamed J, Alhamadani A. Department of Biomedical Sciences, Faculty of Allied Health Sciences, Universiti Kebangsaan Malaysia (UKM), Julan Raja Muda Abdul Aziz, 50300 Kuala Lumpur, Malaysia.

(22) http://acam.typepad.com/blog/2009/09/selling-the-vitamins-dont-work-myth-whats-the-real-story.html September 02, 2009 Selling the "Vitamins Don't Work" Myth: What's the Real Story? by John Pittman, MD

(23) http://www.pharmapal.com/pharmapal/pdf/selenase.pdf Selenase from BioSyn

(24) http://www.biomedcentral.com/content/pdf/cc5109.pdf
Seleno-enzymes and seleno-compounds: the two faces of selenium by Xavier Forceville

(25) http://ccforum.com/content/10/6/180 BioMed Central. Selenium protects cells and inhibits many inflammatory cell mechanisms through antioxidant seleno-enzymes.

CHAPTER 33

Selenium for Hashimoto's Thyroiditis

Susan has Hashimoto's Thyroiditis, an autoimmune thyroid disorder causing fatigue, puffy face and muscle weakness. For the past year, she had been under the care of other doctors who started her on Synthroid, the most widely used thyroid medication. Later, her doctors re-tested the thyroid antibody levels (TPO thyroid peroxidase and thyroglobulin antibodies). The disturbing thing was that her antibodies kept climbing higher on each follow up lab test. The doctors had no explanation, so she came to see me, asking if there was anything else that could be done.

Selenium Can Decrease Antibody Levels

As it turns out, a trace mineral called selenium plays an important role in thyroid. Selenium deficiency has been implicated in the etiology of Hashimoto's Thyroiditis, and selenium supplementation has been found beneficial.

Three Selenium Studies Show Benefits of Selenium for Hashimoto's Thyroiditis

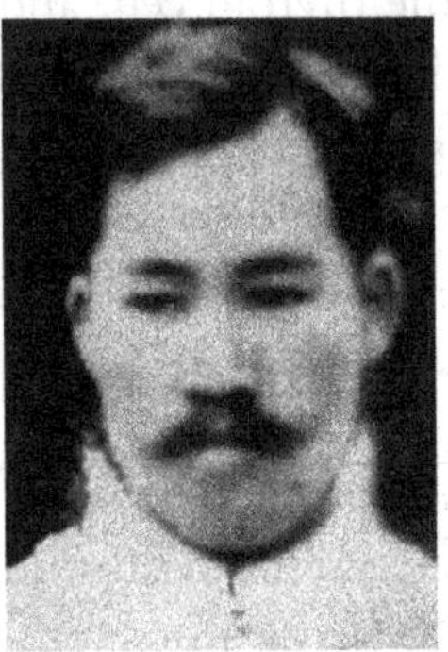

1912 Photograph of Dr. Hakaru Hashimoto, credited with the discovery of Hashimoto's Thyroiditis. Source: reprinted in: Hashimoto K. My Father and his Teachers. Endocr J. 49, 4, 389-91. 2002. Author Unknown. Public domain photo Courtesy of wikimedia commons.

The first study by Mazokopakis from Crete was published in the 2007 Thyroid Journal.(1) This study reported a 21 per cent reduction in TPO antibodies after one year of seleno-methionine supplements (200 mcg per day). A second study from Germany in the 2002 Journal of

Clinical Endocrinology & Metabolism showed a 40 per cent reduction in antibody levels after selenium supplementation with 9 of 36 (25%) patients completely normalizing their antibody levels.(2) A third study done in Turkey by Omer Turker et al. was published in the 2006 Journal of Endocrinology. (5) They showed a 30 per cent decrease in anti-thyroid antibodies after three months of L-seleno-methionine supplementation at 200 mcg per day in women with Hashimoto's Thyroiditis. The starting average Thyroid Peroxidase (TPO) antibodies of 803 and after three months the average was 572.

Why is Selenium So Important for Thyroid Function?

Recent advances in research into thyroid cell physiology shows that selenium is very important for thyroid function. (3-4)(11-12) There are at least 30 selenium dependent proteins, including the glutathione peroxidase enzyme, and the Iodothyronine deiodinases enzyme (this is the one that converts thyroxine (T4) to bioactive (T3). These proteins all need selenium as a co-factor in order to function properly. The selenoprotein, glutathione peroxidase, protects thyroid cells from damage by hydrogen peroxide (H2O2) produced by the thyroid cell. H2O2 is needed as a normal step in thyroid hormone production. However, excess hydrogen peroxide (H202) can damage the thyroid cell. In the event of selenium deficiency, the glutathione peroxidase enzyme cannot do its job protecting the thyroid cell, and the thyroid cells are damaged by excess H2O2.(11-12) The current theory is that this damaged cell material is then recognized by the immune system as foreign, leading to Hashimoto's autoimmune disease.

Back to the Patient

Susan was started on selenomethionine 200 mcg per day. In addition, her thyroid medication was switched from Synthroid to natural desiccated thyroid. Three months later Susan returned for follow up labs which showed a decline in her thyroid antibody levels. Although not all patients will see a dramatic decline in antibody levels, I have found that many patients will benefit from selenium supplementation.

Thyroid Testing and Treatment

A good thyroid testing protocol includes the following lab values, Thyroid Stimulating Hormone (TSH), Free T3 (tri-iodiodothyronine), Free T4, Thyroid Peroxidase (TPO) Antibodies, Thyroglobulin (Tgb) Antibodies, selenium level, and iodine level. The thyroid panel is usually part of a larger evaluation with additional lab tests tailored to the clinical history and examination. A good thyroid treatment protocol uses natural desiccated thyroid medication such as Nature-Throid from RLC labs. Dosage for natural desiccated thyroid medication varies, based on residual thyroid function, body weight, starting thyroid labs, and other variables.

Selenium Safety or Toxicity Depends on Dosage

Although Selenium is an inexpensive mineral supplement available without a prescription at the health food store, I would recommend working closely with your physician if you are considering selenium supplementation. Although selenium is generally considered safe at standard doses, very high dosage can cause selenium toxicity. In addition, your physician will determine if you need thyroid medication, the type and dosage of the medication, etc. By the way, for those looking for a food source for selenium, Brazil Nuts are high in selenium.

Testing and Treatment in Hashimoto's Thyroiditis

Thyroid function in Hashimoto's Thyroiditis can have a variable course, with thyroid function varying, and the thyroid medication dosage may vary as thyroid function changes. Lab studies at any one time may show low, normal or high thyroid function in patients with elevated antibody levels and Hashimoto's thyroid disease. Dr. David Brownstein's protocols are excellent recommendations regarding thyroid testing and treatment. See his book, "Overcoming Thyroid Disorders" 2nd Edition which shows how a holistic treatment program can effectively treat Hashimoto's Disease. His book, Overcoming Thyroid Disorders provides information on safe and effective natural therapies with over 30 actual case studies. The book contains information on: Natural

Thyroid Hormone, Bioidentical Natural Hormones, Diet, Vitamins and Minerals Important for Thyroid Function.(7)

Web Sites with Reliable Information about Selenium for Hashimoto's

Janie Bowthorpe's book and the Stop the Thyroid Madness Blog is an excellent source of reliable information. Mary Shomon's, Thyroid web site and newsletter is also an excellent source of reliable information. Beware and avoid anonymous message boards that may give false or incorrect information about selenium. One question to ask about information on anonymous message boards: Is the information backed up by citations or references in the peer reviewed medical literature? If not, then it may not be reliable information.

For references see web site: www.bioidenticalhormones101.com

References for Chapter 33. Selenium for Hashimoto's Thyroiditis

(1) http://www.ncbi.nlm.nih.gov/pubmed/17696828
Thyroid. 2007 Jul;17(7):609-12. Effects of 12 months treatment with L-selenomethionine on serum anti-TPO Levels in Patients with Hashimoto's thyroiditis. Mazokopakis EE, Papadakis JA, Papadomanolaki MG, Batistakis AG, Giannakopoulos TG, Protopapadakis EE, Ganotakis ES. Department of Internal Medicine, University Hospital of Heraklion, Crete, Greece.

(2) http://jcem.endojournals.org/cgi/content/full/87/4/1687
The Journal of Clinical Endocrinology & Metabolism Vol. 87, No. 4 1687-1691, 2002 Selenium supplementation in patients with autoimmune thyroiditis decreases thyroid peroxidase antibodies concentrations. Gärtner R, Gasnier BC, Dietrich JW, Krebs B, Angstwurm MW. Department of Endocrinology, Medizinische Klinik Innenstadt, University of Munich, D-80336 Munich, Germany.

(3) http://www.ncbi.nlm.nih.gov/pubmed/12487769
Thyroid. 2002 Oct;12(10):867-78.The impact of iron and selenium deficiencies on iodine and thyroid metabolism: biochemistry and relevance to public health. Zimmermann MB, Köhrle J.Laboratory

for Human Nutrition, Swiss Federal Institute of Technology, Zürich, Switzerland.

(4) http://nuclmed.web.auth.gr/magazine/eng/jan07/8.pdf Hashimoto's thyroiditis and the role of selenium. Current concepts. by Hellenic in the Journal of Nuclear Medicine January—April 2007 Review Article

(5) http://joe.endocrinology-journals.org/cgi/content/full/190/1/151 Journal of Endocrinology (2006) 190, 151-156. Selenium treatment in autoimmune thyroiditis: 9-month follow-up with variable doses Omer Turker et al Thyroidology Unit, Department of Nuclear Medicine, GATA Haydarpasa, Istanbul, Turkey

(6) http://edrv.endojournals.org/cgi/content/abstract/26/7/944 Endocrine Reviews 26 (7): 944-984, 2005 Selenium, the Thyroid, and the Endocrine System by J. Köhrle, F. Jakob, B. Contempré and J. E. Dumont Institut für Experimentelle Endokrinologie (J.K.), Charité Universitätsmedizin Berlin, Humboldt Universität, D-10098 Berlin, Germany;

(7) https://www.drbrownstein.com/bookstore_Thyroid.php David Brownstein,M.D. Overcoming Thyroid Disorders, 2nd Edition, Medical Alternatives Press, Inc.

(8) http://lpi.oregonstate.edu/infocenter/minerals/selenium/ Selenium Page. Linus Pauling Institute Micronutrient Research for Optimum Health

(9) http://www.stopthethyroidmadness.com/blog/ Stop the Thyroid Madness Blog Janie Bowthorpe

(10) http://thyroid.about.com/bio/Mary-Shomon-350.htm Mary Shomon Thyroid Web Site

(11) http://www.ncbi.nlm.nih.gov/pmc/articles/PMC2721352/ Biologics. 2008 June; 2(2): 265-273. Selenium and thyroid autoimmunity Roberto Negro

(12) http://jn.nutrition.org/content/127/6/1214.full Dietary Iodine and Selenium Interact To Affect Thyroid Hormone Metabolism of Rats by Christine S. Hotz, Dennis W. fitzpatrick, Keith D. Trick, and Mary R. L'Abbé

Section Nine: Your Drug May Be The Problem. Are You Taking A Bad Drug?

CHAPTER 34

Fosamax Induced Bilateral Femur Fractures

I received this letter from a lady who suffered bilateral mid-femur fractures after ten years of taking the anti-osteoporosis drug, Fosamax™ (Alendronate):

> *Dear Dr. Dach,*
>
> *I am a femur-fracture survivor . . . bilateral. The right leg broke in March, the left one in July, 2009. I also suffered a compression fracture at L1 in May.*
>
> *I was given Fosamax™ 10 years ago as a preventive measure. Now I am worse than I would have been 20 years down the road. I cannot begin to tell you that there are women breaking a leg everyday! And they do not know why. It was through the fact, that the orthopedic doctor who took my emergency case on the first leg, had just received some information about the bilateral fractures. If you held my x-ray up against several other women's, you could not tell us apart!*
>
> *I hope you continue to write and correspond about this important subject. My life has been taken away from me in a way that I never dreamed would happen.*
>
> *Thank You, VS.*

My Reply to VS—These Are Bad Drugs

Dear VS,

Thanks coming forward to share your story of Fosamax induced Femur Fractures. As you know, this type of fracture is very unusual, and only occurs in abnormal bone. This is called "**pathological fracture**" and is caused by change in bone quality induced by Fosamax™. These pathological mid femur fractures heal very poorly even with the best of treatment. Fosamax™, Actonel™, Boniva™ and all the bisphosphonates work by killing the osteoclast bone cells. This creates pathologic abnormalities in bone architecture that leads to increased bone density on the DEXA scan. Paradoxically, this dense bone is weaker, brittle and prone to pathological fracture at the mid-shaft level of the femur. A fracture at this mid—femur location is highly characteristic of a Fosamax induced fracture. We have been hoodwinked by the Sally Fields Television ads and deceitful marketing campaigns. **These are bad drugs.** I predict that as mid-femur pathologic fractures become more common, people will start to wake up, and eventually these drugs will be banned. VS, I am very sorry that this happened, and hopefully your efforts will educate others about this pitfall.

Sincerely, Jeffrey Dach MD

Reports of Spontaneous Mid Femur Fracture on Fosamax

Clarita Odvina MD reported nine cases of spontaneous femur fracture on Fosamax™ (Alendronate). (2) Dr. Goh, a doctor in Singapore, identified nine more cases in his 2007 report of subtrochanteric femur fractures with minimal trauma in women on long term Fosamax. (3) Joseph M Lane MD reported 15 cases of spontaneous femur fracture in women on Fosamax (Alendronate). His report appeared in the New England Journal March 20, 2008. (4) Dr. Lane found that "*ten of the 15 patients were found to share a* ***unique radiographic pattern****, defined as a simple transverse or oblique (30°) fracture with beaking of the cortex and diffuse cortical thickening of the proximal femoral shaft.*" (4)

More Case Reports from Jennifer Schneider MD

These additional case reports were published in 2009 Geriatrics by Jennifer Schneider MD (1):

> *"A 66-year old, previously healthy woman developed a spontaneous stress fracture of her right foot, which eventually healed. Nine months later she took a step in her bedroom and collapsed to the floor. An x-ray revealed a nontraumatic fracture of her right femur. She underwent surgery with placement of an intramedullary rod. Her physician told her she had most likely had a stress fracture, which became a completed fracture. A bone scan done shortly after her surgery revealed a stress fracture of her left femur. Some months later she underwent prophylactic rodding of the left femur. The patient had been on alendronate for 7 years.*
>
> *A 65-year woman visiting Europe stepped off the bottom step of a van and collapsed. An x-ray revealed a nontraumatic fracture of her left femur. She had been experiencing a dull ache in her left femur for some months. The patient underwent placement of an intramedullary rod. One year later she developed a dull ache in her right femur. A bone scan showed a stress fracture in the right femur. A bone specialist recommended prophylactic rodding of the right femur, which was done. The patient had been on alendronate for 9 years.*
>
> *A 59-year-old-woman took a step, her right leg gave out, and she fell to the ground as she heard her leg break. Her femur was fractured. The orthopedic surgeon on call told her, "We don't usually see this type of fracture without trauma." For the preceding year she'd experienced pain in her right thigh, which was severe enough to cause limping. An x-ray had been negative, and her primary care physician thought she had fibromyalgia. She had been on alendronate for more than 5 years." endquote Dr Jennifer Schneider. (1)*

Drug Companies Fight Back Attempting to Exonerate Fosamax

The drug companies are aware of this problem, and are fighting back by paying doctors to deny the link between fosamax and pathological fracture of the femur. An example is this study of the Danish National Bone Registry: (6)

"Something is Rotten in Denmark"

The title is: Subtrochanteric and Diaphyseal Femur Fractures in Patients Treated With Alendronate: A Register-Based National Cohort Study by Bo Abrahamsen in the June 2009 Journal of Bone and Mineral Research. The author says, *"Recent reports have found long-term Alendronate use to be common in patients with subtrochanteric or proximal diaphyseal femur fracture, raising concerns that these fractures could be a consequence of excessive suppression of bone turnover." (6)*

Fosamax Doubles the Risk of Subtrochanteric Fracture

Even though the Danish Registry data actually showed the Fosamax™ (alendronate) group had an increased incidence of subtrochanteric fractures (2.9 vs. 1.6 per 1000 patient years), nonetheless, Dr. Bo Abrahamsen concluded the cause was osteoporosis and **NOT the Drug**!! Here is the author's conclusion: *"Subtrochanteric/diaphyseal femur fractures . . . are best classified as osteoporotic fractures."* In my opinion, this conclusion is not only wrong, it is blatantly wrong. These mid-femur fractures are NOT osteoporotic fractures. This is blatantly obvious. I will explain why below.

Authors On Drug Company Pay Roll

Here is a list of author's competing interests:

> *Dr. Abrahamsen receives consultancy fees from Nycomed and Novartis, research grants from Roche, and speaker's fees from Servier, Eli Lilly, and MSD. Dr. Eiken receives speaker fees from Nycomed, Roche, and Servier. Dr. Eastell receives research funding or consultation honoraria from Amgen, AstraZeneca, Aventis, Eli Lilly, GlaxoSmithKline, Hologic, Interleukin Genetics, Kyphon, Lilly, Maxygen, Nastech Pharmaceuticals, Nestle Research Center, New Zealand Milk Limited, Novartis, Novo-Nordisk, Ono Pharma, Organon, Osteologix, Paraxel, Pfizer, Procter & Gamble, Roche Diagnostics, Sanofi-aventis, Servier, Shire, Transpharma Medical Limited, Unilever, and Unipath.*

Sound familiar?

Fosamax™ Induced Fractures have a UNIQUE Radiographic Appearance

Joseph M Lane MD reported a unique radiographic pattern of these Fosamax induced fractures.(4) This means these spontaneous mid-femur fractures are pathological fractures induced by the drug, and virtually **NEVER** happen unless the patient is on a bisphosphonate drug like Fosamax™.

The Anatomy Dictates that the Femoral Neck Will Fracture First

Osteoporotic fractures present most commonly as compression fractures of the vertebral bodies, or as femoral neck fractures. Even in cases of severe osteoporosis, the femur never spontaneously fractures at the mid femur level simply because the anatomy dictates that the femoral neck will fracture first. I have known this from personal experience as a radiologist for thirty years reading X-Rays of fracture cases. A spontaneous mid-femur fracture is extremely rare and indicates a pathologic fracture caused by a drug or disease process.

Fosamax Same Unique Pattern As Rare Genetic Bone Disease of Toulouse Lautrec

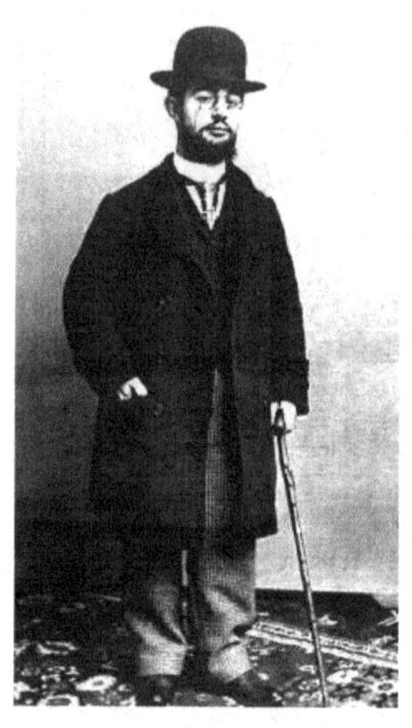

Henri de Toulouse-Lautrec, one of the greatest painters of the Post-Impressionist period. 1864—1901. Note short stature caused by spontaneous bilateral mid-femur fractures as a child from genetic bone disease called pycnodysostosis

Another important observation is the similarity between Fosamax™ induced femur fractures and a rare genetic bone disease, Pycnodysostosis, also called Toulouse Lautrec's Disease.(7-8) This genetic disease causes malfunctioning osteoclasts, the same mode of action of the drug, Fosamax™. The famous French Impressionist artist, Toulouse Lautrec suffered bilateral femur fractures as a child which never healed properly resulting in short stature, as shown in old photographs.(8) Lautrec's femur fractures had the same unique radiographic appearance described by Dr Joseph Lane for Fosamax™ induced femur fracture.(7-8)

Summary: Fosamax™ induced mid-femur fractures have a unique radiographic appearance, and share this unique appearance with a rare genetic bone disease (Toulouse Lautrec's Disease). Therefore, these mid-femur fractures are not typical osteoporotic fractures, they are a distinct form of pathologic fracture induced by the drugs, Fosamax, Actonel and Boniva. These are "Bad Drugs" that should be banned or severely curtailed.

References for Chapter 34. Fosamax™ Induced Femur Fractures

(1) http://www.jenniferschneider.com/articles/Bisphosphonates.pdf Bisphosphonates and low-impact femoral fractures: Current evidence on alendronate-fracture risk by Jennifer P. Schneider, MD, PhD. Geriatrics.2009;64(1):18-23.

(2) http://jcem.endojournals.org/cgi/content/full/90/3/1294 The Journal of Clinical Endocrinology & Metabolism Vol. 90,

No. 3 1294-1301 Severely Suppressed Bone Turnover: A Potential Complication of Alendronate Therapy Clarita V. Odvina, Joseph E. Zerwekh, D. Sudhaker Rao, Naim Maalouf, Frank A. Gottschalk and Charles Y. C. Pak

(3) http://www.jbjs.org.uk/cgi/content/abstract/89-B/3/349 Journal of Bone and Joint Surgery—British Volume, Vol 89-B, Issue 3, 349-353. Subtrochanteric insufficiency fractures in patients on alendronate therapy A CAUTION, S.-K. Goh et al.

(4) http://content.nejm.org/cgi/content/full/358/12/1304 NEJM Volume 358:1304-1306 March 20, 2008 Number 12. Atypical Fractures of the Femoral Diaphysis in Postmenopausal Women Taking Alendronate Brett A. Lenart, B.S. Dean G. Lorich, M.D. Joseph M. Lane, M.D. Weill Cornell Medical College New York, NY 10021

(5) http://www.medpagetoday.com/MeetingCoverage/ASBMR/10904 Alendronate Exonerated in 'Atypical' Femoral Fractures By Michael Smith, North American Correspondent, MedPage Today. September 15, 2008 Reviewed by Robert Jasmer, MD; Associate Clinical Professor of Medicine, University of California, San Francisco.

(6) http://onlinelibrary.wiley.com/doi/10.1359/jbmr.081247/pdf J BMR, Volume 24, Number 6, 2009, Subtrochanteric and Diaphyseal Femur Fractures in Patients Treated With Alendronate: A Register-Based National Cohort Study Bo Abrahamsen,1 Pia Eiken,2 and Richard Eastell

(7) http://hormones.gr/preview.php?c_id=38 Pycnodysostosis: Toulouse-Lautrec's and Aesop's disease? By Christos S. Bartsocas. HORMONES 2002, 1(4):260-262

(8) http://www.ncbi.nlm.nih.gov/pmc/articles/PMC1811887/?tool=pubmed Proc R Soc Med. 1970 Aug; 63(8):800-5. Toulouse-Lautrec—triumph over infirmity. Cawthorne T.

CHAPTER 35

Fosamax™ for Pre-Osteoporosis, A Bad Idea

A number of patients have recently told me their primary care doctors started them on Fosamax™ for "pre-osteoporosis" a condition less severe than full blown osteoporosis, also called "osteopenia". This is a very bad idea. Osteopenia is defined by the DEXA T-Score (see below).

DEXA Scan T-Score Definition of Osteopenia	
	DEXA Scan T-Score
Normal Bone Density	Above -2.0
Osteopenia (Pre-Osteoporosis)	-2.0 to -2.5
Osteoporosis	-2.5 to -3.5

Problem One: The Fosamax™ (Alendronate) medical study for FDA approval failed to show any benefit for the Osteopenia Group. Fracture rates actually went up for the Osteopenia Group. This data was published by Cummings in JAMA in 1998 (this is called the F.I.T. study, which stands for Fracture Intervention Trial).(8)

Problem Two: Bisphosphonates drugs like Fosamax have severe adverse side effects of jaw necrosis (OJN), spontaneous femur fracture, atrial fibrillation (a heart rhythm disturbance), and severe bone and joint pain. Another common adverse effect is esophageal erosion, heartburn and esophageal reflux.(10)

Fosamax, A Bad Drug in Litigation—How to Recognize a Bad Drug?

One of the early warning signs of a bad drug is ongoing drug litigation for adverse side effects. This calls the drug into question as a **BAD DRUG**. Fosamax drug litigation began August 2009 against Merck by plaintiff, Shirley Boles, age 71, who suffered ONJ (osteonecrosis of the jaw) allegedly from Fosamax. OJN, osteonecrosis of the jaw, is a well known adverse side effect of Fosamax, which has been heavily documented in the dental and oral surgery medical literature. Merck faces an onslaught of more than 900 cases awaiting litigation. (2-5)

Spontaneous Femur Fracture Induced by Fosamax

Another warning sign of a **BAD DRUG** is spontaneous femur fracture (with no trauma) that occur in women on Fosamax. A number of these embarrassing reports have appeared in the New England Journal of Medicine and the Orthopedic Surgery medical literature.(9)(13)(14) Two more embarrassing studies came out at the 2010 American Academy of Orthopaedic Surgeons (AAOS) Meeting showing Fosamax disturbs bone formation, and implicates Fosamax in spontaneous mid-femur fractures (without trauma). These reports came from the Hospital for Special Surgery (HSS) and Columbia University Medical Center. (11)

FDA Warning Letters—Another Red Flag

Another sign of a **BAD DRUG** is the FDA Warning letter.(1) Physicians received such an FDA warning letter telling them about severe, incapacitating bone and joint pain caused by Fosamax. What causes this pain? No answer there. I would suggest underlying stress fracture as the cause for the severe bone pain. Another FDA safety announcement was made March 10, 2010 (12),and another FDA warning letter was sent to physicians on October 12, 2010, warning about "*Possible increased risk of thigh bone fracture with bisphosphonates*".(18-19)(25) The drug companies have not yet explained why this "wonder drug" intended to prevent fractures actually causes spontaneous femur fractures.

Consumer Complaints Against Fosamax

Another warning sign of a bad drug is the number of consumer complaints on message boards which can be seen by anyone with an internet connection. You are encouraged to perform an internet search of the key words where you will find hundreds of consumer complaints.(6)

Why is Fosamax a BAD Drug?

There is no question that bisphosphonates drugs increase bone density as measured on the DEXA scan. I would be the first to admit this. I have seen it routinely. So, one might ask, why are these "Bad Drugs"? The answer is the following: The increased bone density is cosmetic and does not equate with stronger bone. This is deceptive. Simply put, the bisphosphonate drugs create pathologic bone that is weak and brittle, prone to spontaneous fracture and osteo-necrosis. The drug actually does the reverse of what it is intended to do.

FDA Says Osteoporosis Drugs Cause Femur Fractures—The Perfect Storm

For years, I have been warning patients, friends and family members about the adverse effects of osteoporosis drugs. Finally, after years of dragging their feet, the FDA issued a news release on Oct 13, 2010 warning of "possible" risk of femur fractures caused by the osteoporosis drugs such as Fosamax™, Boniva™, and Actonel™. (18-19) They also added a new warning label recommended by a the Bone Task Force assigned to examine this issue.(20-21) The Task Force found that almost all women suffering from atypical fractures of the mid femur were on bisphosphonate osteoporosis drugs like Fosamax™, Actonel™, and Boniva™. (21) (Note: The task force consists of experts of the American Society of Bone and Mineral Research). This same ASBMR task force previously issued a 2007 report on these same osteoporosis drugs causing osteonecrosis of the jaw (OJN).(26) This is a condition in which the jaw bone literally "falls apart", usually after a dental procedure. When a drug adverse effect is identical to the underlying disease the drug is supposed to treat, we have "the perfect storm". Osteoporosis drugs are marketed and sold as fracture preventive, and are not supposed to cause fractures. Yet, we now have evidence that this class of drugs not only weakens bones, they also cause spontaneous femur fractures. This is a very bad thing, and indicates a very profound problem with the drug.

Dr Susan Ott Reports on Stress Fractures Induced by Bisphosphonates

At a 2010 medical meeting, of the Bone Society (ASBMR) in Toronto, Susan Ott MD presented data on atypical femur fractures induced by osteoporosis drugs like Fosamax. (27) She reviewed X-Rays and data from a large California HMO called Kaiser Permanente. Over a three year period, Kaiser HMO doctors reported 135 atypical femur fractures out of a total of 16,000 broken femurs. Almost all of the 135 patients were on bisphosphonate drugs (96.4%), similar to Fosamax. Dr. Ott reported these atypical fractures have a characteristic X-ray appearance, and may occur bilaterally. The fracture is typically through the mid-shaft of the femur, and the outer bony margin typically thickened, indicating a stress fracture. These fractures occur spontaneously, on their own, with no fall or traumatic event. Patients typically report pain in the area for weeks or months before the actual fracture. Dr. Ott reported an incidence of 0.25 % for atypical mid femur fractures in patients on bisphosphonate drugs for 12 years. Dr Ott is not the first to describe the link between Fosamax and femur fractures. A 2009 report from Sweden by Dr. Aspberger disclosed that the incidence of mid femur stress fracture is **50 times higher** for patients on bisphosphonates drugs compared to untreated women (0.1% vs. 0.002 %). (39)

Stress Fractures from Osteoporosis Drugs

Dr Isaacs from Australia reported Aug 2010 that bisphosphonate drugs cause insufficiency fractures of the femur (also called stress fractures). (28) Dr Isaacs reviewed X-rays of one hundred consecutive patients suffering from spontaneous femur fracture. Some cases occurred before and some after the availability of bisphosphonate drugs. He found X-Ray evidence of pre-existing stress fractures in all 41 patients taking bisphosphonate drugs. However, before the bisphosphonate era, in the group **NOT TAKING** bisphosphonates, there were no pre-existing stress fractures seen in any of the twenty one patients in this group. These patients had their spontaneous femur fracture before the bisphosphonate era. Dr. Isaacs suggested that bisphosphonate drugs cause damage and weakens bone, making it susceptible to painful stress fracture, the initiating lesion later progressing to complete femur fracture. This explains the prodromal pain before the spontaneous femur fracture.

What is the Next Step—A Black Box Warning or Ban the Drug?

The recent medical literature has been inundated with case reports and population studies linking bisphosphonate drugs like Fosamax and Actonel to atypical mid-femur fractures, as well as stress fractures. The message is fairly obvious that there is something dreadfully wrong here. When we have a drug that causes the same disease it is intended to prevent, we have the "perfect storm". Drug manufacturers use ghost-writers to manipulate data from clinical trials to make the drug look good, and clinicians can deny the obvious when patients come in with fractures while on the drug, blaming the fracture on underlying osteoporosis, and not an adverse effect of the osteoporosis drug. My prediction is that most educated patients and doctors will abandon this bisphosphonate family of osteoporosis drugs, and the FDA will eventually issue a Black Box Warning or perhaps a ban on the drug. When this happens, we can say goodbye to another "bad drug".

Bad Drug Warning
Bisphosphonate osteoporosis drugs have had several FDA warning letters and are in drug litigation for adverse effects. Rather than make bones stronger, these drugs actually weaken the bone, causing stress fractures and spontaneous femur fractures. Jaw bone disintegration from these drugs has also been reported. In the future, it is likely this class of drugs will either be banned, or will fall into disuse.

Reverse Osteoporosis Naturally-Our Program

Rather than use a "Bad Drug", like the bisphosphonates such as Fosamax, a far better solution for reversing osteoporosis is a combined program of lifestyle modification, diet, nutrition, exercise and bio-identical hormone supplementation.

Reverse Osteoporosis Naturally Without Drugs
1) Modify diet to an alkaline diet which halts the calcium loss associated with acid excretion. The calcium is pulled from the bones and used as a buffering agent for acid excretion. Test with home pH strips to determine success of alkalinization program.
2) Nutritional supplement with high quality calcium product containing bioavailable calcium, magnesium, boron, strontium, and Vitamin K.
3) Test for, and optimize Vitamin D and Magnesium levels.
4) Engage in a regular weight bearing exercise program, as tolerated.
5) Test for, and optimize hormone levels for estradiol, progesterone, testosterone, and DHEA.

For more on Bad Drugs, see my previous e-book, Natural Medicine 101 which can be found at www.naturalmedicine101.com.

For references and links, see my web site: www.bioidenticalhormones101.com

Chapter 35. Fosamax™ for Pre-Osteoporosis, a Bad Idea

(1) http://www.newsinferno.com/archives/2326
Actonel, Fosamax, other Osteoporosis Drugs Draw FDA Pain Warning. Date Published: Monday, January 7th, 2008

(2) http://www.theage.com.au/world/down-to-the-bone-20090807-ecwy.html Down to the bone RAY MOYNIHAN August 8, 2009

(3) http://www.fiercepharma.com/story/bellwether-fosomax-trial-starts-today/2009-08-10 Bellwether Fosamax trial starts today August 10, 2009 by Tracy Staton. Fierce Pharma.

(4) http://www.bloomberg.com/apps/news?pid=20601103&sid=aN.O.OLorMnc Merck Faces First Trial of Claim That Fosamax Attacks Jawbone By Thom Weidlich and Margaret Cronin Fisk Bloomberg News

(5) http://www.youhavealawyer.com/blog/2008/08/21/fosamax-lawsuits-pile-up/ Fosamax Lawsuits Continue to Pile Up Against Merck August 21st, 2008 by Austin Kirk

(6) http://www.consumeraffairs.com/rx/fosamax.html consumer complaints about Fosamax

(7) http://www.fda.gov/Drugs/DrugSafety/PostmarketDrugSafetyInformationforPatientsandProviders/ucm124165.htm Information for Healthcare Professionals: Bisphosphonates (marketed as Actonel, Actonel+Ca, Aredia, Boniva, Didronel, Fosamax, Fosamax+D, Reclast, Skelid, and Zometa) FDA ALERT [1/7/2008]:

(8) http://jama.ama-assn.org/content/280/24/2077.full
Effect of Alendronate on Risk of Fracture in Women With Low Bone Density but Without Vertebral Fractures Results From the Fracture Intervention Trial Steven R. Cummings, MD et al. for the Fracture Intervention Trial Research Group JAMA. 1998;280(24):2077-2082

(9) http://www.nejm.org/doi/full/10.1056/NEJMc0707493
Atypical Fractures of the Femoral Diaphysis in Postmenopausal Women Taking Alendronate Brett A. Lenart, B.S. Dean G. Lorich, M.D.Joseph M. Lane, M.D. N Engl J Med 2008; 358:1304-1306March 20, 2008

(10) http://blogs.consumerreports.org/health/2010/03/safety-news-on-fosamax-and-boniva-should-you-still-take-fosamax-or-boniva-to-strengthen-bones-.html March 12, 2010 Should you still take Fosamax or Boniva to strengthen bones? By Alan Cassels. Consumer Reports Health Blog.

(11) http://www6.aaos.org/news/pemr/releases/release.cfm?releasenum=877
Quantity vs. Quality: Long-Term se of Bone-Building Osteoporosis Drugs May Affect Quality and Structural Integrity of Bone. Studies find possible links between prolonged bisphosphonate treatments and

atypical fractures in post-menopausal women. NEW ORLEANS, LA. Lauren Pearson 03/10/2010.2010 Annual Meeting of the American Academy of Orthopaedic Surgeons (AAOS).

(12) http://www.fda.gov/Drugs/DrugSafety/PostmarketDrugSafetyInformationforPatientsandProviders/ucm203891.htm FDA Drug Safety Communication: Ongoing safety review of oral bisphosphonates and atypical subtrochanteric femur fractures. 03-10-2010

(13) http://jcem.endojournals.org/cgi/content/full/90/3/1294 The Journal of Clinical Endocrinology & Metabolism Vol. 90, No. 3 1294-1301 Severely Suppressed Bone Turnover: A Potential Complication of Alendronate Therapy Clarita V. Odvina, Joseph E. Zerwekh, D. Sudhaker Rao, Naim Maalouf, Frank A. Gottschalk and Charles Y. C. Pak

(14) http://www.jbjs.org.uk/cgi/content/abstract/89-B/3/349 Journal of Bone and Joint Surgery—British Volume, Vol 89-B, Issue 3, 349-353. Subtrochanteric insufficiency fractures in patients on alendronate therapy A CAUTION, S.-K. Goh et al.

(15) http://jcem.endojournals.org/cgi/content/full/90/3/1294 The Journal of Clinical Endocrinology & Metabolism Vol. 90, No. 3 1294-1301 Severely Suppressed Bone Turnover: A Potential Complication of Alendronate Therapy Clarita V. Odvina, Joseph E. Zerwekh, D. Sudhaker Rao, Naim Maalouf, Frank A. Gottschalk and Charles Y. C. Pak

(16) http://www.jbjs.org.uk/cgi/content/abstract/89-B/3/349 Journal of Bone and Joint Surgery—British Volume, Vol 89-B, Issue 3, 349-353. Subtrochanteric insufficiency fractures in patients on alendronate therapy A CAUTION, S.-K. Goh et al.

(17) http://content.nejm.org/cgi/content/full/358/12/1304 NEJM Volume 358:1304-1306 March 20, 2008 Number 12. Atypical Fractures of the Femoral Diaphysis in Postmenopausal Women Taking

Alendronate Brett A. Lenart, B.S. Dean G. Lorich, M.D. Joseph M. Lane, M.D. Weill Cornell Medical College New York, NY 10021

(18) http://www.fda.gov/NewsEvents/Newsroom/PressAnnouncements/ucm229171.htm FDA NEWS RELEASE Oct. 13, 2010. FDA: Possible increased risk of thigh bone fracture with bisphosphonates. Labeling change adds warning about possible risks of long-term use of osteoporosis drugs

(19) http://online.wsj.com/article/BT-CO-20101013-710300.html Wall Street Journal. OCTOBER 13, 2010, FDA Warns On Risk Of Thigh Bone Fractures With Bisphosphonates Drugs. FDA: Possible increased risk of thigh bone fracture with bisphosphonates

(20) http://www.fda.gov/Drugs/DrugSafety/ucm225681.htm FDA Statement on ASBMR report: Possible Increased Risk of Certain Types of Thigh Bone Fractures with Long-Term Bisphosphonates Use. 9/14/2010. FDA appreciates the report from the American Society of Bone and Mineral Research's (ASBMR's) expert Task Force

(21) http://www.ncbi.nlm.nih.gov/pubmed/20842676 J Bone Miner Res. 2010 Nov;25(11):2267-94. Atypical subtrochanteric and diaphyseal femoral fractures: report of a task force of the American Society for Bone and Mineral Research. Shane E et al.

(22) http://www.asbmr.org/about/pressreleases/detail.aspx?cid=a68f2b70-a117-4094-9f6f-b5993c6a6149 JBMR Publishes ASBMR Task Force Report on Atypical Femoral Fractures.September 14, 2010 Panel Says May be Related to Unusual Thigh Bone Fractures When Used Long Term Expert Panel Calls for Additional Product Labeling, International Patient Registry

(23) http://www.pharmacist.com/AM/Template.cfm?Section=Pharmacy_News&template=/CM/ContentDisplay.cfm&ContentID=24482 FDA warns of femoral fracture risk with bisphosphonates

(24) http://www.aafp.org/online/en/home/publications/news/news-now/clinical-care-research/20101018bisphosphonatelabel.html AAFP.

FDA Warns Docs, Patients of Femoral Fracture Risk Linked to Some Bisphosphonates Long-term Use Suggests Need for Periodic Bone Density Reassessment 10/18/2010

(25) http://www.empr.com/bisphosphonates-labeling-updated-to-include-atypical-fractures-warning/article/180939/ Bisphosphonates labeling updated to include atypical fractures warning October 13, 2010

(26) http://www.ncbi.nlm.nih.gov/pubmed/17663640
J Bone Miner Res. 2007 Oct;22(10):1479-91. Bisphosphonate-associated osteonecrosis of the jaw: report of a task force of the American Society for Bone and Mineral Research. Khosla S et al.

(27) http://www.medpagetoday.com/MeetingCoverage/ASBMR/22859
Analysis Adds to Evidence of Unusual Fractures. By Michael Smith, North American Correspondent, MedPage Today Published: October 20, 2010 Reviewed by Zalman S. Agus, MD

(28) http://www.ncbi.nlm.nih.gov/pubmed/20809164
Clin Orthop Relat Res. 2010 Dec;468(12):3384-92. Femoral Insufficiency Fractures Associated with Prolonged Bisphosphonate Therapy. Isaacs JD, Shidiak L, Harris IA, Szomor ZL. The St George and Sutherland Hospital Orthopaedic Departments, Sydney, NSW, Australia,

(29) http://www.ncbi.nlm.nih.gov/pubmed/20425089
Curr Osteoporos Rep. 2010 Mar;8(1):34-9. Atypical subtrochanteric and femoral shaft fractures and possible association with bisphosphonates. Nieves JW et al.

(30) http://www.ncbi.nlm.nih.gov/pubmed/20524451
J Med Assoc Thai. 2010 May;93(5):620-4. Bilateral atypical femoral fractures after long-term alendronate therapy: a case report. Bamrungsong T, Pongchaiyakul C.

(31) http://jama.ama-assn.org/cgi/reprint/304/13/1480.pdf
JAMA. 2010;304(13):1480-1484 Atypical Fractures as a Potential

Complication of Long-term Bisphosphonate Therapy. By Deborah E. Sellmeyer

(32) http://www.ncbi.nlm.nih.gov/pubmed/20489100
AJR Am J Roentgenol. 2010 Jun;194(6):1581-6. Subtrochanteric femoral fractures in patients receiving long-term alendronate therapy: imaging features. Chan SS, Rosenberg ZS, Chan K, Capeci C.

(33) http://www.ncbi.nlm.nih.gov/pubmed/20954650
Orthopedics. 2010 Oct 11;33(10). doi: 10.3928/01477447-20100826-31. Bilateral simultaneous femoral diaphyseal fractures in a patient with long-term ibandronate use. Patel VC, Lazzarini AM.

(34) http://www.ncbi.nlm.nih.gov/pubmed/20436006
J Bone Joint Surg Br. 2010 May;92(5):679-86. A rational approach to management of alendronate-related subtrochanteric fractures.Das De S, Setiobudi T et al

(35) http://www.ncbi.nlm.nih.gov/pmc/articles/PMC2917569 Acta Orthop. 2010 August; 81(4): 460-462. Histology of an undisplaced femoral fatigue fracture in association with bisphosphonate treatment Frozen bone with remodelling at the crack Per Aspenberg, Jörg Schilcher, and Anna Fahlgren

(36) http://www.ncbi.nlm.nih.gov/pubmed/20374333
Int J Rheum Dis. 2009 Jul;12(2):149-54. Bilateral atypical femoral diaphyseal fractures in a patient treated with alendronate sodium. Lee JK.J. K. Lee Orthopedic and Traumatology, Petaling Jaya, Selangor, Malaysia.

(37) http://www.ncbi.nlm.nih.gov/pubmed/19670917
Drug Saf. 2009;32(9):775-85. Low-energy femoral fractures associated with the long-term use of bisphosphonates: a case series from a Swiss university hospital. Ing-Lorenzini K, Desmeules J, Plachta O, Suva D, Dayer P, Peter R.

(38) http://www.ncbi.nlm.nih.gov/pubmed/18448990
J Orthop Trauma. 2008 May-Jun;22(5):346-50. Low-energy femoral

shaft fractures associated with alendronate use. Neviaser AS, Lane JM, Lenart BA, Edobor-Osula F, Lorich DG.
Hospital for Special Surgery, New York, NY, USA.

(39) http://www.ncbi.nlm.nih.gov/pmc/articles/PMC2823197/
Acta Orthop. 2009 August 7; 80(4): 413-415. Incidence of stress fractures of the femoral shaft in women treated with bisphosphonate Jörg Schilcher and Per Aspenberg Department of Orthopedics, AIM/IKE, Faculty of Health Science, Linköping University, Linköping, Sweden

(40) http://www.ncbi.nlm.nih.gov/pubmed/18222447
Injury. 2008 Feb;39(2):224-31. An emerging pattern of subtrochanteric stress fractures: a long-term complication of alendronate therapy? Kwek EB, Goh SK, et al.

(41) http://www.nejm.org/doi/full/10.1056/NEJMc0707493
Correspondence. Atypical Fractures of the Femoral Diaphysis in Postmenopausal Women Taking Alendronate N Engl J Med 2008; 358:1304-1306 March 20, 2008 Brett A. Lenart, B.S. Dean G. Lorich, M.D. Joseph M. Lane, M.D. Weill Cornell Medical College, New York, NY 10021

CHAPTER 36

Heartburn, GE Reflux (GERD), and Acid Blocker Drugs

No Flame Schematic Diagram, courtesy of Wikimedia Commons.

A July 2009 study of Acid Blocker Drugs shocked the medical community, reporting the drugs actually caused the symptoms they are supposed to treat.(1) The study recruited normal healthy volunteers who had no symptoms. These volunteers were then given Acid Blocker drugs for a few weeks, and then stopped the drug. Upon stopping the Acid Blocker drug, more than 40% of the volunteers reported heartburn and acid regurgitation, symptoms they never had until after they stopped the Acid Blocker drug. (These drugs are Prolisec™, Nexium™ Aciphex™, Protonix™, and are also called PPI's for Proton Pump Inhibitors). Dr. Christine Reimer the author, said her study revealed "*unrecognized aspects of Acid Blocker—PPI drug withdrawal with acid rebound*".

The Acid Blocker Drug Merry-Go-Round

For the typical heartburn relieved with acid blocker drugs, symptoms return with a vengeance when the drug is stopped. This withdrawal effect is the hallmark of an addictive drug, in this case caused by "rebound acid hyper secretion" with increased gastric acid production. The worsening heartburn pain forces the victim to immediately go back on the PPI acid blocker drug, and continue indefinitely into the future. (3-6)

Windfall Profits from An Addictive Drug

With 5% of the population taking acid blocker PPI drugs, this represents a blockbuster profit for the drug companies. Ask any street corner drug dealer, and they will tell you the best business is the addictive drug business, the clients always return for more.

PPI's Are As Safe As Placebo

Your doctor probably tells you acid blocker drugs are safe, with no adverse effects. An article in a mainstream medical journal (AAFP) says," *The frequency of adverse effects associated with PPIs is similar to that of placebo*". (50)This is not exactly true as you will see below.

Adverse Effects of PPI Acid Blocker Usage

The adverse effects of Acid Blocker Drugs are related to the profound reduction in gastric acid. They really do their job well, reducing stomach acid to virtually nothing. Most of the adverse effects of PPI's are related to the fact that stomach acid is needed for digestion and absorption of key nutrients such as vitamin B12, calcium, iron and the amino acids. Long term use of PPI drugs is associated with increased risk for hip fracture (7), B12 deficiency (8), amino acid deficiency, and iron deficiency anemia. One study showed reduced cognition from PPI's.(12) Secondly, Gastric Acid serves as a defensive barrier to invading bacterial organisms and kills any ingested bacteria, before it can overwhelm the body's defenses. With stomach acid turned off by the PPI drug, these bacteria are free to invade the GI tract and body. This results in increased incidence of pneumonia, as well as Clostridia Difficile Entero-Colitis in patients on PPI's.(9-10)

PPI Drugs Cause Gastric Polyps, Paralysis of the Stomach and Gut Dysmotility

Dr A Breck McKay, in a letter to the British Medical Journal, said: "*long term use of PPIs cause gastroparesis, delayed total gut dysmotility and bloating*".(14)

Patients suffer acute, explosive, exacerbation of their gastritis and reflux, on attempted cessation of the PPIs. While the PPI drugs block acid production, these drugs actually stimulate hormones like gastrin, cholecystokinin, and glucagon, which in turn stimulate growth of acid producing cells to massively increase and thus, are able to produce large quantities of acid, suddenly, when inhibition from the acid blocker PPI drug stops.(18) Nonetheless, PPI drugs are handed out freely, like candy. Dr. Yeomans advised physicians not to "over-react" to concerns about the biological effects of inhibiting acid secretion with proton pump inhibitors. (19)

Warning—PPI drugs
Anti-Acid drugs known as proton pump inhibitors (PPI's) may produce worsening symptoms of heart burn, and increased acid production as a rebound phenomenon upon discontinuing the drug. Chronic use of PPI drugs can lead to B12 deficiency, osteoporosis, and immune dysfunction with increased incidence of pneumonia and Clostridia Enterocolitis.

What Causes GE Reflux and Acid Heartburn?

The cause of reflux is well known. Firstly, there is a mechanical problem with the lower esophageal sphincter (valve) which allows gastric contents to go back up into the lower esophagus, causing irritation, damage and heartburn pain. Turning off gastric acid with a blocker drug will relieve the symptoms, but does not address the underlying mechanical problems.

As a radiologist for 30 years, a large part of my job was taking pictures of GE reflux with barium X-rays. I never saw reflux when the patient was standing up. We were able to induce GE reflux before our eyes merely by placing the patient down in the supine position with the motorized table controls. Now, with the patient in the supine position (lying down) turned back and forth on the table, we then see the reflux on the x-ray fluoroscopic screen, with the barium contrast spilling up from the stomach into the esophagus.

Stay Standing Up or Sitting Up For Three Hours After a Meal.

Whenever I saw the GE reflux, I would then inform the patient they have reflux, and that it is important to stay standing up or sitting up for three hours after they eat a meal. GE reflux cannot occur in the standing or sitting position. After three hours, the stomach should be empty, so it should be safe sleep for the night.

Eradicate the Helicobacter Pylori

Secondly, there may be a co-existing bacterial infection in the stomach called H. Pylori.(41-42) This may be detected with testing. We routinely use the H Pylori breath test which is a sophisticated way to non-invasively make the diagnosis of H Pylori infection.(46) Eradiction of the H Pylori infection with antibiotics is an important step to ending the heartburn/reflux and getting off the PPI Merry Go Round. Thirdly, lifestyle and dietary modifications are essential to ending the heartburn. Avoid spicy foods, eat smaller meals, do not lie down after meals, and stay standing or sitting up for three hours after a meal.

Mastic Gum—an Ancient Remedy—Kills H. Pylori

Mastic Gum is an old remedy used for centuries as a chewable gum effective against H Pylori. This is readily available at the health food store. An excellent article on Gum Mastic by Karina L. Gordin appears in the October issue of the Townsend Letter. She interviewed Dr Leo Galland who recommended Mastic Gum in capsule form (1000 mg twice a day) to a patient with gastritis. Not only did the gastritis clear up, underlying ulcerative colitis also went into full remission. A 1998 landmark article in the New England Journal of Medicine on Mastic Gum, showing activity against H Pylori, is largely responsive for renewed interest in this old remedy. (58-62)

The H. Pylori Story, The Nobel Prize and The Eradication of Gastric Ulcers

The 2005 Nobel prize for Medicine was awarded to two Australian pathologists, Barry J. Marshall and J. Robin Warren for the recognition of H. Pylori infection as the causative agent in gastric and duodenal ulcers.(45) With this great discovery, medical science could now cure gastric and duodenal ulcers by eradicating the H Pylori bacterial infection. This is done with "Triple Therapy" consisting of two antibiotics and a PPI acid blocker drug.(42-44) Once the ulcer is cured, treatment is discontinued.

Changes During My Radiology Career

When I started out as at the beginning of my career as a radiologist in 1976, Gastric and Duodenal ulcers were quite common, and a large part of my job was using X-ray imaging to make the diagnosis, and I found many of these ulcers back in the old days using the barium Upper GI. This is no longer the case. Triple therapy for H. Pylori has made gastric and duodenal ulcers ancient history, these are now quite rare, an ancient relic of the past, destined for the medical museum.

For more information on the importance of stomach acid, see the book by Jonathan Wright, "Why Stomach Acid is Good for You: Natural Relief from Heartburn, Indigestion, Reflux and GERD".(27) Dr. Wright pioneered the routine clinical measurement of stomach acid using the Heidelberg capsule, and has written extensively on the clinical syndrome of low gastric acid (21-27)

For references and links, see my web site: www.bioidenticalhormones101.com

References for Chapter 36. Heartburn and Acid Blockers, Getting Off the Merry Go Round

(1) http://www.gastrojournal.org/article/S0016-5085(09)00522-8/fulltext Gasteroenterology, Vol 137, Issue 1, P 80-87 (July 2009). Proton-Pump Inhibitor Therapy Induces Acid-Related Symptoms in Healthy Volunteers After Withdrawal of Therapy, Christina Reimer et al.

(2) http://www.gastrojournal.org/article/S0016-5085(09)00780-X/fulltext Evidence That Proton-Pump Inhibitor Therapy Induces the Symptoms it Is Used to Treat, 01 June 2009 Kenneth E.L. McColl, Derek Gillen Gastroenterology July 2009 (Vol. 137, Issue 1, Pages 20-22)

(3) http://www.ncbi.nlm.nih.gov/pubmed/10848649 Aliment Pharmacol Ther. 2000 Jun;14(6):651-68. Potential Gastrointestinal Effects of

Long-term Acid Suppression with Proton Pump Inhibitors. Laine L, Ahnen D, McClain C, Solcia E, Walsh JH.

(4) http://www.gastro.org/wmspage.cfm?parm1=7371
Science News—Acid-Reducing Medicines May Lead to Dependency. Data suggests proton pump inhibitors can induce acid-related symptoms in healthy adults

(5) http://heartburn.about.com/b/2009/07/01/256382.htm
PPIs May Induce Reflux Symptoms & Become Addictive—Wednesday July 1, 2009

(6) http://www.medicinenet.com/script/main/art.asp?articlekey=101718
Study: Acid Reflux Drugs Cause Rebound Symptoms

(7) http://jama.ama-assn.org/cgi/content/abstract/296/24/2947
Long-term Proton Pump Inhibitor Therapy and Risk of Hip Fracture. Yu-Xiao Yang et al. JAMA. 2006;296:2947-2953.

(8) http://www.annals.org/cgi/content/abstract/120/3/211
Omeprazole Therapy Causes Malabsorption of Cyanocobalamin (Vitamin B12) Stefan P. Marcuard; Lisa Albernaz; and Prabhaker G. Khazanie—Annals of Internal Med February 1994, Volume 120. Issue 3, Pages 211-215

(9) http://archinte.ama-assn.org/cgi/content/abstract/167/9/950
Gulmez SE, Holm A, Frederiksen H, Jensen TG, Pedersen C, Hallas J. Use of proton pump inhibitors and the risk of community-acquired pneumonia: a population-based case-control study. Arch Intern Med 2007;167:950-5.

(10) http://www.medicine.ox.ac.uk/bandolier/booth/Pharmacy/PPIcdiff.html Proton pump inhibitors and Clostridium difficile. R Cunningham et al. Proton pump inhibitors as a risk factor for Clostridium difficile diarrhoea. Journal of Hospital Infection 2003 54: 243-245.

(11) http://jama.ama-assn.org/cgi/content/abstract/301/20/2120
Shoshana J. Herzig et al. Acid-Suppressive Medication Use and the Risk for Hospital-Acquired Pneumonia. JAMA 301 (20): 2120-2128.

(12) http://www.ncbi.nlm.nih.gov/pubmed/17661965
Boustani, M. The Association Between Cognition and Histamine-2 Receptor Antagonists in African Americans. Journal of the American Geriatrics Society, August 2007; Vol 55: pp. 1248

(13) http://www.bmj.com/cgi/content/full/336/7634/2
BMJ 2008;336:2-3 (5 January), Overprescribing proton pump inhibitors—Is expensive and not evidence based.

(14) http://www.bmj.com/cgi/eletters/336/7634/2#185858
Letters to BMJ. side effects with long term use of the proton pump inhibitors (PPIs). Dr A Breck McKay

(15) http://myweb.lsbu.ac.uk/dirt/museum/margaret/722-255-2320420.jpg
http://myweb.lsbu.ac.uk/dirt/museum/728-3212a.html
Images of gastric ulcers.

(16) http://www.pubmedcentral.nih.gov/articlerender.fcgi?tool=pubmed&pubmedid=19379513 BMC Gastroenterol. 2009; 9: 25. Published 2009 April 20. Decreasing incidence of peptic ulcer complications after the introduction of the proton pump inhibitors, a study of the Swedish population from 1974-2002. Michael Hermansson et al.

(17) http://www.pubmedcentral.nih.gov/articlerender.fcgi?tool=pubmed&pubmedid=17521422 Arthritis Res Ther. 2007; 9(3): R52. 2007 May 23. Vonkeman et al.; Proton-pump inhibitors are associated with a reduced risk for bleeding and perforated gastroduodenal ulcers attributable to non-steroidal anti-inflammatory drugs: a nested case-control study. Harald E Vonkeman et al.

(18) http://www.ncbi.nlm.nih.gov/pubmed/12904157
Expert Opin Drug Saf. 2002 May;1(1):29-38. Long-term safety of proton pump inhibitors: risks of gastric neoplasia and infections. Waldum HL, Brenna E, Sandvik AK.

(19) http://www.ncbi.nlm.nih.gov/pubmed/10735918
Aliment Pharmacol Ther. 2000 Mar;14(3):267-71. Personal review: alarmism or legitimate concerns about long-term suppression of gastric acid secretion? Yeomans ND, Dent J. Department of Medicine, Western Hospital, Melbourne, Australia.

(20) http://www.ncbi.nlm.nih.gov/pubmed/16433886
Basic Clin Pharmacol Toxicol. 2006 Jan;98(1):4-19. Consequences of long-term proton pump blockade: insights from studies of patients with gastrinomas. Jensen RT.

(21) http://www.pubmedcentral.nih.gov/articlerender.fcgi?artid=1930240
Can Med Assoc J. 1970 May 23; 102(10): 1087-1089. Tubeless gastric analysis with a radiotelemetering pill (Heidelberg capsule).M. R. Andres, Jr and J. R. Bingham

(22) http://www.phcapsule.com/
The Heidelberg pH Diagnostic System is a State-of-the-Art Diagnostic Tool for Measuring the pH Levels in the Digestive Tract.

(23) http://www.vrp.com/articles.aspx?ProdID=art784&zTYPE=2
Why Stomach Acid is Good For You (The Gray Man) By Jonathan Wright, MD, and Lane Lenard, PhD, Book published by M. Evans and Company, Inc. (November 25, 2001)

(24) http://www.tahoma-clinic.com/aging2.shtml
Jonathan Wright on Stomach Acid, Tahoma Clinic.

(25) http://www.ahha.org/AntacidsArticle.htm
Age and Antacids: A Double Whammy Against Your Body's Optimal Health. This article was published in the March, 2007 issue of the Dr. Jonathan V. Wright's Clinical Nutrition & Healing newsletter.

(26) http://www.healthfreedom.net/index.php?option=com content&task=view&id=873 Stomach Trouble: Too Little Acid? Are Antacids and acid blockers curing—or causing—stomach troubles? Book by Jonathan Wright MD.

(27) http://www.amazon.com/Why-Stomach-Acid-Good-You/dp/0871319314/ref=ntt_at_ep_dpi_1 Why Stomach Acid is Good for You: Natural Relief from Heartburn, Indigestion, Reflux and GERD by Jonathan Wright, M. Evans and Company, Inc. (November 25, 2001)

(28) http://www.gilbertguide.com/articles/stomaching-stomach-acid-a-simple-solution/ Stomaching Stomach Acid: A Simple Solution. One simple trick is taking a half teaspoon of organic apple cider vinegar in half a cup of water before meals to stop acid reflux.

(29) http://www.ncbi.nlm.nih.gov/pubmed/7286584 Gastroenterology. 1981 Dec;81(6):1068-71. Role of gastric acid in food iron absorption. Skikne BS, Lynch SR, Cook JD.

(30) http://www.annals.org/cgi/content/abstract/120/3/211 Omeprazole Therapy Causes Malabsorption of Cyanocobalamin (Vitamin B12) Stefan P. Marcuard; Lisa Albernaz; and Prabhaker G. Khazanie Annal of Internal Med February 1994 Volume 120 Issue 3 Pages 211-215

(31) http://www.cmaj.ca/cgi/content/full/172/4/450-a
CMAJ, February 15, 2005; 172 (4). Cobalamin deficiency in elderly patients—Jonathan E. Prousky Associate Dean of Clinical Education, Chief Naturopathic Medical Officer, The Canadian College of Naturopathic Medicine, Toronto, Ont.

(32) http://www.jacn.org/cgi/content/abstract/13/6/584
Journal of the American College of Nutrition, Vol 13, Issue 6 584-591, 1994 by American College of Nutrition CLINICAL TRIAL. Effect of hypochlorhydria due to omeprazole treatment or atrophic gastritis on protein-bound vitamin B12 absorption J. R. Saltzman et al.

(33) http://jama.ama-assn.org/cgi/content/summary/278/20/1659-a Gastric Hypochlorhydria and Achlorhydria in Older Adults-Reply Aryeh Hurwitz, MD; Constance Ruhl, MD, MPH University of Kansas Medical Center Kansas City JAMA. 1997;278(20):1659-1660.

(34) http://www.ncbi.nlm.nih.gov/pubmed/11316140
A J Gastro (2001) 96, 1014-1018; Helicobacter pylori infection

and serum ferritin: a population-based study among 1806 adults in Germany. Gabriele Berg et al.

(35) http://www.springerlink.com/content/jw39wenkbfp1mra0/ Eur J Pediatr. 2003 Mar;162(3):177-9. Refractory iron-deficiency anaemia due to silent Helicobacter pylori gastritis in children.Kostaki M, Fessatou S, Karpathios T.

(36) http://www.townsendletter.com/July2004/unseenepidemic0704.htm The unseen epidemic: the linked syndromes of achlorhydria and atrophic gastritis. Townsend Letter for Doctors and Patients, July, 2004 by Nigel Plummer

(37) http://www.ncbi.nlm.nih.gov/pubmed/15029091 Encephale. 2003 Nov-Dec;29(6):560-5. Psychiatric manifestations of vitamin B12 deficiency: a case report] Antibodies to parietal cells were positive in the serum and antibodies to intrinsic factor were negative.

(38) http://www.ncbi.nlm.nih.gov/pubmed/8598839 N Engl J Med. 1996 Apr 18;334(16):1018-22. Atrophic gastritis and Helicobacter pylori infection in patients with reflux esophagitis treated with omeprazole or fundoplication. Kuipers EJ et al.

(39) http://www.pubmedcentral.nih.gov/articlerender.fcgi?tool=pubmed&pubmedid=14684569 Gut. 2004 January; 53(1):12-20. Cure of Helicobacter pylori infection in patients with reflux oesophagitis treated with long term omeprazole reverses gastritis without exacerbation of reflux disease: results of a randomised controlled trial. E J Kuipers et al.

(40) http://www.ncbi.nlm.nih.gov/pubmed/16508317 Gerontology. 2006;52(2):99-106. Effect of Helicobacter pylori eradication on the outcome of reflux esophagitis and chronic gastritis in the elderly. A randomized, multicenter, eight-month study. Pilotto A et al.

(41) http://www.pubmedcentral.nih.gov/articlerender.fcgi?artid=1140724 MedGenMed. 2004; 6(1): 19. 2004 February 18. Eradication of Helicobacter pylori: A Clinical Update—Marco Romano, MD and Antonio Cuomo, MD

(42) http://www.ncbi.nlm.nih.gov/pubmed/11860399
Aliment Pharmacol Ther. 2002 Feb;16(2):167-80. Current concepts in the management of Helicobacter pylori infection—the Maastricht 2-2000 Consensus Report. Malfertheiner P et al.

(43) http://nobelprize.org/nobel_prizes/medicine/laureates/2005/index.html
The Nobel Prize in Physiology or Medicine 2005 to Barry J. Marshall, J. Robin Warren for their discovery of the bacterium Helicobacter pylori and its role in gastritis and peptic ulcer disease.

(44) http://www.ncbi.nlm.nih.gov/pubmed/2593958
Med J Aust. 1989 Oct 16;151(8):435-9. The 14C-urea breath-test for the detection of gastric Campylobacter pylori infection. Surveyor I et al.

(45) http://www.ncbi.nlm.nih.gov/pubmed/10882957
Gastrointest Endosc. 2000 Jul;52(1):20-6 Noninvasive tests as a substitute for histology in the diagnosis of Helicobacter pylori infection. Hahn M et al.

(46) http://gut.bmj.com/cgi/eletters/53/1/5
BMJ Letter. H pylori infection and reflux oesophagitis—Jannis Kountouras,

(47) http://www.pubmedcentral.nih.gov/articlerender.fcgi?artid=2266058
J Clin Biochem Nutr. 2008 March; 42(2): 71-75. Proton Pump Inhibitors and Gastritis—Masayuki Suzuki et al.

(48) http://www.aafp.org/afp/20020715/273.html
Proton Pump Inhibitors: An Update 2002 by the American Academy of Family Physicians. Bruce T. Vanderhoff et al.

(49) http://www.ncbi.nlm.nih.gov/pubmed/9679031
Gastroenterology. 1998 Aug;115(2):268-74. Serum ferritin, hemoglobin, and Helicobacter pylori infection: a seroepidemiologic survey comprising 2794 Danish adults. Milman N et al.

(50) http://www.ncbi.nlm.nih.gov/pubmed/10577329
Ann Intern Med. 1999 Nov 2;131(9):668-72. Reversal of iron

deficiency anemia after Helicobacter pylori eradication in patients with asymptomatic gastritis. Annibale B et al.

(51) http://www.wjgnet.com/1007-9327/13/5380.asp
World J Gastroenterol 2007 October 28; 13(40): 5380-5383 Effects of H pylori therapy on erythrocytic and iron parameters in iron deficiency anemia patients with H pylori-positive chronic gastristis Lun-Hua Chen, He-Sheng Luo

(52) http://www.ncbi.nlm.nih.gov/pubmed/17211708
Dig Dis Sci. 2007 Feb;52(2):405-10. Ferritin, vitamin B(12), folate, and zinc levels in children infected with Helicobacter pylori. Akcam M et al.

(53) http://www.ncbi.nlm.nih.gov/pubmed/12827006
J Pediatr Gastroenterol Nutr. 2003 Jul;37(1):53-62. Correlation between Helicobacter pylori infection and vitamin C levels in whole blood, plasma, and gastric juice, and the pH of gastric juice in Korean children. Park JH, Kim SY, Kim DW, Lee WG, Rhee KH, Youn HS. Department of Pediatrics

(54) http://www.johnshopkinshealthalerts.com/reports/digestive_health/869-1.html Digestive Health Special Report—The H. Pylori Story. Jophns Hopkins Health Alert.

(55) European Journal of Dermatology. Volume 19, Numéro 5, 431-44, September-October 2009, Review article Ana C Hernando-Harder, Nina Booken, Sergij Goerdt, Manfred V Singer, Hermann Harder

(56) Al-Habbal MJ, Al-Habbal Z, Huwez FU. A double-blind controlled clinical trial of mastic and placebo in the treatment of duodenal ulcer. Clin Exp Pharmacol Physiol. 1984 Sep-Oct;11(5):541-4.

(57) Huwez FU, Al-Habbal MJ. Mastic in treatment of benign gastric ulcers. Gastroenterol Jpn. 1986 Jun;21(3):273-4.

(58) http://content.nejm.org/cgi/content/extract/339/26/1946 NEJM Volume 339:1946 December 24, 1998 Number 26 Mastic Gum Kills Helicobacter pylori

(59) http://www.healthandwellnessfoundation.org/monographs/helicobacter_pylori.pdf Helicobacter pylori Eradication: Are there Alternatives to Antibiotics? Alan R. Gaby, MD

(60) http://www.koreamed.org/SearchBasic.php?DT=1&RID=474823 Korean J Gastroenterol. 2003 Apr;41(4):277-283. Korean. The Effect of Mastic Gum on Helicobacter pylori-infected Gastritis. Roe IH, Nam SW, Myung NH, Kim JT, Shin JH., Korea.

(61) http://aac.asm.org/cgi/content/full/51/2/551 Antimicrobial Agents and Chemotherapy, February 2007, p. 551-559, Vol. 51, No. 2 In Vitro and In Vivo Activities of Chios Mastic Gum Extracts and Constituents against Helicobacter pylori Sotirios Paraschos et al.

(62) http://www.ultrawellness.com/blog/heart-burn-and-acid-reflux Three simple steps to eliminate heart burn and acid reflux by Mark Hyman MD, UltraWellness.

(63) http://www.youtube.com/watch?v=ORY1cUB_k6M
Three Simple Steps to Eliminate Heartburn and Acid Reflux by Mark Hyman MD, Video on You Tube. UltraWellness blog.

CHAPTER 37

SSRI Antidepressants Are No Better Than Placebo, Says JAMA

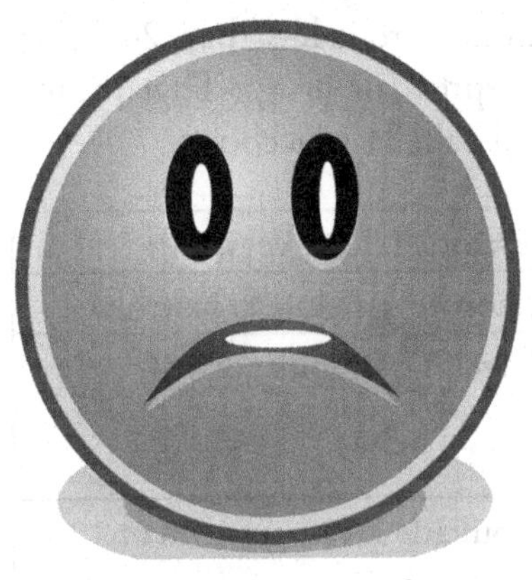

Sad Face Icon, courtesy of Tango Desktop Project and Wikimedia Commons

Getting Off SSRI Anti-Depressant Drugs

A study published in JAMA on Jan 5, 2010 reported that SSRI antidepressants are no better than placebo for most cases of depression. (1) The authors reviewed 30 years of data and concluded that "*the benefit of antidepressant medication compared with placebo may be minimal or nonexistent in patients with mild or moderate symptoms*". Of course, this is old news, and reminds me of the famous scene in 1942 film, Casablanca starring Humphrey Bogart and Ingrid Bergman where the game is always rigged. When Rick asks, "*why is the casino being closed down*"? The French Captain replies with the famous line: "*I am Shocked, Shocked . . . to find gambling here . . . . Here are your winnings . . . Oh thank you.*" You must see the video clip on You Tube. (12)

Better than Placebo for Severe Depression

I should add that the study found SSRI antidepressants work better than placebo for severe depression. This is not surprising, since virtually any psycho-stimulant can be found useful for the most severely depressed patient.

Is Depression Really a Medical Disease?

Medically speaking, the term "Depression" is a vague constellation of feelings and symptoms scored by a questionnaire called the Hamilton Depression Score. There are a number of handy on-line tools for taking the Hamilton Depression Score Questionnaire. For the short 17-item version of the Hamilton questionnaire, scores can range from 0 to 54. Hamilton scores between 0 and 6 are normal. Scores between 7 and 17 indicate mild depression, scores between 18 and 24 indicate moderate depression, and scores over 24 indicate severe depression. According to the Jan 5 JAMA study, if the Hamilton score is less than 24, then placebo is just as effective as SSRI antidepressant drugs. That means the SSRI drug is as effective as a sugar pill called a placebo.

Hamilton Depression Score Questions (short version):	
Mood	Are you sad, hopeless, helpless, worthless?
Feeling of Guilt	Do you have feelings of guilt, or self reproach?
Suicide	Do you have Suicide ideas, gestures or attempts?
Insomnia	Do you have difficulty falling asleep, staying asleep?
Work and Activities	Do you have thoughts and feelings of fatigue or weakness? related to activities, or decreased or stopped activities or working because of present illness?
Slowness	Do you have Slowness of thought and speech; Do you have difficulty concentrating; slow movements?
AGITATION	Do you have Fidgeting, Playing with hands, hair, etc, Moving about, can't sit still. Hand ringing, nail biting, hair-pulling, biting of lips etc?
ANXIETY	Do you have tension and irritability, Worrying, Apprehension, Fears expressed?
ANXIETY: SOMATIC	Do you have dry mouth, wind, indigestion, diarrhea, cramps, belching.—Cardio-vascular: palpitations, headaches. hyperventilation, sighing. Urinary frequency—Sweating?

SOMATIC SYMPTOMS: GASTROINTESTINAL	Do you have loss of appetite, require laxatives or medication for bowels, or medication for gastro-intestinal symptoms?
SOMATIC SYMPTOMS: GENERAL	Do you have Heaviness in limbs, back or head? Backaches, headache, muscle aches. Loss of energy and fatigability?
GENITAL SYMPTOMS	Do you have loss of libido, menstrual disturbances?
HYPOCHONDRIASIS	Do you have preoccupation with your health?
LOSS OF WEIGHT	Do you have weight loss from depression?
INSIGHT	Acknowledges or denies being depressed?

Overlapping Symptoms—Is it Really Depression?

As is obvious, many of these feelings or symptoms are somewhat subjective and rather vague, so depression scoring is not an exact science and can be manipulated according to the agenda of the research or questioner. As you can see, many of these Hamilton symptoms overlap with real medical diseases. For example, inflammatory bowel disease patients would score positive for the GI symptoms even though they may not be clinically "depressed". Somatic symptoms of fatigue and muscle pain may overlap with fibromyalgia and hypothyroid symptoms. Slowness of thought and speech could overlap with a low thyroid condition or a neurological disorder such as B12 deficiency. Patients in chronic severe pain contemplating suicide may not necessarily indicate clinical "depression". Obviously, these patients need pain relief rather than an SSRI antidepressant.

Hormonal Imbalance Symptoms Overlap with Many of the Hamilton Symptoms

Many women with hormonal imbalance related to pre-menopause or post menopausal transitions will have mood disorders and symptoms which overlap with many of the symptoms on the Hamilton Depression

Score. For example, estrogen deficiency is a well known cause of anxiety, a symptom listed on Hamilton Depression Score. However, it would be a mistake to treat a woman with estrogen deficiency with an SSRI antidepressant.

The syndrome Premenstrual Dysphoric Disorder is commonly treated by mainstream physicians with SSRI antidepressants. (39) This is an error, and a practice that should be halted. These patients would be best served by treating them with progesterone, the hormone missing in this disorder. With the Jan 5, 2010 JAMA article, we now have evidence that Premenstrual Dysphoric Disorder and other common forms of hormonal imbalance are poorly served by SSRI antidepressants. Using SSRI's is simply the wrong way. The benefit of SSRI antidepressants for this group is the same as the benefit from placebo. Rather than give them SSRI antidepressants, this group of women with PMS, estrogen deficiency or progesterone deficiency should be properly evaluated, and then treated with bioidentical hormones to address their underlying problem. We have noted considerable success using cyclic natural progesterone in this group of women with PMS and other hormonal imbalances. In my opinion, natural progesterone is a far better form of treatment with none of the adverse side effects associated with SSRI antidepressants.

Adverse Side Effects of Antidepressants—Placebos Have NONE

When SSRI antidepressants are found equally effective compared to placebo, the next question relates to adverse side effects. By definition, placebos have no adverse side effects. However, this is not true for SSRI antidepressants which have the following adverse effects: Sexual dysfunction, weight gain and sleep disturbance are the most troubling adverse effects of SSRI anti-depressant therapy.(42-44) The most common side effects associated with SSRI antidepressants are nausea, headache, nervousness, insomnia and sexual dysfunction. When I examine these patients in my office, they usually demonstrate dilated pupils and hyperactive reflexes. The long term SSRI users may have irreversible neurological changes, and many are simply "burned out" from chronic over-stimulation of the nervous system.

SSRI Antidepressants and Suicide Risk

Another troubling adverse effect of SSRI antidepressants is increased suicide first reported by Teicher in 1990.(40) According to David Healy's book, "Let Them Eat Prozac", the original clinical trial data was manipulated by moving the suicide cases from the treatment arm over to the placebo arm of the study.(41) This manipulated data was then submitted to the FDA who conveniently looked the other way. This disturbing information was presented at a Cornell University Mar 25, 2009 talk by David Healy which can be seen on a You Tube video. (42)

The Army and Military Suicide from SSRIs Antidepressant Use

Another striking finding is the unprecedented increased suicide rate in the military with widespread use of SSRI's and other psycho active drugs in the Army. Again this is a rather sad commentary, and another nail in the coffin for SSRI drugs as more harmful than helpful.(34-36)

For references and links, see my web site: www.bioidenticalhormones101.com

References for Chapter 37. SSRI Antidepressants No Better Than Placebo Says JAMA

(1) http://jama.ama-assn.org/cgi/content/short/303/1/47?home Antidepressant Drug Effects and Depression Severity A Patient-Level Meta-analysis by Jay C. Fournier et al. JAMA. 2010;303(1):47-53.

(2) http://www.plosmedicine.org/article/info:doi/10.1371/journal.pmed.0050045 Initial Severity and Antidepressant Benefits: February 26, 2008 A Meta-Analysis of Data Submitted to the Food and Drug Administration. Irving Kirsch et al.

(3) http://www.psychologytoday.com/blog/charting-the-depths/201001/depression-treatment-we-need-better-not-simply-more Depression treatment: We need better not simply more Getting more people into treatment for depression is not enough. Psychology Today. January 5, 2010

(4) http://www.nytimes.com/2010/01/06/health/views/06depress.html?hp New York Times. Popular Drugs May Help Only Severe Depression By BENEDICT CAREY. January 5, 2010

(5) http://online.wsj.com/article/SB10001424052748703436504574640641607761408.html?mod=rss_Health Wall Street Journal. Jan 6, 2010. Effectiveness of Antidepressants Varies Widely By Jennifer Doorden

(6) http://www.upenn.edu/pennnews/article.php?id=1791 Penn Study Shows Antidepressants Work Best for Severe Depression, Provide Little to No Benefit Otherwise. January 05, 2010

(7) http://www.pharmalot.com/2010/01/antidepressants-dont-help-mild-depression-analysis/ Antidepressants Don't Help Mild Depression: Study. Pharmalot.

(8) http://www.minddisorders.com/Flu-Inv/Hamilton-Depression-Scale.html Online Hamilton Depression Score. 17—item version of Questionnaire

(9) http://www.cure4you.dk/960/HAMD-17%20Grid%20version%20-%20English.pdf On-Line Hamilton rating scale for depression 17 questions

(10) http://www.real-depression-help.com/hamilton-depression-scale.html online HMD questionaire—quick score for depression—adjusted for layman

(11) http://www.psy-world.com/online_hamd.htm online HMD questionaire—quick score for depression—classic printable version

(12) http://www.youtube.com/watch?v=-Gf8NK1WAOc Casablanca is a 1942 film—Captain Louis Renault. I am shocked—shocked—to find that gambling is going on in here!

(13) http://www.psy-world.com/ssri_problems.htm Problems associated with long term treatment with selective serotonin reuptake inhibitors by Chantal Moret and Mike Isaac

(14) http://depressioncell.com/article.asp?articleid=73575
The Antidepressant Dilemma—antidepressants have limited-to-zero efficacy for those with mild depression.

(15) http://www.pharmalot.com/2010/01/antidepressants-dont-help-mild-depression-analysis/ Antidepressants Don't Help Mild Depression: Study By Ed Silverman. January 5th, 2010

(16) http://www.furiousseasons.com/archives/2010/01/study_antidepressants_ineffective_for_mild_moderate_depression.html
Furious Seasons:Study: Anti-Depressants Ineffective For Mild, Moderate Depression

(17) http://www.time.com/time/health/article/0,8599,1717306,00.html
Antidepressants Hardly Help By Laura London Feb. 26, 2008 Time Magazine

(18) http://www.srmhp.org/0201/media-watch.html
Antidepressant-Placebo Debate in the Media—Balanced Coverage or Placebo Hype?

(19) http://www.guardian.co.uk/education/2002/jun/20/research.highereducation Burne, J. (2002, June 20). Make-believe medicine. The Guardian.

(20) http://www.ncbi.nlm.nih.gov/pubmed/15627852
Gaudiano, B. A., & Herbert, J. D. (2003). Methodological issues in clinical trials of antidepressant medications: Perspectives from psychotherapy outcome research. Psychother Psychosom 2005;74:17-25.

(21) http://www.ncbi.nlm.nih.gov/pubmed/8279933
Kessler, R. C., McGonagle, K. A., Zhao, S., Nelson, C. B., Hughes, M., Eshleman, S., et al. (1994). Lifetime and 12-month prevalence of DSM-III-R psychiatric disorders in the United States: Results from the national comorbidity survey. Archives of General Psychiatry, 51, 8-19.

(22) http://www.ncbi.nlm.nih.gov/pubmed/11799341
Khan, A., Leventhal, R. M., Khan, S., & Brown, W. A. (2002). Severity of depression and response to antidepressants and placebo: An analysis of the Food and Drug Administration database. Journal of Clinical Psychopharmacology, 22, 40-45.

(23) http://journals.apa.org/prevention/volume5/pre0050023a.html Kirsch, I., Moore, T. J., Scoboria, A., & Nicholls, S. S. (2002). The emperor's new drugs: An analysis of antidepressant medication data submitted to the U.S. Food and Drug Administration. Prevention & Treatment, 5, art. 23.

(24) http://journals.apa.org/prevention/volume1/pre0010002a.html. Kirsch, I., & Sapirstein, G. (1998). Listening to Prozac but hearing placebo: A meta-analysis of antidepressant medication. Prevention & Treatment, 1, art. 0002a. Retrieved February 1, 2003, from

(25) http://journals.apa.org/prevention/volume1/pre0010006c.html. Klein, D. F. (1998). Listening to meta-analysis but hearing bias. Prevention & Treatment, 1,

(26) http://www.ncbi.nlm.nih.gov/pubmed/10773176
Leber, P. (2000). The use of placebo control groups in the assessment of psychiatric drugs: An historical context. Biological Psychiatry, 47, 699-706.

(27) http://www.ncbi.nlm.nih.gov/pubmed/11772700
Leuchter, A. F., Cook, I. A., Witte, E. A., Morgan, M., & Abrams, M. (2002). Changes in brain function of depressed subjects during treatment with placebo. American Journal of Psychiatry, 159, 122-129.

(28) http://www.ncbi.nlm.nih.gov/pubmed/11986125
Mayberg, H. S., Silva, J. A., Brannan, S. K., Tekell, J. L., Mahurin, R. K., McGinnis, S., & Jerabek, P. A. (2002). The functional neuroanatomy of the placebo effect. American Journal of Psychiatry, 159, 728-737.

(29) http://www.thomasjmoore.com/pages/prozpop.html.
Moore, T. J. (1999, October 17). No prescription for happiness. Boston Globe, E01.

(30) http://www.ncbi.nlm.nih.gov/pubmed/14974002
Moncrieff, J., Wessely, S., & Hardy, R. Active placebos versus antidepressants for depression (Cochrane Review). The Cochrane Library, Cochrane Database Syst Rev. 2004;(1):CD003012.

(31) http://ajp.psychiatryonline.org/cgi/content/full/157/3/327 Quitkin, F. M., Rabkin, J. G., Gerald, J., Davis, J. M., & Klein, D. F. (2000). Validity of clinical trials of antidepressants. American Journal of Psychiatry, 157, 327-337.

(32) http://www.cs.ucl.ac.uk/staff/M.Sewell/faq/publishing-research/Rosenthal1979.pdf Rosenthal, R. (1979). The "file drawer problem" and tolerance for null results. Psychological Bulletin, 1979, V86, 638-641.

(33) http://www.washingtonpost.com/ac2/wp-dyn/A42930-2002May6.
Vedantam, S. (2002, May 7). Against depression, a sugar pill is hard to beat. Washington Post

(34) http://www.time.com/time/nation/article/0,8599,1811858,00.html
America's Medicated Army—By Mark Thompson Thursday, Jun. 05, 2008

(35) http://ajp.psychiatryonline.org/cgi/content/abstract/ajp;164/7/1044
R.D. Gibbons, C.H. Brown, K. Hur, S.M. Marcus, D.K. Bhaumik, and J.J. Mann, "Relationship Between Antidepressants And Suicide Attempts: An Analysis of the Veterans Health Administration Data Sets," American Journal of Psychiatry 164 (2007): 1044-1049.

(36) http://www.ncbi.nlm.nih.gov/pmc/articles/PMC2909461/ Valenstein M, Kim HM, Ganoczy D, McCarthy JF, Zivin K, Austin KL, Hoggatt K, Eisenberg D, Piette JD, Blow FC, Olfson M. Higher-risk periods for suicide among VA patients receiving depression treatment: prioritizing

suicide prevention efforts. Journal of Affective Disorders, 2009 Jan;112(1-3):50-8.

(37) http://www.ncbi.nlm.nih.gov/pubmed/18541308
M. Raja, A. Azzoni, and A.E. Koukopoulos, "Psychopharmacological treatment before suicide attempt among patients admitted to a Psychiatric Intensive Care Unit," Journal of Affective Disorders 113 (2009): 37-44.

(38) http://iospress.metapress.com/content/5p66t6645226x742/ Peter R. Breggin, Antidepressant-induced suicide, violence and mania: Risks for military personnel,Journal The International Journal of Risk and Safety in Medicine, Volume 22, Nu

(39) http://www.aafp.org/afp/2002/1001/p1239.html
Diagnosis and Treatment of Premenstrual Dysphoric Disorder by SUBHASH C. BHATIA, M.D., and SHASHI K. BHATIA, M.D. Am Fam Physician. 2002 Oct 1;66(7):1239-1249.

(40) http://www.ncbi.nlm.nih.gov/pubmed/2301661
Am J Psychiatry 1990; 147:207-210 Emergence of intense suicidal preoccupation during fluoxetine treatment. MH Teicher, C Glod and JO Cole

(41) http://www.healyprozac.com/booksale-healy.pdf
Let Them Eat Prozac: The Unhealthy Relationship Between the Pharmaceutical Industry and Depression by David Healy, NYU Press (June 1, 2004)

(42) http://www.youtube.com/watch?v=X53r3zTQJNk
The Future of Medical Care. David Healy, psychiatrist and Cardiff University professor addresses the question: Can Industrialized and Marketized Healthcare be Made Universally Available? (Mar 25, 2009 at Cornell University)

(43) http://www.ncbi.nlm.nih.gov/pmc/articles/PMC181155/ Prim Care Companion J Clin Psychiatry. 2001 February; 3(1):22-27. SSRI

Antidepressant Medications: Adverse Effects and Tolerability by James M. Ferguson, M.D.

(44) http://www.psy-world.com/SSRI_problems.pdf
http://www.ncbi.nlm.nih.gov/pubmed/18635702/
J Psychopharmacol. 2009 Nov;23(8):967-74. Problems associated with long-term treatment with selective serotonin reuptake inhibitors. Moret C, Isaac M, Briley M.

CHAPTER 38

Getting Off Statin Drug Stories

Statin drugs such as Lipitor™ and Crestor™ are used to lower cholesterol levels. These are a few case stories of patients on these types of drugs.

Case Number One, Martha

Fifty Five year old Martha is, healthy, and never had heart disease. Nonetheless, for the past five years, Martha has been taking a statin drug for "high cholesterol" under the care of "the top cardiologist" in South Florida. Martha has also been under my care, taking a bioidentical hormone program for menopausal symptoms, and doing very well. Every six months, we run a lab panel which always shows low cholesterol of 170, courtesy of her statin anti-cholesterol drug. The drugs lower cholesterol levels, of that there is no doubt.

Just Ask Judith Walsh MD in JAMA

And, every time Martha comes into the office to review her lab results, I print out a 2004 JAMA article by Judith Walsh, MD who reviewed thirteen statin drug clinical trials from 1966 to 2003.(1) Dr. Judith Walsh concludes in her JAMA article that cholesterol lowering drugs provide no health benefit for women. I give Martha a copy of the JAMA article and, at the same time, explain to her that no woman should be on a statin drug. Lowering cholesterol with a statin drug has no health benefit for women, that's a fact, and public information readily available.

Important Point
Statin Cholesterol lowering drugs provide no health benefit for women, according to a review of statin drug studies by Judith Walsh MD published in JAMA.

Playing Games With Statin Drugs

Every six months I recommend to Martha stopping the statin drug, and every six month, her cardiologist puts her back on the statin drug. This has been going on for three years now.

Finally Success At Convincing Martha to Stop the Statin Drug

Finally this last time, Martha seems more receptive to idea that the statin drug is harming her and not helping her. She is sitting in my office recounting multiple health problems for which she sees numerous doctors: back pain, asthma, sinus infections, skin problems, and allergies. I suggested to Martha the possibility that many of her health problems are caused by the low cholesterol from the statin drug. Martha finally sees the light, goes home and tosses the bottle of pills into the garbage can.

Feeling Better

About a week later, Martha called me and reported, "*I feel so much better off that statin drug, thank you so much!*". Stopping the statin drug produced an immediate improvement.

Believing in the Propaganda

This case illustrates the difficulty in convincing patients to stop their statin drug. It is difficult to counter the drug company propaganda, and convince these patients they are harming their health with the statin drugs. Many continue to believe in the myth that cholesterol causes heart disease, and they go on to become statin drug medical victims. I see them every day. When we have a success like Martha, who finally gets off her statin drug, this is a cause for celebration.

Case Number Two—Roger

Roger is a seventy one year old retired executive, and an avid tennis player. He has no history of coronary artery disease and has always been healthy. Two years ago, his cardiologist said his cholesterol of

210 was “too high”, and prescribed a statin anti-cholesterol drug. A year later, Roger’s tennis game deteriorated, he found his timing and balance was off, and he lost every game to players who could never beat him before.

Adverse Effects of the Statin Drug

I suggested to Roger that the decline in his tennis game was most likely an adverse effect of the statin drug on his muscle and nerve function causing loss of balance and coordination. I recommended stopping the statin anti-cholesterol drug. At first, Roger resisted and said his wife wanted him to take the statin drug because she thought it was “good medical care”, and she (mistakenly) believed that lower cholesterol was somehow preventive of heart disease.

How to Counter the Propaganda: A Book For You

In order to counter the drug company cholesterol propaganda, I gave Roger a copy of the book, “Fat and Cholesterol are Good for You”, by Uffe Ravnskov MD PhD.(2) This book reviews the medical studies which supposedly show that cholesterol is the cause of heart disease, and reveals that these studies do no such thing. This is a medical myth. Neither cholesterol consumption nor cholesterol blood levels cause heart disease. Similarly, many medical studies demonstrate that anti-cholesterol drugs work very well to reduce cholesterol levels, however, this treatment does not prolong life and makes most people sick with adverse side effects.

Statin Drugs For the Elderly?

Another important point made to Roger while sitting in my office is that a number of studies in the elderly (over the age of 70) revealed low cholesterol levels are not associated with health, and are a “robust predictor” of increased mortality, while higher cholesterol levels are associated with improved survival.(6-9) This “reverse epidemiology” or “lipid paradox” for the elderly is also true for other subgroups such as patients with chronic kidney failure on dialysis, congestive heart failure, chronic obstructive lung disease, and cancer survivors, in which lowering cholesterol is associated with increased mortality, and higher cholesterol improves survival.(10)

Seeing the Light

Roger was amazed and his eyes practically popped out of his head when he "saw the light". The statin drugs were turning him another medical victim. Once Roger learned the truth about the "cholesterol causes heart disease" myth, he took his statin drug bottle and threw it into the garbage can. Two weeks later, off the statin drug, Roger was back to his old self, prancing about the tennis court like a gazelle, and winning every game with ease.

Are You Still a Believer in Anti-Cholesterol Drugs?

If you are still a believer in Statin Drugs, take a look at this primary prevention study published July 2010 in the Archives of Internal Medicine by Dr. Ray.(3) He reviewed 11 statin drug clinical trials with 65,229 participants followed for approximately 244,000 person-years. The astounding results showed the statin drug group all-cause mortality was **THE SAME** as the placebo group! (3) The statin drug group had no health benefits over placebo!!! This article was published in the mainstream medical literature!!

Important Point
For men who do not have underlying heart disease, taking a statin drug to lower cholesterol provides no health benefit. They have same mortality rate as those taking a placebo drug. In other words: no benefit.

How About Heart Attack Victims? What's Their Cholesterol?

If cholesterol was truly the cause of heart attacks, then one would expect heart attack victims to reveal the high cholesterol causing their heart attack. They found the opposite. Heart attack victims have low cholesterol. A study analyzed 137,000 admissions for coronary artery disease from 541 US hospitals, and found mean cholesterol was only 174. This is low, not high. (4) In addition, if high cholesterol was truly the cause of heart attacks, one would expect heart attack victims with the highest cholesterol to have the worst prognosis, and lowest cholesterol to have the best prognosis. They don't. A study from Henry Ford Hospital in Detroit showed that three years after a heart attack, the patients with lowest cholesterol had the highest mortality (14% vs. 7 %). (5)

Important point:
Patients entering the hospital with a heart attack have low cholesterol, not high cholesterol, on average. In patients after their first heart attack, follow up studies show higher mortality for lower cholesterol levels. Patients with higher cholesterol levels live longer.

Conclusion:

The cholesterol theory of heart disease is a myth maintained by drug company propaganda to support massive profits from cholesterol lowering drugs. For most patients, this class of drugs provides no health benefit in terms of prolonging life, while causing harm from adverse side effects. Avoid becoming a victim of the statin drug propaganda machine.

References for Chapter 38. Getting Off Statin Drug Stories

(1) http://jama.ama-assn.org/content/291/18/2243
JAMA. 2004;291(18):2243-2252. Drug Treatment of Hyperlipidemia in Women
Judith M. E. Walsh, MD, MPH; Michael Pignone, MD, MPH

(2) Fat and Cholesterol are Good for You, Uffe Ravnskov GB Publishing (January 26, 2009)

(3) http://archinte.ama-assn.org/cgi/content/abstract/170/12/1024
Statins and All-Cause Mortality in High-Risk Primary Prevention A Meta-analysis of 11 Randomized Controlled Trials Involving 65 229 Participants. Kausik K. Ray, MD, MPhil, FACC, FESC; Sreenivasa Rao Kondapally Seshasai, MD, MPhil; Sebhat Erqou, MD, MPhil,

PhD; Peter Sever, PhD, FRCP, FESC; J. Wouter Jukema, MD, PhD; Ian Ford, PhD; Naveed Sattar, FRCPath. Arch Intern Med. 2010;170(12):1024-1031.

(4) http://www.ahjonline.com/article/S0002-8703(08)00717-5/abstract
AHJ Volume 157, Issue 1, Pages 111-117.e2 (January 2009) Lipid levels in patients hospitalized with coronary artery disease: An analysis of 136,905 hospitalizations in Get With The Guidelines. Amit Sachdeva, MD et al.

(5) http://www.ncbi.nlm.nih.gov/pubmed/19437396
Cardiol J. 2009;16(3):227-33. Low admission LDL-cholesterol is associated with increased 3-year all-cause mortality in patients with non ST segment elevation myocardial infarction. Al-Mallah MH, Hatahet H, Cavalcante JL, Khanal S.

(6) http://www.ncbi.nlm.nih.gov/pubmed/11502313
Cholesterol and all-cause mortality in elderly people from the Honolulu. Heart Program: a cohort study. The Lancet Volume 358, Issue 9279, August 4, 2001, pp. 351-355. Irwin J Schatz MD, Kamal Masaki MD, Katsuhiko Yano MD, Randi Chen MS, Beatriz L Rodriguez MD and J David Curb MD

(7) http://www.ncbi.nlm.nih.gov/pubmed/12834520
J Am Geriatr Soc. 2003 Jul;51(7):991-6.Low total cholesterol and increased risk of dying: are low levels clinical warning signs in the elderly? Results from the Italian Longitudinal Study on Aging. Brescianini S, Maggi S, Farchi G, Mariotti S, Di Carlo A, Baldereschi M, Inzitari D; ILSA Group.

(8) http://www.ncbi.nlm.nih.gov/pubmed/15673344
J Am Geriatr Soc. 2005 Feb;53(2):219-26. Relationship between plasma lipids and all-cause mortality in nondemented elderly. Schupf N, Costa R, Luchsinger J, Tang MX, Lee JH, Mayeux R.

(9) http://www.ncbi.nlm.nih.gov/pubmed/20470020
Scand J Prim Health Care. 2010 Jun;28(2):121-7. Serum total cholesterol levels and all-cause mortality in a home-dwelling elderly

population: a six-year follow-up. Tuikkala P, Hartikainen S, Korhonen MJ, Lavikainen P, Kettunen R, Sulkava R, Enlund H.

(10) http://www.drhoffman.com/downloads/Lipids.pdf
Lipids in aging and chronic illness impact on survival, Kovesdy, C.P. Kalantar-Zadeh, K. Arch Med Sci 2007; 3, 4A: S74-S80

Section Ten: Preventing and Reversing Heart Disease

CHAPTER 39

Heart Disease, Ascorbate, Lysine and Linus Pauling

The Steam Roller is Not Joking

I once had a conversation with a cardiologist friend of mine in which I casually mentioned the Linus Pauling Theory of heart disease, and the idea that non-toxic nutritional supplements such as vitamin C and two amino acids could prevent and reverse heart disease. The response from my cardiologist friend was hearty laughter that anyone would even suggest such a nonsensical idea, and surely you must be joking? My cardiologist friend and the rest of the mainstream medical system has no clue about the steamroller coming to health care aimed at the huge profits from diagnosis and treatment of heart disease, a multibillion dollar industry in the US. The Cardiac Catheterization Lab and Cardiac Bypass Surgery Programs will be flattened, the first casualties of the internet revolution, providing information about a safe and cheap program of nutritional supplements to reverse heart disease, the Linus Pauling Protocol. Time has come for the old dinosaurs to go. In the near future, thanks to Linus Pauling, heart disease will become a curiosity of the past, like the disappearance of gastric ulcers after the invention of antacids and antibiotics.

The Linus Pauling Protocol—Vitamin C

Vitamin C Deficiency Has Major Impact on Collagen Production

Ascorbate, also called Vitamin C, is required to make a protein called collagen which is the major component of connective tissues. The lack of Vitamin C is a deficiency disease called Scurvy. Why is Collagen Important? Collagen is the most abundant protein in the body. Collagen is the structural protein used to make connective tissues, bones, teeth, hair, and arteries. Strong collagen is important for a strong body. Basic medical science tells us that Vitamin C is required for strong collagen. How does this work? Vitamin C is required for lysyl hydroxylase, an enzyme responsible for attaching the lysine residues together on adjacent collagen strands. (38) Vitamin C deficiency results in weakened collagen strands caused by disrupted lysine cross linking. The resulting weakened collagen results in widespread problems in the connective tissues, bones, teeth, skin, hair, arteries, etc. (35, 38, 39,42)

Full Blown Scurvy—Collagen Falls Apart

In the full blown Vitamin C deficiency disease called Scurvy, the structural elements of the body literally fall apart. Collagen is broken down and not replaced. The joints wear out, the small arteries begin to crack and degenerate, the skin shows easy bruising and bleeding as small vessels rupture throughout the body, and the teeth may loosen and fall out.

Linus Pauling: Heart Disease is a Chronic Scurvy Condition

Linus Pauling was unquestionably the greatest scientist of the twentieth century. All of modern biochemistry and molecular biology chemistry is based on Linus Pauling's work, especially his discovery and elucidation of the chemical bond. Pauling is the only scientist to be awarded two unshared Nobel prizes. Pauling's later years were devoted to study of heart disease, and in 1989 he published "A Unified Theory of Human Cardiovascular Disease," in which he states that atherosclerotic plaques in heart disease are actually part of a repair process, to repair the arterial damage caused by chronic vitamin C deficiency. (15) In essence, Pauling said that heart disease is a manifestation of chronic scurvy, and atherosclerotic plaque is a mechanism evolved to repair or patch blood vessels and arteries damaged by chronic vitamin C deficiency. Linus Pauling also said that atherosclerotic plaque formation can be prevented or reversed with vitamin C, lysine and proline. These are nutritional supplements available at any health food store for a few dollars.

Atherosclerotic Plaques Found at Maximal Mechanical Stress

Atherosclerotic plaques are not found randomly distributed throughout the arterial tree, rather distribution is restricted to sites of high mechanical stress such as bifurcations, and areas of motion such as the surface of the heart (coronary arteries). In the early 1950's, a Canadian, G. C. Willis, MD, made these same observations, and they have been confirmed by 60 years of coronary and peripheral arteriography at major medical centers. (1-4)

Exposed Lysine Crosslinks from Damaged Collagen is Site of LipoProtein (a) attachment and Plaque Formation

Imagine stepping on your garden hose a thousand times a day. You will soon notice cracks in the wall of the garden hose. This is the same process that happens in the artery. As these cracks open up, the collagen strands in the wall of the artery are teased apart. The collagen strands are normally bound together with lysine crosslinks which are now teased apart and exposed to the circulating blood stream. The Lysine residues look like little flags waving from the damaged collagen strand. The exposed Lysine strands are available for binding to circulating Lipoprotein (a), a special form of cholesterol that has lysine receptors, and is known to increase heart disease risk. This attachment of lipoprotein (a) to the free lysine residues of damaged collagen initiates the atherosclerotic process. Over time, this process builds larger plaque deposits which eventually narrow the inner diameter of the artery causing a blockage, or leads to plaque rupture and thrombosis, a catastrophic event which may cause heart attack or sudden death. Animal experiments in genetically modified "knocked out" mice with no lysine binding sites on lipoprotein (a) show a fivefold reduction in atherosclerotic plaque formation.(50-51)

Animals Make Vitamin C, But You Can't

We humans cannot make vitamin C in our liver as all other animals do. We humans had a genetic mutation in our ancestry 50 million years ago which "knocked out" the final enzyme in the hepatic synthesis of vitamin C. The missing enzyme is called GLO (gulano lactone oxidase).

Primates such as gorillas, chimpanzees and orangutans also share this same GLO mutation and cannot make vitamin C. In addition, all primates share with us humans the same susceptibility to develop heart disease.

All Animals Can Make Vitamin C, but the Guinea Pig Can't

Except for humans and primates, all other animals have the three enzymes in the liver which can synthesize vitamin C from glucose (a simple sugar). One major exception is the guinea pig, which is really a rodent and not a pig. The guinea pig, for some unexplained reason, shares with humans the GLO genetic mutation and also lacks the GLO enzyme just like we do. This makes the guinea pig an ideal experimental model for human diseases. By the way, although animals that make vitamin C never get heart disease, the guinea pig which lacks the ability to synthesize vitamin C, **DOES GET HEART DISEASE**.

Animals That Make Vitamin C, Don't Get Atherosclerotic Heart Disease

I thought this was worth repeating. (note: here I am referring to atherosclerotic vascular heart disease in animals. Dogs and Cats **DO** succumb to other common types of heart disease such as cardiomyopathy and heart worm etc.)

Animals That Don't Make Vitamin C, Do Get Atherosclerotic Heart Disease

This should be starting to become clear now.

Animal Scientific Support for the Pauling Unified Theory

As mentioned above, guinea pigs are especially well suited to study atherosclerosis because guinea pigs are unable to make their own vitamin C, and in addition, they develop atherosclerotic plaques similar to those found in humans. G. C. Willis, a Canadian doctor, conducted research with guinea pigs in the 1950's showing that guinea pigs deprived of dietary vitamin C developed atherosclerotic plaques, while guinea pigs given plentiful vitamin C were protected. (52) In addition, guinea pigs fed a vitamin C deficient diet had elevated Lipoprotein (a) levels along with increased atherosclerotic plaque formation in the arteries. (53)

Similar findings were demonstrated in genetically engineered mice lacking the GLO enzyme. The GLO deficient mice fed a vitamin C deficient diet developed atherosclerotic plaques in the aorta with characteristic deranged collagen crosslinking. GLO deficient mice fed vitamin C were protected. (38)(54)

Human Studies Supporting the Linus Pauling Theory

Optometrist, Dr. Sydney Bush's retinal artery observations support the Pauling theory. Using modern equipment to non-invasively photograph the retinal arteries of the eye before and after Vitamin C supplementation in humans, Dr. Bush has documented reversal of atherosclerotic plaque with Vitamin C supplementation. (54) Coronary Calcium Score studies also support the Pauling Theory with favorable results after treatment with Vitamin C and Lysine. (55) Anecdotal case evidence of reversal of heart disease can be found in the medical literature and documented in Owen Fonorow's book.(56) In these cases, advanced heart disease regresses after supplementation with the Linus Pauling Protocol. This is highly significant because the natural course of heart disease is progression, and any intervention that alters the natural course of a disease process is highly significant.

Message boards are a source of anecdotal cases reports supporting the Linus Pauling Protocol. The Track Your Plaque Message Boards have documented many cases of regression of atherosclerotic disease with protocols which include vitamin C as well as other nutritional supplements. (58) Why no drug company sponsored double blind placebo controlled studies? Since there are no patents involved for natural supplements, and no drugs involved, no drug company would ever invest the 250 million dollars to fund such a study with no potential for financial return.

The Physician's Health Study—Don't Waste Your Money On Vitamins!!

Using public funds, the NIH (National Institute of Health) funded a large study called The Physicians' Health Study II which evaluated Vitamins C and E in heart disease and was published Nov. 9, 2008 in JAMA by Howard D. Sesso.(59) The study found that Vitamin C and E did not prevent mortality from heart disease; results which are completely opposite to massive previously published research and anecdotal case reports. A closer look shows a few glaring errors in study design. The Linus Pauling Protocol was not followed. The dosage of vitamin C was set too low, at one tenth the dosage recommended by the Linus Pauling protocol, and lysine was not provided. While the Sesso study showed no mortality benefit, many previous studies such as the Enstrom Study showed a striking a 42% reduction in cardiovascular mortality and a 35% reduction in all-cause mortality over 6 years for those with the highest vitamin C intake. (60) The Paul Knecht study showed a 25% reduction in Heart Disease risk with daily 700 mg Vitamin C.(61) Two medical studies from Japan and Finland showed that Vitamin C reduces risk for stroke, an example of atherosclerosis involving the cerebral arteries.(62-63) There are many more like these.

Since favorable results would be financially destructive to the drug and hospital industries, a cynic might suggest that vested interests were at work in Sesso's study intending to discredit vitamin C (as documented many times in the past with examples of corporate influence in medical research). It is not difficult to design a medical study to fail. I regard this as merely another example of the information war waged by corporate mainstream medicine against natural medicine. Enstrom showed that increasing vitamin C intake had a dramatic 40% reduction in mortality benefit which exceeds any statin drug study ever conducted.

Linus Pauling Protocol for Prevention and Reversal of Plaque

If heart disease is chronic scurvy, caused by chronic vitamin C deficiency, then it makes sense to supplement with vitamin C in the amounts needed to make strong collagen and prevent arterial damage from mechanical stress. In addition, Pauling devised a clever yet simple method to address the issue of Lipoprotein (a) attaching to the lysine residues on the damaged collagen fibers in the arterial wall. He recommended supplementing with 2-4 grams of lysine per day. The additional lysine in the blood stream attaches to the receptor sites on the lipoprotein (a) molecules, inactivating the lipoprotein (a) and preventing it from attaching to the arterial wall. This prevents the initiation of the atherosclerotic process. In addition, Vitamin C and Lysine are both important precursors for building strong collagen which makes strong arteries. In addition to Lysine, some of the collagen crosslinking is done with another amino acid called Proline, so proline was also added to the treatment protocol.

A good book on the Linus Pauling protocol is "Practicing Medicine Without a License", by Owen Fonorow, dedicated to the 1992 Linus Pauling Protocol for prevention and reversal of heart disease.(64-66) Another excellent book on the subject of Vitamin C and heart disease is, "Stop America's #1 Killer", by Thomas Levy MD, JD.(67) Another excellent resource for prevention and reversal of heart disease is the William Davis MD, "Track Your Plaque" blog and web site.(58)

What is the Linus Pauling Protocol?

Linus Pauling Protocol for Prevention and Reversal of Heart Disease
1) L-Ascorbate (Vitamin C) 5-6 grams a day in divided doses 2) L-Lysine 5 grams a day in divided doses 3) L-Proline 2-3 grams a day in divided doses 4) The Tocotrienol form of Vitamin E.

These supplements can be obtained at any the health food store as tablets or capsules for 40 to 50 dollars a month.

Opposition to the Linus Pauling Protocol by Mainstream Medicine

If you are facing the prospects of coronary artery bypass surgery, you might ask the obvious question: Why hasn't my cardiologist told me about this information and started me on the Linus Pauling Protocol? Most cardiologists either don't know about it or ignore it because of the information war going on between mainstream medicine and natural medicine. Cardiologists read medical journals which regularly run incorrect and biased articles saying Vitamin C is useless for prevention and reversal of heart disease, such as the 2008 Sesso study. Diagnosing and treating heart disease with expensive tests and procedures such as coronary angiography, angioplasty, stenting and bypass operations is the most profitable part of hospital big business. That's why hospitals compete and fight with each other over the rights to expand and build larger cardiac cath labs and cardiac bypass operation programs. These programs are huge money makers for the national hospital system.

What would happen if there was a cheap and effective way to reverse and prevent heart disease, (ie. the Linus Pauling Protocol)? Heart disease would become an uncommon illness. With fewer heart patients to treat, the multi-million dollar cardiac catheter labs and cardiac bypass programs at your local hospital would become obsolete and disappear. This would be a financial catastrophe for mainstream medicine.

No More Construction Cranes?

With so much money and vested interest at stake, you can imagine why it is not prudent for a cardiologist to bring up the benefits of the Linus Pauling Protocol in friendly conversation while lunching in the Doctor's Dining Hall. That would be an instant ticket off the medical staff roster and out the hospital door, and the end of a lucrative cardiology practice. What cardiologist in their right mind would do that? It is easier for the mainstream cardiologists to simply laugh it off as a joke and go back to the Cardiac Catheter Lab, do more procedures and make some money to pay their bills. I certainly would.

Financial Disclosure: I have no financial interest in any Vitamin C products, books or web sites mentioned in this article. For references and links, see my web site: www.bioidenticalhormones101.com

References for Chapter 39. Heart Disease, Ascorbate, Lysine and Linus Pauling

(1) http://www.vitamincfoundation.org/pdfs/WillisGround.pdf An Experimental Study of the Intimal Ground Substance in Atherosclerosis, G.C. Willis, Canad. M. A. J. Vol 69, 1953, p. 17-22

(2) http://www.vitamincfoundation.org/pdfs/WillisSerial.pdf Serial Arteriography in Atherosclerosis, G. C. Willis, A. W. Light, W.S. Cow, Canad. M. A. J. Dec 1954, Vol 71, 1954, p. 562-568

(3) http://www.vitamincfoundation.org/pdfs/WillisTissue.pdf Ascorbic Acid Content of Human Arterial Tissue, G. C. Willis, S. Fishman, Canad. M. A. J., April 1, 1955, Vol 72, Pg 500-503

(4) http://www.vitamincfoundation.org/pdfs/WillisAthero.pdf The Reversibility of Atherosclerosis, G. C. Willis, Canad. M. A. J., July 15, 1957, Voll 77., Pg 106-109

(5) http://www.vitamincfoundation.org/pdfs/ CAPILLARY RUPTURE WITH INTIMAL HEMORRHAGE IN THE CAUSATION OF CEREBRAL VASCULAR LESIONS, J. C. Paterson, Arch Path, Vol 29, 1940, Pg 345-354

(6) http://www.vitamincfoundation.org/pdfs/ Some Factors In The Causation of Intimal Hemorrhages in the Precipitation of Coronary Thrombi, J. C. Paterson, Canad. M. A. J., Feb 1941, Pg 114-120

(7) http://www.pubmedcentral.nih.gov/articlerender.fcgi?artid=1435897 Nutr Metab (Lond). 2006; 3: 17. Guinea pigs: A suitable animal model to study lipoprotein metabolism, atherosclerosis and inflammation by Maria Luz Fernandez and Jeff S Volek

(8) http://jn.nutrition.org/cgi/content/full/131/1/10 Journal of Nutrition. 2001;131:10-20. Guinea Pigs as Models for Cholesterol and Lipoprotein Metabolism by Maria Luz

(9) http://ci.nii.ac.jp/naid/110002603577/
Japanese circulation journal Vol.35, No.12(19711200) pp. 1559-1565 EXPERIMENTAL ATHEROSCLEROSIS WITH ASCORBIC ACID DEFICIENCY by FUJITANI TAKAO et al.

(10) http://www.pnas.org/content/87/23/9388.full.pdf Immunological evidence for the accumulation of lipoprotein(a) in the atherosclerotic lesion of the hypoascorbemic guinea pig. M Rath, L Pauling—Proceedings of the National Academy of Sciences, 1990—National Acad Sciences. Vol. 87, pp. 9388-9390, December 1990

(11) http://www.pnas.org/content/87/16/6204.full.pdf
Hypothesis: lipoprotein (a) is a surrogate for ascorbate. M Rath, L Pauling—Proceedings of the National Academy of Sciences 1990

(12) http://www.pubmedcentral.nih.gov/articlerender.fcgi?tool=pubmed&pubmedid=2143582 Proc Natl Acad Sci U S A. 1990 August; 87(16): 6204-6207. PMCID: PMC54501 Hypothesis: lipoprotein(a) is a surrogate for ascorbate. M Rath and L Pauling

(13) http://faculty.washington.edu/ely/paulinglysine.html
Journal of Orthomolecular Medicine, 6(3-4): 144-46, 1991. Case Report: Lysine/Ascorbate-Related Amelioration of Angina Pectoris by Linus Pauling

(14) http://www.orthomed.org/jom/jom.htm
Case Report: Lysine/Ascorbate-Related Amelioration of Angina Pectoris by Linus Pauling

(15) http://orthomolecular.org/library/jom/1992/pdf/1992-v07n01-p005.pdf A Unified Theory of Human Cardiovascular Disease Leading the Way to the Abolition of This Disease as a Cause for Human Mortality M Rath, L Pauling—J Ortho Med, 1992—

(16) http://www.americanhearthealthservices.com/images/Cellular_Essentials.pdf J App Nut, Vol 48, N 3, 1996 Nutritional Supplement Program Halts Progression of early coronary atherosclerosis

Documented by UltraFast Computed Tomography by Matthias Rath, M.D. and Aleksandra Niedzwiecki, Ph.D.

(17) http://www.ncbi.nlm.nih.gov/pubmed/1588941
Mol Cell Biochem. 1992 Apr;111(1-2):41-7. Protective role of ascorbic acid against lipid peroxidation and myocardial injury. Chakrabarty S, Nandi A, Mukhopadhyay CK, Chatterjee IB. Department of Biochemistry, University College of Science, Calcutta, India.

(18) http://www.ncbi.nlm.nih.gov/pubmed/11500168 Atherosclerosis. 2001 Sep;158(1):1-12. Hyperglycemia-induced ascorbic acid deficiency promotes endothelial dysfunction and the development of atherosclerosis.Price KD, Price CS, Reynolds RD.

(19) http://www.ajcn.org/cgi/reprint/23/1/27.pdf
Am J Clin Nutr. 1970 Jan;23(1):27-30. Ascorbic acid and atherosclerosis.Shaffer CF.

(20) http://jama.ama-assn.org/cgi/content/full/2008.600
Vitamins E and C in the Prevention of Cardiovascular Disease in Men. The Physicians' Health Study II Randomized Controlled Trial—JAMA-EXPRESS, Howard D. Sesso et al. JAMA. 2008;300(18):2123-2133.

(21) http://circ.ahajournals.org/cgi/content/full/105/12/1396 Vitamin C, Collagen, and Cracks in the Plaque, by Peter Libby, MD; Masanori Aikawa, MD PhD. Circulation. 2002;105:1396-1398

(22) http://www.ncbi.nlm.nih.gov/pubmed/1591317
Epidemiology. 1992 May;3(3):194-202. Vitamin C intake and mortality among a sample of the United States population.Enstrom JE, Kanim LE, Klein MA.School of Public Health, University of California, Los Angeles 90024.

(23) http://www.ajcn.org/cgi/content/full/80/6/1508
8-1520, December 2004. Antioxidant vitamins and coronary heart disease risk: a pooled analysis of 9 cohorts. Paul Knekt et al.

(24) http://www.pubmedcentral.nih.gov/articlerender.fcgi?tool=pubmed&pubmedid=15117714 Am J Public Health. 2004 May; 94(5): 870-875. Vitamin C Deficiency and Depletion in the United States: The Third National Health and Nutrition Examination Survey, 1988 to 1994 Jeffrey S Hampl, et al.

(25) http://www.internetwks.com/owen/TheoryPaper.htm The Unified Theory, The Long Neglected Theory of Cardiovascular and Heart Disease By Owen Richard Fonorow 2002

(26) http://www.internetwks.com/owen/ Health Articles by Owen Fonorow, Orthomolecular Naturopath (Orthomopath) 1996-2008 Owen Fonorow.

(27) http://practicingmedicinewithoutalicense.com/protocol/excerpt_chp7.pdf Chapter 7 Practicing Medicine WIthout a License, Owen Fonorow, summary of Pauling therapy to reverse heart disease

(28) http://www.vitamincfoundation.org/ Vitamin C Foundation, Owen Fonorow

(29) http://www.nutritionreview.org/library/collagen.connection.html Linus Pauling's Unified Theory of Human Cardiovascular Disease. The Collagen Connection Jim English and Hyla Cass, MD

(30) http://www.orthomolecular.org/library/jom/1992/pdf/1992-v07n03-p153.pdf Reducing the Risk for Cardiovascular Disease with Nutritional Supplements M Rath.

(31) http://www.chestjournal.org/cgi/content/abstract/121/5/1589 Chest. 2002;121:1589-1594. Elevated Serum Lipoprotein(a) Level Is an Independent Marker of Severity of Thoracic Aortic Atherosclerosis Marcel Peltier, MD et al.

(32) http://www.ncbi.nlm.nih.gov/pubmed/2528948 Arteriosclerosis. 1989 Sep-Oct;9(5):579-92. Detection and quantification of lipoprotein(a) in the arterial wall of 107 coronary bypass patients. Rath M, Niendorf A, Reblin T, Dietel M, Krebber HJ, Beisiegel U.

(33) http://www.ncbi.nlm.nih.gov/pubmed/7605357
Atherosclerosis. 1995 Mar;113(2):179-88. Extraction of lipoprotein(a), apo B, and apo E from fresh human arterial wall and atherosclerotic plaques.Reblin T et al.

(34) http://www.jlr.org/cgi/reprint/32/2/317
Journal of Lipid Research Volume 32, 1991 317 Quantification of apo[a] and apoB in human atherosclerotic lesions by Judith M. Pepin et al.

(35) http://www.pubmedcentral.nih.gov/articlerender.fcgi?rendertype=abstract&artid=508329 J Clin Invest. 1997 September 15; 100(6): 1493-1500. Lipoprotein(a) vascular accumulation in mice. In vivo analysis of the role of lysine binding sites using recombinant adenovirus by S D Hughes et al.

(36) http://www-personal.umich.edu/~egatenby/collagen%20eyre%20chapter.pdf collagen and lysine crosslinking images.

(37) http://www.ncbi.nlm.nih.gov/pubmed/10572964
Biochim Biophys Acta. 1999 Oct 18;1472(1-2):408-11. Random nucleotide substitutions in primate nonfunctional gene for L-gulono-gamma-lactone oxidase, the missing enzyme in L-ascorbic acid biosynthesis. Ohta Y, Nishikimi M.

(38) http://www.jbc.org/cgi/content/abstract/269/18/13685
J. Biol. Chem., Vol. 269, Issue 18, 13685-13688, 05, 1994 Cloning and chromosomal mapping of the human nonfunctional gene for L—gulono-gamma-lactone oxidase, the enzyme for L-ascorbic acid biosynthesis missing in man. by M Nishikimi et al.

(39) http://www.pnas.org/content/97/2/841.full PNAS January 18, 2000 vol. 97 no. 2 841-846 Aortic wall damage in mice unable to synthesize ascorbic acid by Nobuyo Maeda et al.

(40) http://www.ncbi.nlm.nih.gov/pubmed/3008449
Yale J Biol Med. 1985 Nov-Dec;58(6):553-9. Regulation of collagen biosynthesis by ascorbic acid: a review. by Pinnell SR.

(41) http://www.jci.org/articles/view/119565
Published in Volume 100, Issue 3 J. Clin. Invest. 100(3): 558-564 (1997). Modification of apolipoprotein(a) lysine binding site reduces atherosclerosis in transgenic mice. N W Boonmark et al.

(42) http://www.knockoutscience.com/showabstract.php?pmid=9239402
J Clin Invest (1997) 100: 558-64. Modification of apolipoprotein(a) lysine binding site reduces atherosclerosis in transgenic mice by NW Boonmark et al.

(43) http://www.ohiolink.edu/etd/send-pdf.cgi/Person%20Margaret%20M.pdf?acc_num=ysu1196173663 Collagen consists of three polypeptide chains, termed alpha chains, which are arranged in a parallel triple helix.

(44) http://www.cqs.com/cvd.htm
A Simple Preventive and Therapy for Cardiovascular Disease (CVD) Jonathan Campbell, Health Consultant Natural Therapies for Chronic Illness & Health Maintenance

(45) http://www.lef.org/Vitamins-Supplements/Item02117/L-Proline-L-Lysine.html L-Proline, L-Lysine 275 mg/275 mg, 120 tablets Item Catalog Number: 2117 $14.16. Life Extension Vitamin Compnay.

(46) http://www.hullcontactlensclinic.co.uk/cardior.htm CardioRetinometry Dr. Sydney J Bush. PhD. DOpt. (IOSc. London) Optic nerve heads (Disc) Before Vitamin C 2002, After Vitamin C 2004,

(47) http://www.bmj.com/cgi/eletters/329/7457/79#68348
CardioRetinometry 23 July 2004 Sydney J Bush, Optometrist. CardioRetinometrist 20-22 Brook St. HULL HU2 8LA

(48) http://www.ncbi.nlm.nih.gov/pubmed/14703305
Inai Y et al. (2003), "The Whole Structure of the Human Non-Functional L-Guluno-gamma-Lactone Oxidase Gene—the Gene Responsible for Scurvy—and the Evolution of Repetitive Sequences Thereon," J Nutr Sci Vitaminology 49:315-319.

(49) http://www.jbc.org/cgi/content/abstract/267/30/21967
J. Biol. Chem., Vol. 267, Issue 30, 21967-21972, Oct, 1992. Guinea pigs possess a highly mutated gene for L-gulono-gamma-lactone oxidase, the key enzyme for L-ascorbic acid biosynthesis missing in this species. M Nishikimi, T Kawai and K Yagi

(50) http://www.cdc.gov/mmwr/preview/mmwrhtml/mm4830a1.htm
MMWR Weekly—Decline in CVD Death Rates, Achievements in Public Health, 1900-1999: Decline in Deaths from Heart Disease and Stroke—United States, 1900-1999

(51) http://www.vitamincfoundation.org/forum/index.php
Vitamin C Foundation Message Board

(52) http://www.jci.org/articles/view/119565
Modification of apolipoprotein(a) lysine binding site reduces atherosclerosis in transgenic mice.J Clin Invest. 1997;100(3):558-564. N W Boonmark, X J Lou, Z J Yang, K Schwartz, J L Zhang, E M Rubin and R M Lawn

(53) http://www.ncbi.nlm.nih.gov/pmc/articles/PMC1823880/
Can Med Assoc J. 1957 July 15; 77(2): 106-109. The Reversibility of Atherosclerosis by G. C. Willis.

(54) http://ci.nii.ac.jp/naid/110002603577/
EXPERIMENTAL ATHEROSCLEROSIS WITH ASCORBIC ACID DEFICIENCY by FUJITANI TAKAO Japanese circulation journal 35(12), 1559-1565, 1971-12 Japanese Circulation Society

(55) http://www.pnas.org/content/97/2/841.full
PNAS January 18, 2000 vol. 97 no. 2 841-846. Aortic wall damage in mice unable to synthesize ascorbic acid. Nobuyo Maeda et al.

(56) http://www.hullcontactlensclinic.co.uk/cardior.htm CardioRetinometry. Dr. Sydney J Bush. PhD. DOpt. (IOSc. London)

(57) http://www.americanhearthealthservices.com/images/Cellular Essentials.pdf J Applied Nutrition, V48, N3, 1996. Nutritional

Supplement Program Halts Progression of Early Coronary Atherosclerosis Documented by Ultrafast Computed Tomggraphy. Matthias Rath, M.D. and Aleksandra Niedzwiecki, Ph.D.

(58) http://www.orthomolecular.org/library/jom/1991/pdf/1991-v06n03&04-p144.pdf Case Report: Lysine/Ascorbate-Related Amelioration of Angina Pectoris Linus Pauling. Journal of Orthomolecular Medicine Vol. 6, Nos. 3 & 4, 1991

(59) http://www.trackyourplaque.com/
Track Your Plaque Web Site by William Davis MD.

(60) http://jama.ama-assn.org/cgi/content/full/2008.600
JAMA. 2008;300(18):2123-2133. Vitamins E and C in the Prevention of Cardiovascular Disease in Men. The Physicians' Health Study II Randomized Controlled Trial. Howard D. Sesso et al.

(61) http://www.ncbi.nlm.nih.gov/pubmed/1591317
Epidemiology. 1992 May;3(3):194-202. Vitamin C intake and mortality among a sample of the United States population. Enstrom JE, Kanim LE, Klein MA.

(62) http://www.ajcn.org/content/80/6/1508.full
American Journal of Clinical Nutrition, Vol. 80, No. 6, 1508-1520, December 2004. Antioxidant vitamins and coronary heart disease risk: a pooled analysis of 9 cohorts. Paul Knekt et al.

(63) http://stroke.ahajournals.org/cgi/content/full/31/10/2287 Stroke. 2000;31:2287-2294 Serum Vitamin C Concentration Was Inversely Associated With Subsequent 20-Year Incidence of Stroke in a Japanese Rural Community. The Shibata Study

(64) http://stroke.ahajournals.org/cgi/reprint/33/6/1568.pdf
Plasma Vitamin C Modifies the Association Between Hypertension and Risk of Stroke S. Kurl, MD; T.P. Tuomainen, MD; J.A. Laukkanen, MD; K. Nyyssönen, PhD; T. Lakka, MD, PhD; J. Sivenius, MD, PhD; J.T. Salonen, MD, PhD, MscPH

(65) http://practicingmedicinewithoutalicense.com/ Practicing Medicine Without A License? The Story of the Pauling Therapy for Heart Disease By Owen Fonorow with Sally Jewell Copyright 2008

(66) http://www.google.com/patents?hl=en&lr=&vid=USPAT5278189&id=GlwiAAAAEBAJ&oi=fnd&printsec=abstract#v=onepage&q&f=false United States Patent 5,278,189 Rath et al. Jan. 11, 1994 PREVENTION AND TREATMENT OF OCCLUSIVE CARDIOVASCULAR DISEASE WITH ASCORBATE AND SUBSTANCES THAT INHIBIT THE BINDING OF LIPOPROTEIN (A)

(67) http://orthomolecular.org/library/jom/1992/pdf/1992-v07n01-p005.pdf A Unified Theory of Human Cardiovascular Disease Leading the Way to the Abolition of This Disease as a Cause for Human Mortality Matthias Rath M.D. and Linus Pauling Ph.D. Journal of Orthomolecular Medicine Vol. 7, No. 1, 1992

(68) http://www.livonlabs.com/cgi-bin/htmlos.cgi/LV/apps/stop-americas-killer.html Stop America's #1 Killer by Thomas E. Levy, MD, JD (2006)

CHAPTER 40

Cholesterol Lowering Statin Drugs for Women, Just Say No

A Woman on Crestor™ With Leg Muscle Pain

Sally, a 56 year old retired real estate agent, came to see me in the office with the chief complaint of hot flashes, night sweats, mood disturbance and weight gain which are all fairly typical post-menopausal symptoms. In addition, leg pain for the past 3 months prevented exercising. An MRI scan of the Lumbar Spine to evaluate the leg pain showed only a bulging disk and was otherwise negative. About 6 months ago, Sally's cholesterol was 245, and her cardiologist prescribed a cholesterol lowering statin drug, Crestor™. Sally has no history of heart disease, does not smoke, eats a healthy diet, and takes a few vitamins, and doesn't supplement with CoEnzyme Q-10. I explained to Sally that her leg pain was a well known adverse side effect of Crestor™, a statin drug which lowers cholesterol, and this is a valid reason for stopping the drug.(41) The leg muscle pain is caused by statin drug depletion of Co-enzyme Q-10, a substance critical for energy production in the muscle cells.(42-44) I suggested to Sally that she supplement with Co-Enzyme Q-10, and strongly recommended stopping the statin drug.

The New Cholesterol Guidelines—What is elevated cholesterol?

When I was a medical student in 1976, normal cholesterol was 240 mg/dl. However, this was changed in 1993 by new guidelines. Above 240 is high, from 200-240 is borderline high and below 200 is desirable (see below chart).

New Blood Cholesterol Guidelines as of 1993 (1-3)	
Above 240 mg/dl	High
From 200-240 mg/dl	Borderline High
Below 200 mg/dl	Desirable.

These new cholesterol guidelines came from a committee of nine doctors, eight of whom were receiving money from statin drug companies, a blatant conflict of interests. In addition, there was no science behind this revision. (1-3) A 2006 article in the Annals of Internal Medicine argues that there is **NO EVIDENCE** to support the target numbers outlined by the Cholesterol Guidelines panel, challenging the mainstream medical belief that lower cholesterol levels are always better.(45) A 2004 petition letter to the NIH by thirty prominent MD's complains about the faulty 1993 Cholesterol Guidelines and asks for a revision. (46)

A number of prominent experts in the field have been critical of the new guidelines.

Mary Enig says cholesterol and heart disease is a "Phoney Issue"(4): "*Blood cholesterol levels between 200 and 240 mg/dl are **normal**. These levels have always been **normal**. In older women, serum cholesterol levels greatly above these numbers are also **quite normal**, and in fact they have been shown to be associated with longevity. Since 1984, however, in the United States and other parts of the western world, these normal numbers have been treated as if they were an indication of a disease in progress or a potential for disease in the future. For women, a total cholesterol result 240 should not be considered elevated. This is quite normal for women and compatible with good health.*" (4)

No Female Should Ever Take a Statin Drug

The obvious message here is that NO woman should ever be prescribed statin drugs for elevated cholesterol. Dr. Colin Rose says, "*There are no statin trials with even the slightest hint of a mortality benefit in women and women should be told so*".(5) In other words, statin drugs don't work for women. Yes, statin drugs work quite well at lowering cholesterol levels, but this does not equate with improved health or longer life span.

Let me repeat that so this is very clear: **No female should ever take a statin drug to lower cholesterol for primary prevention of heart disease.** These drugs do not provide a health benefit for women. Women who take Lipitor or any other statin drug to lower cholesterol do not live any longer than women who do not take the drug. There is no benefit in terms of prolonging life for women. On the other hand, statin drugs carry numerous adverse effects such as muscle pain, cognitive impairment, neuropathy, congestive heart failure, transient global amnesia, dementia, cancer and erectile dysfunction (impotence) and CoQ10 depletion. (47-49)

Why Do Cardiologists Give Statin Drugs to Women?

You might be asking yourself the question: In spite of the lack of health benefit and known adverse effects, why do cardiologists and mainstream doctors continue to prescribe statin drugs for women? The answer is mainstream doctors and cardiologists succumb to the drug company "spin" from the drug reps and the medical journals slanted in favor of statin drugs downplaying adverse effects. In addition, the mainstream doctors yield to their patients' demand for statin drugs created by celebrity television drug ads.

Are You Still Not Convinced?

Mary Enig writes: "*No study has shown a significant reduction in mortality in women treated with statins. The University of British Columbia Therapeutics Initiative came to the same conclusion, with the finding that statins offer no benefit to women for prevention of heart disease.*" (6) (7)

Are you still not convinced that women should NOT take Statin Drugs? Don't take my word for it. Take the word of Judith Walsh MD who wrote this in JAMA article entitled, Treatment of Hyperlipidemia in Women: "*For women without cardiovascular disease, lipid lowering does not affect total or CHD (Cardiovascular Heart Disease) mortality. Lipid lowering may reduce CHD events, but current evidence is insufficient to determine this conclusively. For women with known cardiovascular disease, treatment of hyperlipidemia is effective in reducing CHD events,* CHD *mortality, nonfatal myocardial infarction, and revascularization, but it does not affect total mortality."*(8) **Translation:** Cholesterol lowering with statin drugs does not reduce total mortality in women, PERIOD. It doesn't reduce mortality in women without heart disease, called primary prevention. It doesn't reduce mortality in women with heart disease, called secondary prevention.

Still not convinced? Then read this article by Malcolm McKendrick, a doctor in England, in the British Medical Journal, May 2007, entitled: "Should Women be Offered Cholesterol Lowering Drugs? NO" . . . "*To date, none of the large trials of secondary prevention with statins has shown a reduction in overall mortality in women. Perhaps more critically, the primary prevention trials have shown neither an overall mortality benefit, nor even a reduction in cardiovascular end points in women. This raises the important question whether women should be prescribed statins at all.* ***I believe that the answer is clearly no.***"(50) Note: Secondary prevention means women with known heart disease. Primary prevention means women without known heart disease.

Still not convinced? Then read this June 2007 article by Electra Kaczorowski, of the National Women's Health Network: "*There is currently no indication that women of any age or any risk level will benefit from taking statins to prevent CHD and other heart conditions—yet this is precisely how statins are being marketed to women.* "(9)

Still not convinced? Are statin drugs good for anybody? Read this 2003 review article by Joel Kauffman PhD, in which he points out the best statin trial, the HPS Simvastatin Study (50), had an absolute reduction of all cause mortality of only 0.38% per year, a result inferior to that obtained with less expensive buffered aspirin.(10)(50)

Still not convinced? Then read this article by Harriett Rosenberg from Women and Health Protection June 2007, "Do Cholesterol Lowering Drugs Benefit Women? Evidence for Caution: Women and Statin Use", by Harriet Rosenberg: "*Our review of these fields identifies a troubling disjuncture between the widespread use of statin medication for women and the evidence base for that usage. What we found instead was evidence for caution.*"(11)

Still not convinced? Then read this Jan 2007 Lancet article by Harvard trained MD, John Abramson, "Are lipid-lowering guidelines Evidence-Based? ". (14) "*No studies have shown statin cholesterol-lowering drugs to be effective neither for women at any age, nor for men 69 years of age or older, who do not already have heart disease or diabetes. Better than fifty adults have to take a cholesterol-lowering drug for one patient to avoid a mortal heart attack, and that figure only applies to high-risk patients. There is a vanishing benefit to lowering cholesterol for healthy adults.*" (14) Dr. John Abramson joined with thirty MD's in a 2004 letter to the NIH calling for a complete revision of the faulty cholesterol treatment guidelines. Can't convince your doctor NOT TO prescribe statin drugs for you? Print out this chapter and give it to your doctor.

For references and links, see my web site: www.bioidenticalhormones101.com

References for Chapter 40. Cholesterol Lowering Statin Drugs for Women, Just Say No

(1) http://www.postgradmed.com/issues/2002/08_02/pearlman.shtml The new cholesterol guidelines, Applying them in clinical practice, Brian L. Pearlman. Vol 112, N 2, Aug 2002, Postgraduate Medicine

(2) http://hp2010.nhlbihin.net/ncep_slds/atpiii/slide25.htm The new cholesterol guidelines

(3) http://www.usatoday.com/news/health/2004-10-16-panel-conflict-of-interest_x.htm USA Today, 2004, Cholesterol guidelines become a morality play the Associated Press

(4) http://www.westonaprice.org/know-your-fats/538-cholesterol-and-heart-disease-a-phony-issue?qh=YToyOntpOjA7czo0OiJlbmlnIjtpOjE7czo1OiJlbmlnZSI7fQ%3D%3D Cholesterol and Heart Disease: A Phony Issue. by Mary G. Enig, PhD June 30 2001, at www.westonprice.com

(5) http://www.cmaj.ca/cgi/content/full/173/10/1207-a Questioning the benefits of statins Eddie Vos and Colin P. Rose, CMAJ • November 8, 2005; 173 (10). doi:10.1503/cmaj.1050120.

(6) http://www.westonaprice.org/moderndiseases/statin.html Dangers of Statin Drugs: What You Haven't Been Told About Popular Cholesterol-Lowering Medicines By Sally Fallon and Mary G. Enig, PhD

(7) http://www.ti.ubc.ca/pages/letter48.htm
Therapeutics Initiative, Do Statins have a Role in Primary Prevention? There were 10,990 women in the primary prevention trials (28% of the total). Only coronary events were reported for women, but when these were pooled they were not reduced by statin therapy, RR 0.98 [0.85-1.12]. Thus the coronary benefit in primary prevention trials appears to be limited to men, RR 0.74 [0.68-0.81], ARR 2.0%, NNT 50 for 3 to 5 years.

(8) http://jama.ama-assn.org/cgi/content/abstract/291/18/2243 Drug Treatment of Hyperlipidemia in Women Judith M. E. Walsh, MD, MPH; Michael Pignone, MD, MPH JAMA. 2004;291:2243-2252.

(9) http://www.nwhn.org/newsletter/article.cfm?content_id=134 Women's Health Activist May/ June 2007: Exploring Statins: What Does the Evidence Say? By Electra Kaczorowski, National Women's Health Network

(10) http://www.laleva.org/eng/2004/04/statin_drugs_-_a_critical_review_of_the_riskbenefit_clinical_research.html Statin Drugs: A Critical Review of the Risk/Benefit Clinical Research, Joel M. Kauffman, Ph.D. Professor of Chemistry Emeritus USP Philadelphia, PA, USA 9 Dec 2003. Also see: http://www.healthyskepticism.org/global/library/item/11630

(11) http://www.whp-apsf.ca/pdf/statinsEvidenceCaution.pdf Evidence for Caution: Women and statin use By Harriet Rosenberg Danielle Allard Women and Health Protection June 2007

(12) http://www.health-heart.org/malpractice.pdf
LETTER TO THE EDITOR: Statins for women, elderly: Malpractice? Nutrition, Metabolism & Cardiovascular Diseases (2007) 17, e19ee20 Eddie Vos 127 Courser Rd, Sutton (Qc),

(13) http://www.lewrockwell.com/sardi/sardi69.html
Who Will Tell the People? It Isn't Cholesterol! by Bill Sardi

(14) http://overdosedamerica.com/articles.php
Lancet: Vol 369 January 20, 2007 Are lipid-lowering guidelines evidence-based? J Abramson and JM Wright

(15) http://www.health-fx.net/eBook.pdf
The Hidden Truth About Cholesterol-Lowering Drugs, by Shane Ellison, MS, Organic Chemistry

(16) http://www.nytimes.com/2008/01/17/business/17drug.html
New Questions on Treating Cholesterol, By ALEX BERENSON, New York Times January 17, 2008

(17) http://www.lewrockwell.com/sardi/sardi79.html
Government Health Agencies Complicit in Cholesterol Ruse by Bill Sardi on Lew Rockwell.com

(18) http://pharmamkting.blogspot.com/2008/01/should-i-stop-taking-zetia.html Pharma Marketing Blog by Shaun McIver, of Streamlogics, Inc discussion of Zetia Enhance trial.

(19) http://blogs.wsj.com/health/2008/01/14/zetia-doesnt-enhance-zocor/
January 14, 2008, 9:11 am Zetia Doesn't Enhance Zocor Posted by Shirley S. Wang Wall Street Journal

(20) http://www.youtube.com/watch?v=kBfWybm0218
Vytorin video AD on You Tube 30 sec, Humorous clothes which look like the food. These ads have been pulled from national television.

(21) http://energycommerce.house.gov/Press_110/110-ltr.010708.Pfizer.Jarvik.pdf Letter from John Dingel Mich to CEO of Pfizer asking for records on Jarvik and Lipitor, celebrity endorsement of Lipitor Ads.

(22) http://blogs.wsj.com/health/2008/01/16/congress-investigates-vytorin-ads/ Wall Street Journal January 16, 2008, 3:44 pm Congress Investigates Vytorin Ads Posted by Anna Wilde Mathews

(23) http://blogs.wsj.com/health/2008/01/07/congress-to-pfizer-why-is-robert-jarvik-the-lipitor-man/ January 7, 2008, Wall Street Journal,

Congress to Pfizer: Why is Robert Jarvik the Lipitor Man? Posted by Shirley S. Wang

(24) http://video.search.yahoo.com/video/play?vid=1298285495&vw=g&b=0&pos=4&p=lipitor&fr=yfp-t-501
Lipitor Ad with Robert Jarvik 60 seconds. This ad has been pulled and no longer shown on national television.

(25) http://www.nytimes.com/2008/01/17/business/17drug.html
New Questions on Treating Cholesterol By ALEX BERENSON Published: January 17, 2008. NY Times.

(26) http://www.jpands.org/vol10no3/colpo.pdf
LDL Cholesterol, Bad Cholesterol or Bad Science by Anthony Colpo, Journal of American Physicians and Surgeons Volume 10 Number 3 Fall 2005

(27) http://www.joplink.net/prev/200411/200411_10.pdf
Recurrent Acute Pancreatitis Possibly Induced by Atorvastatin and Rosuvastatin. Is Statin Induced Pancreatitis a Class Effect? JOP. J Pancreas (Online) 2004; 5(6):502-504.

(28) http://www.cmellc.com/geriatrictimes/g040618.html
Statin Adverse Effects: Implications for the Elderly by Beatrice A. Golomb, M.D., Ph.D. Geriatric Times May/June 2004 Vol. V Issue 3. "No survival benefit with statin drugs is seen in elderly patients at high risk for cardiovascular disease (Shepherd et al., 2002). For patients older than 85, benefits may be more attenuated and risks more amplified (Weverling-Rijnsburger et al., 1997). In fact, in this older group, higher cholesterol has been linked observationally to improved survival.

(29) http://www.bmj.com/cgi/content/full/335/7614/285
Preventive health care in elderly people needs rethinking, BMJ 2007;335:285-287 (11 August), "Preventive use of statins shows no overall benefit in elderly people as cardiovascular mortality and morbidity are replaced by cancer".

(30) http://image.thelancet.com/extras/02art8325web.pdf
Pravastatin in elderly individuals at risk of (PROSPER): a randomised controlled trial. THE LANCET • Published online November 19, 2002•

(31) http://www.spacedoc.net/index.html
SpaceDoc, Duane Graveline MD Author of Statin Drugs Side Effects

(32) http://www.thincs.org/index.htm
THINCS The International Society of Cholesterol Sceptics

(33) http://www.jpands.org/vol12no1/kauffman.pdf
Misleading Recent Papers on Statin Drugs in Peer-Reviewed Medical Journals Joel M. Kauffman, Ph.D. Journal of American Physicians and Surgeons Volume 12 Number 1 Spring 2007

(34) http://www.scientificexploration.org/jse/articles/pdf/18.4_bauer.pdf
Science in the 21st Century: Knowledge Monopolies and Research Cartels. Henry H. Bauer. Journal of Scientific Exploration, Vol. 18, No. 4, pp. 643-660, 2004

(35) http://www.ajronline.org/cgi/reprint/151/4/667
Radiologic Appearance of the Jarvik Artificial Heart Implant Its Thoracic Complications AJR 151:667-671, October 1988 Laurie L. Fajardo

(36) http://query.nytimes.com/gst/fullpage.html?res=9A0DE0DC1F3FF93AA15755C0A960948260 The End of Life: Euthanasia and Morality (Oxford University Press, 1986). SUICIDE AND EUTHANASIA Barney Clark's key to turn off artificial heart.

(37) http://www.pubmedcentral.nih.gov/articlerender.fcgi?tool=pubmed&pubmedid=11678788 Statins for primary prevention: at what coronary risk is safety assured? Peter R Jackson Br J Clin Pharmacol. 2001 October; 52(4): 439-446.

(38) http://www.ncbi.nlm.nih.gov/pubmed/16815382?dopt=AbstractPlus Statins act like Vitamin D!! Lancet. 2006 Jul 1;368(9529):83-6. Grimes DS.

(39) http://www.reuters.com/article/governmentFilingsNews/idUSN2525934020080225 Pfizer pulls TV ads with heart expert Jarvik. By Lisa Richwine Mon Feb 25, Reuters

(40) http://www.hc-sc.gc.ca/ahc-asc/media/advisories-avis/_2004/2004_34-eng.php Updated safety information regarding Crestor® Warning 2004-58 November 24, 2004. Canadian Adverse Drug Reaction Monitoring Program (CADRMP)—HEALTH CANADA. Health Canada is advising Canadians about a possible association between Crestor® and rhabdomyolysis, and muscle pain.

(41) http://www.ncbi.nlm.nih.gov/pubmed/14695925 Biofactors. 2003;18(1-4):101-11. The clinical use of HMG CoA-reductase inhibitors and the associated depletion of coenzyme Q10. A review of animal and human publications. Langsjoen PH, Langsjoen AM.

(42) http://www.ncbi.nlm.nih.gov/pubmed/17482884 Mitochondrion. 2007 Jun;7 Suppl:S168-74. Coenzyme Q10 and statins: biochemical and clinical implications. Littarru GP, Langsjoen P.

(43) http://www.ncbi.nlm.nih.gov/pubmed/17493470 Am J Cardiol. 2007 May 15;99(10):1409-12. Effect of coenzyme q10 on myopathic symptoms in patients treated with statins. Caso G, Kelly P, McNurlan MA, Lawson WE.

(44) http://www.annals.org/content/145/7/520.full Ann Intern Med. 2006 Oct 3;145(7):520-30. Narrative review: lack of evidence for recommended low-density lipoprotein treatment targets: a solvable problem. Hayward RA, Hofer TP, Vijan S.

(45) http://cspinet.org/new/pdf/finalnihltr.pdf Petition To The National Institutes of Health Seeking an Independent Review Panel To Re-Evaluate The National Choesterol Education

Program Guidelines, September 23, 2004. Merrill Goozner, Director, Integrity in Science Project, Center for Science in the Public Interest.

(46) http://www.ncbi.nlm.nih.gov/pmc/articles/PMC2849981/
Am J Cardiovasc Drugs. 2008; 8(6): 373-418. Statin Adverse Effects: A Review of the Literature and Evidence for a Mitochondrial Mechanism by Beatrice A. Golomb, M.D., Ph.D.ab and Marcella A. Evans, B.S.ac

(47) http://fampra.oxfordjournals.org/content/19/1/95.full
Family Practice (2002) 19 (1): 95-98. Do lipid-lowering drugs cause erectile dysfunction? A systematic review by Kash Rizvi, John P Hampson and John N Harvey

(48) http://www.ncbi.nlm.nih.gov/pmc/articles/PMC1732626/ Epidemiol Community Health. 2004 December; 58(12): 1047-1051. Lipid lowering drugs prescription and the risk of peripheral neuropathy: an exploratory case-control study using automated databases G. Corrao, A. Zambon, L. Bertu, E. Botteri, O. Leoni, and P. Contiero

(49) http://www.bmj.com/cgi/content/full/334/7601/983
BMJ 2007;334:983 (12 May), Should women be offered cholesterol lowering drugs to prevent cardiovascular disease? No, says Malcolm Kendrick, general practitioner.

(50) http://www.ctsu.ox.ac.uk/~hps/pubs/Lancet%20360;7-22.pdf
http://www.ncbi.nlm.nih.gov/pubmed/12114036 Lancet. 2002 Jul 6;360(9326):7-22. MRC/BHF Heart Protection Study of cholesterol lowering with simvastatin in 20,536 high-risk individuals: a randomised placebo-controlled trial.Heart Protection Study Collaborative Group.

CHAPTER 41

A Choirboy for Cholesterol Turns Disbeliever

Steven Sinatra MD, a board certified cardiologist in Connecticut and popular author, admits he was a cholesterol believer for many years, and even lectured on behalf of statin makers Merck and Pfizer. However, after years of clinical practice, Sinatra had a change of heart. He transformed himself from a choirboy for cholesterol drugs into a disbeliever because of the following observations:

Observations That Show Cholesterol IS NOT the Cause of Heart Disease
(1) Many patients with low cholesterol will go on to develop heart disease.
(2) In many patients with cholesterol above 280, angiograms show normal coronary arteries. They don't have heart disease.
(3) Population studies discredit cholesterol. For example, the French have the highest cholesterol levels in Europe of 250, and they also have lowest incidence of heart disease. On the Greek Island of Crete, average cholesterol is well over 200, yet there was not a single heart attack there in ten years.
(4) Half of all heart attacks occur in people with normal total cholesterol.

A Vending Machine for Statin Drugs?

Steven Sinatra, MD remarked in his writings that drug companies Merck and Pfizer have transformed the medical profession into one big vending machine for statin drugs.(1-4) Dr. Sinatra also informs us that the routine Cholesterol Blood Test ordered by your doctor is now obsolete, and has been replaced by the VAP test, a more sophisticated lipoprotein panel which provides a wealth of useful information absent from the old cholesterol panel. What is this added information?

The VAP Test—LDL Particles—Not All Sizes are Equal

Firstly the VAP Test provides the LDL particle size. Small LDL particle size is the dangerous one associated with increased risk of heart disease. Large buoyant LDL particle size is the safe one, with less heart disease risk. Secondly the VAP includes Lipoprotein (a), a marker of high risk for heart disease risk.

What is the Value of a Total Cholesterol Test?

Sinatra says total cholesterol doesn't mean much unless you have a level over 320 which increases risk of stroke. Reducing cholesterol can be accomplished with weight reduction and increasing dietary fiber. He would not give a statin drug for this unless you are a male with documented heart disease.

Adverse Effects of Low LDL

Sinatra says that statin drugs can drive down LDL, yet low LDL below 80 is associated with adverse side effects of increased risk of cancer, aggression, cerebral bleeding, amnesia, and immune dysfunction.

Just Don't Do It

Here is Dr Sinatra's advice to you if your doctor tells you to take statin based on the standard cholesterol panel:

Dr Sinatra's Advice:
(1) Don't do it. Ask for a VAP test. (2) If you are a 50-75 year old male with increased numbers of small dense LDL particles on a VAP test, then go for the statin drug. It's a good idea. If you are over 75, then don't take a statin drug as the drugs cause increased mortality in the elderly.

(3) If you are a woman, avoid statins, as no statin drug study has ever shown a benefit in all-cause mortality for women by lowering cholesterol, and adverse effects of the drugs are horrendous.

(4) If you have elevated lipoprotein (a), do not take a statin. The drugs don't work for this. Instead use Niacin (B3) 500-2000 mg per day, fish oil 2-3 grams per day, and nattokinase 100 mg per day.

The Greatest Scam Ever

The famous Framingham Study is the foundation and basis of the cholesterol theory of heart disease. This is the idea that elevated cholesterol causes heart disease, and statin drugs reduce cholesterol thereby preventing heart disease. A biochemist and participant in the Framingham study, George Mann, later described this as, *"the greatest 'scientific' deception of the century, and perhaps any century"*.(17)

I Stopped My Statin Drug—Now What?

Once a patient decides to get off statin drugs, the next question is what replaces the statin drug? What lifestyle modifications and nutritional supplements are used to prevent or reverse heart disease? The answer is that an entire program has been devised for this. This program is called "**Track Your Plaque**", and was devised by William Davis MD, a Wisconsin cardiologist. Contained within Dr. Davis's program are lifestyle and diet modifications and targeted supplements based on the VAP—Lipoprotein results. A complete description of this program can be found in Natural Medicine 101.

William Davis MD Warns About the Evil Trio

If total cholesterol is not useful as a predictor of heart disease risk, what is? Firstly, Dr. Davis uses the calcium score as a predictor of heart disease risk. Secondly, there are a few lipoprotein markers on the VAP test which are useful. Dr. Davis tells us the VAP test sometimes reveals an evil trio of lipoprotein abnormalities which are strongly predictive of heart disease risk, often leading to advanced heart disease at an early age.(6)

The Evil Trio of Dr Davis
1) Low HDL—generally less than 50 mg/dl. 2) Small Particle Size LDL—especially if 50% or more of total LDL. 3) Elevated Lipoprotein(a)—an aggressive risk factor by itself.

If you have the "Evil Trio" on your VAP test, rather than robotically prescribe a statin drug, Dr. Davis instead recommends lifestyle modification and key dietary supplements. Davis remarks that some of his greatest heart disease reversals, with reduction in calcium score, have been in patient with this Evil Trio, which responds well to the regimen listed below. Reversal of heart disease is determined by reduction in coronary calcium score (or less of an increase) on follow up scans.

Here is Dr Davis' Program for Reversing Heart Disease and the Evil Trio
1) Niacin—increases HDL, reduces small LDL, and reduces Lp(a) 2) Elimination of wheat, cornstarch, and sugars—Best for reducing small LDL; less potent for Lp(a) reduction. 3) Reduce carbohydrates and increase healthy fats—Like niacin, effective for all three. 4) High-dose fish oil—Higher doses of EPA + DHA 3000 mg per day.

Statin Drug Case Stories: Here are a few statin drug case histories from my office:

Case Number One—Chronic Psoriatic Rash from Statins:

Dan is about 65 with no history of heart disease and has been on a statin drug for a cholesterol of 220 about two years. His major problem is a red raised rash on his forearms, and hands and forehead which looks a lot like psoriasis, present for about 2 years. Dermatologists have been stumped and of no help. Dan's VAP test show large buoyant LDL particles indicating low risk for heart disease. His coronary calcium score was 75th percentile indicating only moderately above average risk of heart disease (50% per centile is average risk). I told Dan that the rash was most likely a reaction to the statin anti-cholesterol drug, and advised a two week trial off the drug to see if the rash resolves. Three weeks later Dan returns to the office, and reports the skin rash is gone.

Case Number Two—Lupus-like Skin Lesion from Statins

Sarah is an 82 year old with no history of heart disease on a statin drug for a cholesterol of 235. She had been to the dermatologist because of skin lesions on her face near the temple areas which were biopsied and reported by the pathologist as inflammation in the skin suggestive of lupus erythematosis (SLE). Sarah is concerned she has Lupus and came to see me for a second opinion. I told Sarah she most definitely did not have Lupus and advised her that the skin eruptions were a reaction to the statin drug. Sarah stopped the statin drug and three weeks later reported the skin had returned to normal.

Case Number Three—Early Alzheimer's from Statins

Lori is a 52 year old post menopausal with chief complaint of memory loss, cognitive dysfunction and severe fatigue. She had no history of heart disease and been on a statin drug for many years for a cholesterol of 230. I advised her to stop the statin drug. However, her cognitive dysfunction and memory loss continued unchanged. Her memory was so bad, she got lost and was unable to find her way to the office for her follow up visit. She wandered around and eventually made her way home A study by Muldoon showed virtual 100% of patients on statin drugs have some element of cognitive impairment, ranging from mild to severe symptoms of amnesia and cognitive dysfunction. (5) I have found this to be the case in actual clinical practice.

Case Number Four—Wheelchair bound non-healing deep infections from statins

Jim is a war veteran and was paralyzed from a roadside bomb many years ago, and has since been wheelchair bound. Although there is no history of heart disease, his doctor placed him on a statin drug for a cholesterol of 245 about two years ago. Shortly thereafter, Jim developed non-healing chronic decubitus infections at the ischial tuberosities (buttocks) at the site of pressure sitting in the wheelchair. Jim has had numerous surgical procedure and drainages, debridement, and multiple courses of antibiotics for these chronic infections which refuse to heal. In this case, the statin drug prevents healing of chronic infection. Jim stopped the statin drug, began an intensive nutritional program to boost immunity and healing ability. Six weeks later he reported considerable improvement.

For references and links, see my web site: www.bioidenticalhormones101.com

References for Chapter 41. A Choirboy for Cholesterol Turns Disbeliever

(1) http://www.spacedoc.net/stephen_sinatra_1
Dr. Stephen Sinatra—From Cholesterol Choirboy to Non-Believer, Spacedoc blog.

(2) http://www.spacedoc.net/stephen_sinatra_2
Dr. Stephen Sinatra—How to Determine if You Really Need a Statin

(3) http://www.spacedoc.net/stephen_sinatra_3
Dr. Stephen Sinatra—Statins, CoQ10, and Carnitine

(4) http://www.townsendletter.com/June2009/June2009.htm Clearing Up the Cholesterol Confusion by Steven Sinatra, MD, Townsend Letter.

(5) http://www.ncbi.nlm.nih.gov/pubmed/10806282 Am J Med. 2000 May;108(7):538-46. Effects of lovastatin on cognitive function and psychological well-being. Muldoon MF, Barger SD, Ryan CM, Flory JD, Lehoczky JP, Matthews KA, Manuck SB.

(6) http://heartscanblog.blogspot.com/2009/05/lethal-lipids.html Lethal lipids-Heart Scan Blog William Davis MD

(7) http://jeffreydach.com/2008/01/27/cholesterol-lowering-statin-drugs-for-women-just-say-no-by-jeffrey-dach-md.aspx Cholesterol Lowering Statin Drugs for Women, Just Say No by Jeffrey Dach MD

(8) http://jeffreydach.com/2008/08/30/cholesterol-lowering-drugs-for-the-elderly-just-say-no-by-jeffrey-dach-md.aspx Cholesterol Lowering Drugs for the Elderly, Bad Idea

(9) http://jeffreydach.com/2008/11/27/heart-disease-ascorbate-lysine-and-linus-pauling-by-jeffrey-dach-md.aspx Heart Disease, Ascorbate, Lysine and Linus Pauling by Jeffrey Dach MD

(10) http://jeffreydach.com/2008/06/26/saving-tim-russert-and-george-carlin-by-jeffrey-dach-md.aspx Saving Tim Russert and George Carlin by Jeffrey Dach MD

(11) http://jeffreydach.com/2007/05/14/lipitor-and-the-dracula-of-modern-technology-by-jeffrey-dach-md.aspx Lipitor and The Dracula of Modern Technology by Jeffrey Dach MD

(12) http://jeffreydach.com/2008/03/27/cat-coronary-calcium-scoring-reversing-heart-disease-by-jeffrey-dach-md.aspx CAT Coronary Calcium Scoring, Reversing Heart Disease by Jeffrey Dach MD

(13) http://jeffreydach.com/2008/04/18/heart-disease-part-two-by-jeffrey-dach-md.aspx Heart Disease Part Two by Jeffrey Dach MD

(14) http://jeffreydach.com/2008/11/14/crestor-jupitor-crp-and-heart-attack—by-jeffffrey-dach-md.aspx Crestor, Jupitor, CRP and Heart Attack by Jeffrey Dach MD

(15) http://jeffreydach.com/2007/05/05/jeffreydachdrdachvitaminc.aspx Vitamin C and Stroke Prevention by Jeffrey Dach MD

(16) http://jeffreydach.com/2009/01/13/cardiac-bypass-angioplasty-and-stenting-by-jeffrey-dach-md.aspx Cardiac Bypass, Angioplasty and Stenting by Jeffrey Dach MD

(17) http://www.cambridgemedscience.org/reports/CholMythCamb.pdf "Saturated fat and cholesterol in the diet are not the cause of coronary heart disease. That myth is the greatest 'scientific' deception of the century, and perhaps any century."—George V. Mann, M.D. Professor of Biochemistry, The Physician's Concise Guide To: The Cholesterol Myth.

SECTION ELEVEN: VITAMINS B5, B6, E AND WHEATGRASS

CHAPTER 42

Pantothenic Acid, Vitamin B5 for Acne

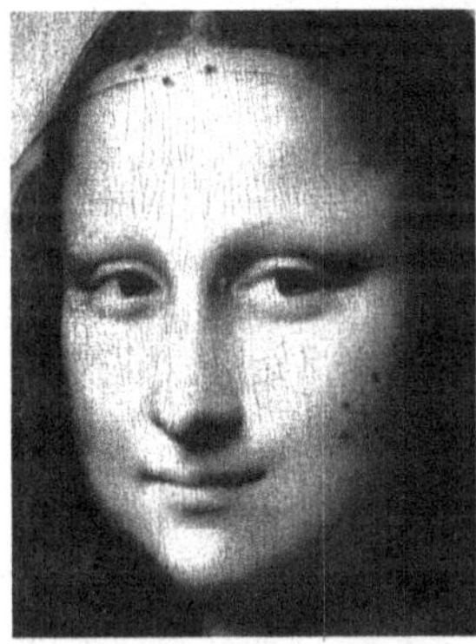

The Mona Lisa with Acne, 1503—1505 by Leonardo da Vinci (1452-1519), Medium Oil on poplar. Louvre Museum Paris

Virtually everyone remembers the frustrating experience of acne with small inflamed dots called pimples or blackheads. For the young woman concerned about self-image, skin complexion is important. One or two strategically placed pimples can be intolerable. For some, acne can progress, leading to scarring and disfigurement, with pitting and nodularity called Acne Vulgaris. While some are spared this chronic ordeal, others endure many years of ineffective treatments by a succession of dermatologists. Although some treatments such as Accutane™ may offer success, there is a price in terms of serious adverse side effects.

What Causes Acne?

Acne is caused by excess oil called sebum which originates in the sebaceous glands at the root of the hair follicles. This oily build may occlude the duct in the skin causing blockage and infection. "Popping the pimple" is a home remedy which forces the occluding plug to pop out of the pore, providing drainage and temporary relief.

Common Causes of Acne

Acne is a common adverse side effect of synthetic birth control pills which mimic testosterone. Elevated testosterone levels in males and females are associated with increased oil production in the skin resulting in acne. A common genetic mutation called atypical CAH (congenital adrenal hyperplasia) causes increased testosterone in females resulting in acne. PCOS (polycystic ovary syndrome) syndrome is associated with increased testosterone production and acne is common. Acne can also be associated with PMS symptoms in the cycling female. When estrogen levels drop suddenly the last week of the cycle, serum binding protein also declines. This liberates free testosterone which may cause PMS related acne for a week or so, until estrogen levels return to normal. Young males may suffer from acne from abundant testosterone production. Below, we make the case for vitamin B5 deficiency as a possible cause for acne.

What are the Acne Treatments?

Traditionally, acne is treated by the dermatologist with various topical cleansers, antibiotics and drugs such as Accutane™. Accutane's most commonly reported adverse side effect is depression which can lead to suicide.(25)

Vitamin B5 Treatment for Acne

In this article we will present to you information about Vitamin B5 (Pantothenic acid) as a treatment for acne. We will explain the role of Vitamin B5 in the metabolism of fats and oils, and how increasing the metabolism of oils will reduce oil accumulation in the skin, and thereby reduce or eliminate acne. Both Accutane™ and Vitamin B5 work by different mechanisms. Accutane™ works by shrinking the sebaceous glands at the root of the hair follicles. However, quite differently, Vitamin B5 works by reducing the oil production of the sebaceous glands. This is done by increasing Coenzyme A (Co-A) which increases the metabolic breakdown of oils by normal activity of cell physiology. (26)

Co-Enzyme A and Pantothenic Acid for Acne—Lit-Hung Leung

I first became aware of the use of Vitamin B5 (also called Pantothenic Acid) as a treatment for acne from an article by Lit-Hung Leung (1997).

(4,5,11,12) In this article, Dr Leung explains that acne can be reduced or eliminated with the use of Vitamin B5, also called Pantothenic acid. Pantothenic acid is a major component of Co-Enzyme A (CoA).(6) CoA is used at the cellular level for fatty acid oxidation and in many other biochemical reactions in the cell. Taking additional B5 increases the amount of Coenzyme A available for use in the cell. The more Co-Enzyme A, the more fatty acids can be metabolized, which means they are oxidized or burned up as energy production. CoEnzyme A is actually a Pantothenic Acid molecule attached to an ADP molecule. ADP is widely available throughout cellular biochemistry as the currency of energy in the cell.

What is Pantethine?

Pantethine is made of two Vitamin B5 molecules linked together with two sulfurs (S-S) in the center. It is well known that the Beta Oxidation of Fatty Acids depends on CoA.(26) If there is a deficiency of Acetyl CoA in the body, oxidation of fatty acids will slow down, and the skin becomes oily resulting in acne. Increasing availability of Acetyl CoA speeds up metabolic breakdown of fatty acids, then converted into cellular energy. Taking vitamin B5, pantothenic acid, is the easiest way to increase acetyl Co A and increase rate of fatty acid metabolism.

Dr Leung's Dosage is Rather Large

Dr. Leung gave his acne patients rather large doses of five to ten grams of Pantothenic Acid per day with considerable improvement in their acne. He reported success with this regimen.

Message Board Discuss Pantethine and B5 for Acne

After reading Dr. Leung's article, I then did an internet search for Acne and B5, and found a large amount of information on message boards posted by people suffering from acne trying various treatments, including pantothenic acid. (9,10) I found that many, but not all, of these acne sufferers had success with vitamin B5 (Pantethine) which did work for many of them. However, a common complaint was that the large amount of pantethine (10 grams) was hard to take, causing gastrointestinal gas and bloating, etc.

L-Carnitine Used as Booster

Obviously, the major difficulty with Dr Leung's Vitamin B5 protocol is the large amount of B5 required. It would be advantageous to reduce the B5 dosage to a more reasonable level. Considering the biochemical pathways involved, this would be possible with the addition of L-Carnitine, which transports fatty acids across the mitochondrial membrane where they can be oxidized. (26-28)

Transport is Rate Limiting Step for Fatty Acid Oxidation

According to the biochemistry of fatty acid oxidation, transport is the **RATE LIMITING STEP** for oxidation of long chain fatty acids. Carnitine transports long-chain acyl groups from fatty acids into the mitochondrial matrix, so that they can be broken down through β-oxidation to acetate to obtain usable energy via the citric acid cycle. (26-28)

Reducing or Eliminating Acne with Pantethine and L Carnitine

Using the modified Leung B5 protocol with Pantethine 750 mg with 250 mg of L Carnitine three times a day, we have noted excellent success rates in reducing or eliminating acne. An added advantage is a good cosmetic result with smaller pore size and smoother skin. The vitamins are safe with no adverse side effects noted.

A College Student with Acne

A college student under my care was making preparations for her upcoming wedding when she noticed some new acne lesions on her face. We immediately began the Pantethine and L-Carnitine. Her acne cleared up immediately, and she was quite pleased. By now, we have a number of satisfied patients who have used this program to clear up acne. I myself have used the program and can report that it works quite well. Since this anti-acne regimen is essentially a fat burning protocol, it is also useful for weight loss as noted in this article. Unlike Accutane™ which may have serious adverse side effects, vitamin B5 has little or no adverse side effects.

Acetyl CoA Important for Cholesterol and Steroid Biosynthesis

Acetyl CoA is the first step in the body's synthesis of Cholesterol. Cholesterol is then used to make all steroidal hormones. Many of the steroidal hormones are made by the adrenal gland, so it is very logical that B5 deficiency can result in a syndrome called adrenal failure, or the inability to synthesis steroidal hormones such as Cortisol. See my previous article on Adrenal Fatigue for more information about this syndrome.

Systemic Lupus and Acetyl CoA Deficiency

Systemic Lupus is an autoimmune disease with no known cause first described in 1851. A blood test for anti-nuclear antibodies is diagnostic. However, a number of features of Lupus suggest a link with steroid hormone synthesis. For example, there is a well know tendency for Lupus to flare up under certain conditions in which there is a greater demand for steroidal hormone biosynthesis, such as puberty, and pregnancy. Females are more affected than males by a ratio of ten to one. Lupus preferentially affects females because they have greater demands for hormone production than do males. These lupus flares seem to correlate with demand for higher levels of hormones. Production of higher hormone levels could deplete the stores of precursor molecules for production of these hormones. The first such precursor molecule is acetyl CoA, so a deficiency in acetyl CoA could be the culprit.

Low Hormone Levels in Lupus

Another feature of female Lupus patients is that when hormone levels are measured, they tend to run low. Irregular menstrual cycles and absent menses is common among lupus patients. Giving hormones to raise levels seems to help. For example, Quality of Life for Lupus patients seems to be ameliorated by DHEA administration, an adrenal hormone precursor. DHEA administration can even reduce the number of Lupus Flares. After menopause when hormone production declines dramatically, there is a reduction in Lupus flares and the disease becomes quiescent. Acne tends to be a common issue for Lupus patients given DHEA, and this would be expected assuming there is an underlying B5/Acetyl CoA deficiency. Administration of B5 along with the DHEA usually resolves the acne. Cortisol production is also decreased in lupus patients, explaining why they do better when treated with steroids.

Drug Induced Lupus

Another interesting feature of Lupus is that the disease can be caused by 70 various drugs. The three most common are procainamide, hydralazine and isoniazid. These drugs have nothing in common except they are metabolized by the acetylation pathway, a connection to Acetyl CoA.

Combined Nutritional Deficiency Disease

The first manifestations of a nutritional deficiency state appear in the skin, joint and connective tissue with various lesions. The vital organs are only involved much later on. For example, deficiency states such as Beri Beri and Scurvy initially spare the vital organs, and first involve the skin and musculoskeletal system. Lupus follows this pattern as well.

In his article, Dr. Leung noted a connection between Systemic Lupus (SLE) and Acetyl CoA deficiency, however he was not the first to suggest giving Pantethine (Vitamin B5) to Lupus patients. There were a number of reports on this in the 1950's. However, early studies seemed to discredit the whole idea of B5 deficiency or acetyl CoA deficiency or a genetic acetylation defect in Lupus. Nonetheless, Leung reported improvement in his lupus patients who supplemented with pantothenic acid. Late stages of Lupus are characterized by specific anti nuclear antibodies (ANA test) which obviously will not be affected by giving pantothenic acid. However, much can be done to improve quality of life of the lupus patient. Perhaps a combined approach supplementing with bioidentical hormones such as estradiol, progesterone, DHEA, Cortef, testosterone as well as vitamin mineral supplementation with pantethine, and others would be the most logical way to help lupus patients get back their health.

Facial Rash of Lupus, Pregnancy and Addison's

Another interesting connection is the appearance of a skin rash on the face in Lupus flares with pregnancy. There can be increased facial skin pigmentation in pregnancy itself (without lupus) called Melasma, also known as chloasma or the mask of pregnancy. Another syndrome is Addison's Disease (adrenal failure) which frequently causes hyper-pigmentation in the face and elsewhere. Characteristic sites are skin creases in the hands, and the inside of the cheek (buccal mucosa). Old scars may darken. All three, Lupus, Pregnancy and Addison's, share the need to stimulate more adrenal steroidal hormones with ACTH (ACTH = adreno cortico stimulating hormone). ACTH is secreted by the pituitary to stimulate more adrenal hormone synthesis. Increased ACTH causes an increase in melanocyte-stimulating hormone (MSH). The MSH induces melanocytes to cause the pigmentation.

A Lupus Patient Tells Her Story

A 45 year old Lupus patient came to see me in the office. She had seen many rheumatologists and specialists over the years with a confirmed diagnosis of Lupus. She appeared under weight and chronically ill, and had absent menses for the last 7 years. Her main complaint was severe chronic fatigue and inability to gain weight. In the past she had been on many of the usual drug treatments for lupus with many adverse effects and no real improvement in quality of life.

Initial testing showed low salivary cortisol, and low serum levels for the other hormones, DHEA, estradiol, progesterone and testosterone. She also had low B12 and Vitamin D levels. She was started on bio-identical hormones, Pantethine (B5), B12 and Vitamin D. About three months after starting treatment, she calls me and states she is feeling much better with improved energy levels, and she just had a normal menstrual period, the first one after seven years of absent menses.

For references and links, see my web site: www.bioidenticalhormones101.com

References for Chapter 42. Pantothenic Acid, B5 for Acne and Lupus

(1) http://www.vilantae.com/index.php
Vilante Home, and Video

(2) http://www.b5acnetreatment.com/2007_03_01_archive.html
Vilante B5 web site

(3) http://www.acnetohealth.com/vitamin-b-5-acne.html
The Vitamin B 5 Acne Theory Debunked

(4) http://deficiencydiseases.com/ Papers on B5 and Acne by Lit-Hung Leung, M.D.

(5) http://www.coenzyme-a.com/acne_vulgaris.html Pantothenic Acid in the Treatment of Acne Vulgaris "A Medical Hypothesis" by Lit-Hung Leung, M.D. The Effect of Pantothenic Acid on Acne Vulgaris

(6) http://www.coenzyme-a.com/research.html Research Articles on Coenzyme A, Pantethine: A Review of their Biochemistry and Therapeutic Applications first published in Alternative Medicine Review, Volume 2, Number 5.

(7) http://www.coenzyme-a.com/research.html Pantothenic Acid in the Treatment of Obesity. "A Medical Hypothesis" by Lit-Hung Leung, M.D. Journal of Orthromolecular Medicine Vol. 12 Number 2, 1997.

(8) http://www.coenzyme-a.com/research.html Coenzyme-ATM "Precursor The Master CoenzymeTM" by Nickolaos D. Skouras, Ph.D.

(9) http://www.acne.org/messageboard/index.php?showtopic=15341 Acne. Org message board . . . nuts and bolts advice on b5.

(10) http://www.ironmagazineforums.com/history/topic/23051-1.html acne b5 accutane message board

(11) http://orthomolecular.org/library/jom/1997/articles/1997-v12n02-p099.shtml The Journal of Orthomolecular Medicine Vol. 12, 2nd Quarter 1997. A Stone that Kills two Birds: How Pantothenic Acid Unveils the Mysteries of Acne Vulgaris and Obesity Lit-Hung Leung. M.D.

(12) http://deficiencydiseases.com/ articles by Lit-Hung Leung on B5 and Acne

(13) http://deficiencydiseases.com/SLE_full_text.pdf
LUPUS ERYTHEMATOSUS: A Combined Deficiency Disease by Lit-Hung Leung, M.D. Formerly Consultant Surgeon, Department of General Surgery, Hong Kong Central Hospital, Hong Kong.

(14) http://www.ncbi.nlm.nih.gov/pubmed/7476595
Med Hypotheses. 1995 Jun;44(6):490-2. Pantothenic acid deficiency as the pathogenesis of acne vulgaris. Leung LH.

(15) http://ezinearticles.com/?Using-Pantothenic-Acid-(Vitamin-B5)-as-an-Acne-Treatment&id=48855 Using Pantothenic Acid (Vitamin B5) as an Acne Treatment By Ryan Bauer

(16) http://www.ncbi.nlm.nih.gov/pubmed/3976557 Am J Clin Nutr. 1985 Mar;41(3):578-89. Effects of supplemental pantothenic acid on wound healing: experimental study in rabbit. Aprahamian M, Dentinger A, Stock-Damgé C, Kouassi JC, Grenier JF.

(17) http://lpi.oregonstate.edu/infocenter/vitamins/pa/ Pantothenic Acid, Linus Pauling Inst. Oregon State.

(18) http://www.bastyrcenter.org/content/view/439/ Nutritional Supplements In The Treatment Of Acne Bastyr University.

(19) http://www.ncbi.nlm.nih.gov/pubmed/13985157
Vestn Dermatol Venerol. 1963 Mar;37:16-20. [Combined treatment of lupus erythematosus patients with resochin and calcium pantothenate.] [Article in Russian] TISHCHENKO LD.

(20) http://www.ncbi.nlm.nih.gov/pubmed/13423891
AMA Arch Derm. 1957 Jun;75(6):845-50.The diagnosis of lupus

erythematosus; probable significance of pantothenate blood levels. SLEPYAN AH, FROST DV, OVERBY LR, FREDRICKSON RL, OSTERBERG AE.

(21) Cochrane, T., Leslie, G. (1952). The treatment of lupus erythematosus with calcium pantothenate and panthenol. J. Invest. Dermat., 18, 365-367.

(22) http://www.journals.elsevierhealth.com/periodicals/ymehy/article/PIIS0306987704000945/abstract Volume 62, Issue 6, Pages 922-924 (June 2004) Systemic lupus erythematosus: a combined deficiency disease. Lit-Hung Leung.

(23) http://www.mitamins.com/library/Concern/Lupus.html Welsh AL. Lupus erythematosus: Treatment by combined use of massive amounts of pantothenic acid and vitamin E. Arch Dermatol Syphilol 1954;70:181-98.

(24) http://archive.food.gov.uk/committees/evm/papers/evm0101.pdf Cochrane T, Leslie G. The treatment of lupus erythematosus with calcium pantothenate and panthenol. J Invest Dermatol 1952;18:365-7.

(25) http://www.accutaneaction.com/adr/index.html
most frequently reported adverse event for Accutane/Roaccutane

(26) http://www.ncbi.nlm.nih.gov/pmc/articles/PMC1217938/?tool=pubmed Biochem J. 1996 December 1; 320(Pt 2): 345-357. Mammalian mitochondrial beta-oxidation.S Eaton, K Bartlett, and M Pourfarzam

(27) http://www.sciencedirect.com/science/article/pii/S0006291X85722322 Fatty Acid β-Oxidation in Peroxisomes and Mitochondria: The First, Unequivocal Evidence for the Involvement of Carnitine in Shuttling Propionyl-CoA from Peroxisomes to Mitochondria. Jakobs B. S. and Wanders R. J. A.

(28) http://oregonstate.edu/dept/biochem/hhmi/hhmiclasses/biochem/lectnoteskga/2kjan14lecturenotes.html Fatty Acid Oxidation-Oregon State University dept of biochemistry.

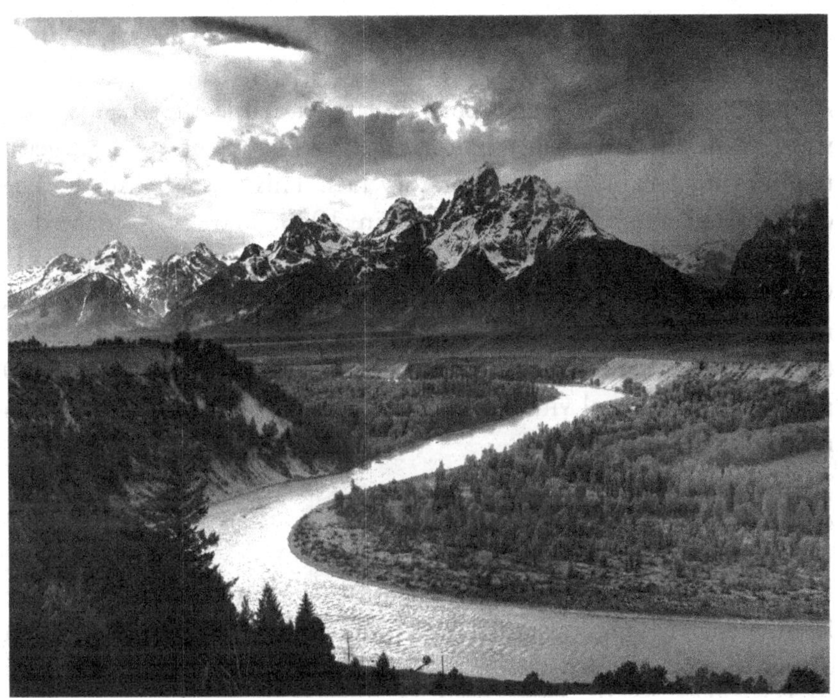

Above Left Image: 1942 Photo by Ansel Adams of The Tetons and the Snake River, Grand Teton National Park, Wyoming. National Archives and Records Administration, US National Park Service.

CHAPTER 43

Vitamin E, Curse or Blessing?

Years ago, when the kids were little, my family went on a rafting trip on the Snake River in Idaho. Everyone enjoyed the river adventure, and we later took a side trip through Coeur D'Alene where we found a dusty second hand book store called the "Book Worm". Inside the store, I found a 1964 copy of "Vitamin E, Your Key to a Healthy Heart" by Herbert Bailey.(49) This was one of the first books that stimulated interest in Vitamin E and sold a million copies.

The History of Vitamin E—Discovered in 1922

About 90 years ago, an obscure researcher named Herbert Evans, was hot on the trail of an unknown dietary ingredient in wheat germ required for fertility in his laboratory rats. This was Vitamin E. The chemical structure was determined in 1938, and Evans named it "tocopherol", a word meaning "to bear young" in ancient Greek. Early work also found Vitamin E prevented muscular dystrophy in young rats fed a vitamin E deficient diet. (46-48). In the 1930's and 1940's, two Canadian cardiologists, Wilfred and Evan Shute treated 30,000 patients with natural vitamin E and reported considerable success in reversing heart disease.(45)

A Medical Conference on Vitamin E

In 2008, I attended the ACAM Medical Meeting in Orlando where Kenny Jialal, MD was awarded the Linus Pauling Medal in recognition of his Vitamin E research.(3-4) Dr. Jialal then took the podium and spoke on Vitamin E, summarizing hundreds of research studies over decades. Some studies were favorable, some were unfavorable, some used one type of vitamin E, and some used another type of vitamin E, some he had no idea which type was used. I think you get the gist. At the end of the hour, Dr Jialal had completely confused my remaining understanding of Vitamin E, transforming the topic into a giant enigma wrapped in a mystery. I left the room with a headache. In this article, we will hopefully remedy the headache, and clear up any confusion about Vitamin E with new insights. First, let's look at some recent doubts about Vitamin E.

New Doubts About Vitamin E, Vitamin E is Deadly!!

You may have seen news reports that Vitamin E is dangerous, deadly and increases mortality. These media stories were based on an article by Edgar Miller in the Jan 2005 Annals of Internal Medicine, a meta-analysis of 19 studies on Vitamin E, concluding that Vitamin E increases mortality. (13-14) Here are a few of the news reports:

News Reports on Vitamin E is Deadly (1-2):
High dose vitamin E death warning, November, 11, 2004 from BBC News: *High doses can be harmful. Elderly people could be risking their lives if they take even moderately high doses of vitamin E, evidence suggests. (1)* **Study: High dose of Vitamin E increases death risk.** By Steve Sternberg, USA TODAY November 10, 2004: *High-dose vitamin E supplements taken daily can increase a person's risk of premature death, researchers said Wednesday. People who take daily doses of 400 international units or higher are about 10% more likely to die of a variety of causes than people who take smaller doses or no vitamin E, according to an analysis of 14 studies conducted between 1993 and 2004. Many of the studies did not specify causes of death, but researchers believe patients died of all the usual causes, including heart disease and cancer.(2)*

The Solution: Use Natural Vitamin E and Avoid Synthetic E

The effect of Miller's Vitamin E article was that many people stopped taking Vitamin E. An excellent rebuttal to Dr Miller by Dr Mark Houston pointed out the type of Vitamin E used in Miller's meta-Analysis was synthetic DL alpha tocopherol. "*None of the 19 studies in Miller's review article included any of the other seven forms of vitamin E, and, in fact, most of them used the synthetic DL alpha tocopherol form.*"(15) It is important to distinguish natural vitamin E from the synthetic Vitamin E which is to be avoided. In addition, Houston recommends a mixture of the 8 types of Vitamin E found in nature.

The Fox Guarding the Henhouse?

Amazingly, another negative Vitamin E study published by Sesso in JAMA Nov 9, 2008 again used the synthetic form of Vitamin E.(9) You would think that doctors are highly intelligent, and would know to use the natural form of vitamin E, when designing such a study. A skeptic might suggest that perhaps the synthetic form was intentionally used to insure failure and discredit vitamin E. Another disturbing fact is that Sesso's negative Vitamin study was sponsored by Wyeth, a drug company with a long history of animosity to natural treatments. The paper also disclosed that the authors were in bed with the drug companies. They received funding from Wyeth, Merck, Bristol Meyer Squibb, Astra Zeneca, Pfizer and Bayer. Dr. Gaziano, the chair of the project, even served as expert witness for Merck, defending the drug company in court. (9) I would say this is another example of "the Fox Guarding the Henhouse".(10)

The Different Types of Vitamin E, Synthetic vs. Natural

Natural vitamin E is in the "D" form (D is for Dextro which is Latin for Right-Handed). Synthetic Vitamin E is a combination of D and L form (i.e. DL). The synthetic form is cheaper, but is not recommended. There are the 8 types of Vitamin E—tocopherols in natures including, alpha, delta, gamma forms. Dr. Jialal says the gamma form is more beneficial than the alpha form.

Evidence that the Natural Form of Vitamin E is Beneficial

Two landmark Vitamin E studies were published in 1993 in the New England Journal of Medicine. Eric Rimm's study showed a 36% reduction in heart disease in men taking the relatively modest 60 IU vitamin E daily in the diet.(41) Meir Stamfer's study showed a 33% reduction in heart attacks in women with the highest dietary vitamin E consumption.(43)

More Studies Showing Benefits of Natural Vitamin E

In 1992, Verlangieri published a study in which natural vitamin E reversed atherosclerosis in a primate model.(27) A 1995 study published in JAMA by Hodis showed Vitamin E caused regression of atherosclerosis on serial coronary angiography. (28) Dr. Hodis concluded with this statement: "*These results indicate an association between supplementary vitamin E intake and angiographically demonstrated reduction in coronary artery lesion progression.*" In 1996, Stephens published his study in Lancet which showed that tocopherol (vitamin E) given to patients with advanced coronary artery disease reduced the risk of non-fatal Myocardial Infarction (MI) by 77%, (but did not decrease total mortality in this study).(37) In 2000, Boaz published a study in Lancet showing that 800 IU/daily of natural Vitamin E reduced heart attacks by 70% over 1.4 years in Hemodialysis patients. (44)

Reversing Carotid Stenosis with Natural Vitamin E

In 1997 Bierenbaum presented data on reversal of atherosclerosis in carotid stenosis with mixed tocopherols and tocotrienols at a meeting in Montreal.(2) The Bierenbaum study was done at the Kenneth Jordan Heart Research Foundation in New Jersey. The five-year study evaluated 50 patients who had stenosis of the carotid artery. One group of 25 patients received 650 mgs of tocotrienols plus tocopherols. The other group of 25 received a placebo. All patients had serial carotid sonography every six months. In the Placebo group, fifteen patients showed worsening of the stenosis, eight remained stable and two showed some improvement. In the Vitamin E Group using Tocotrienol plus tocopherol, three patients showed minor worsening, and 12 remained stable. Ten patients showed regression of stenosis with improvement. (29-32)

Not only is there a difference between synthetic and natural vitamin E, there is also a new form of vitamin E called Tocotrienol which new research suggests is the more biologically useful form. (22) Let's take a look at the Tocotrienol form of Vitamin E:

The 21st Century Form of Vitamin E—Tocotrienol

The Difference Between the Tocopherol and Tocotrienol Forms

Tocotrienol is **IDENTICAL** to Tocopherol except for the three double bonds in the tail. These three double bonds create a kinked configuration of the "tail" which allows the molecule more mobility through lipid membranes. The double bond also indicates a state of electron desaturation, meaning it can accept electrons readily as an antioxidant. The three double bonds represent an "unsaturated" side chain which allows the molecule to penetrate into saturated lipid membrane layers in various target organs. Thus, the tocotrienol form is superior to tocopherol as an antioxidant, serving to reverse lipid peroxidation. About 99% of medical research since the discovery of Vitamin E has been devoted to the tocopherol form, and 1% on the tocotrienol form. This seems to be changing. There are no synthetic forms of tocotrienols available, only natural ones.(5-8)(16-19)(22-25)

Processed Trans-Fats vs. Natural Oils

Remember the difference between Processed Trans-Fats and Natural Oils such as cold pressed olive oil? The unhealthy Trans-Fats have a straight carbon tail because they have been processed, so the Carbons are located on the opposite sides of the double bonds (trans). The healthy natural oils have a curved configuration of the carbon tail because the Carbons are on the same side of the double bond (cis). This difference is called cis-trans isomerism.

Toxic Trans Fats Have Straight Tails—Tocotrienols Have Curved Tail

Similar to the beneficial natural oils, Tocotrienols have a curved carbon tail, giving them more biological activity than the tocopherol counterpart. The Tocotrienol tail is not stationary, but actually vibrates back and forth in space like a pendulum, absorbing energy within the membrane bi-layer. (8)

Health Benefits of Tocotrienol Form of Vitamin E

1) Tocotrienols are protective in stroke-induced injuries. Natural palm tocotrienol complex fed to hypertensive rats led to increased tocotrienols level in the brain, and more protection against stroke-induced injury compared to controls. (50)

2) Tocotrienol reversed atherosclerosis in carotid artery stenosis in a human study by Bierenbaum. (51)

3) Tocotrienols and cholesterol reduction: Gamma tocotrienol inhibit hepatic cholesterol synthesis without interfering with CoQ10 production, thus reducing LDL cholesterol levels safely. (5-7)

Important Point:
The Tocotrienol form of Vitamin E is useful in prevention and reversal of heart disease, stroke and other forms of atherosclerotic vascular disease.

Apo-E Mouse Studies Show Tocotrienol Protects, Tocopherol Does NOT

The Apo-E Mouse Model is a genetically modified mouse that develops atherosclerosis of the aorta. Two separate studies, by Qureshi and another by Black showed that feeding Tocotrienols to the Apo-E mice virtually eliminates atherosclerotic plaque. (38,39) Tocotrienols reduced the atherosclerosis plaque by 98%, an amazing result. On the other hand, Tocopherols had no such beneficial effect in Apo-E mice in the study by Shaish (1999) who found no change in plaque size with Tocopherols. (40)

Reversing Coronary Artery Disease

My previous article discussed the use of high dose Vitamin C, and the amino acid, Lysine, (the Linus Pauling Protocol) for reversing heart disease. Steve Hickey and Hilary Roberts come right out on page 167 of their book, and make the statement, "***Vitamin C and Tocotrienols can reverse coronary artery disease***". (52) They would improve the Linus Pauling Protocol by adding the Tocotrienol form of Vitamin E. Regarding heart disease and atherosclerotic vascular disease, the authors state that "***on the available evidence, the combination of Vitamin C and Tocotrienols could be curative with no known harmful effects.***" (52)

Future Research for the NIH, the Guinea Pig Model:

Tocotrienols clearly prevent atherosclerosis in the Apo-E mouse model. Further research in the guinea pig model should be done. C. G. Willis showed that Vitamin C deprived guinea pigs develop atherosclerotic vascular disease. (see references in Chapter 37) Experiments should be done giving tocotrienols to Vitamin C deprived guinea pigs, and I would predict Tocotrienols would be beneficial, reducing or preventing atherosclerotic plaque formation. In addition, there is a GLO deficient mouse model used to study atherosclerosis. Experiments giving tocotrienols to GLO deficient mice should also be done.

Warning—Vitamin E—Bleeding Precautions
Vitamin E can have a blood thinning effect, so most surgeons and anesthesiologists will ask about Vitamin E use prior to elective surgery, and request that the Vitamin E be discontinued a week in advance of elective surgery to avoid bleeding complications. Increased mortality from high dose vitamin E could be related to bleeding complications.

For references and links, see my web site: www.bioidenticalhormones101.com

References for Chapter 43. Vitamin E, Curse or Blessing?

(1) http://news.bbc.co.uk/1/hi/health/3998847.stm
High dose vitamin E death warning, November 11, 2004, BBC News.

(2) http://www.usatoday.com/news/health/2004-11-10-vitamin-e-risks_x.htm Study: High dose of Vitamin E increases death risk. By Steve Sternberg, USA TODAY 11/10/2004

(3) http://www.ucdmc.ucdavis.edu/ucdavismedicine/issues/fall2008/departments/honors_and_awards.html American College for Advancement in Medicine presented Ishwarlal Jialal with the Linus Pauling Award.

(4) http://www.ucdmc.ucdavis.edu/search/faculty/biodetail.asp?bioid=860
Ishwarlal Jialal, M.D., Ph.D. UC Davis Professor Robert E. Stowell Endowed Chair in Experimental Pathology Director of Laboratory for Atherosclerosis and Metabolic Research Specialty: Pathology and Laboratory Medicine, Biological Chemistry

(5) http://www.drpasswater.com/nutrition_library/tan_1.html
Doctor Tocotrienol Barrie Tan Part One

(6) http://www.drpasswater.com/nutrition_library/tan_2.html Doctor Tocotrienol Barrie Tan Part Two

(7) http://www.acgrace.com/images/stories/acgrace/healthbenefitsbeyondvitamineactivity.pdf Health Benefits Beyond Vitamin E Activity, Solving the Tocotrienol Riddle. Dr. Barrie Tan

(8) http://www.pubmedcentral.nih.gov/articlerender.fcgi?tool=pubmed&pubmedid=17507086 Mol Aspects Med. 2007; 28(5-6): 692-728. Tocotrienols in health and disease: the other half of the natural vitamin E family. Chandan K. Sen, Savita Khanna, and Sashwati Roy

(9) http://jama.ama-assn.org/cgi/content/full/300/18/2123
Vitamins E and C in the Prevention of Cardiovascular Disease in Men. The Physicians' Health Study II Randomized Controlled Trial. Howard D. Sesso et al JAMA. 2008;300(18):2123-2133. November 9, 2008

(10) http://aahf.nonprofitsoapbox.com/index.php?option=com_content&task=view&id=601&Itemid Unfair Attacks on Supplements. The following is an analysis of a recent study on vitamins C and E by the scientific team of the Alliance for Natural Health, our international affiliate. Designed To Fail: A Trial Without Meaning. Contributed by Steve Hickey, Ph.D.; Damien Downing, M.B.B.S.; and Robert Verkerk, Ph.D., Alliance for Natural Health.

(11) http://www.ncbi.nlm.nih.gov/pubmed/16190316
Nutr Rev. 2005 Aug;63(8):290-3. Failure of vitamin E in clinical trials: is gamma-tocopherol the answer? Devaraj S, Jialal I.

(12) http://www.annals.org/cgi/content/full/142/1/75
Vitamin E Supplements: Good in Theory, but Is the Theory Good? E. Robert Greenberg, MD Annals of Internal Medicine 4 January 2005, Vol 142, Issue 1, Pages 75-76

(13) http://www.annals.org/cgi/content/full/142/1/37
High-Dosage Vitamin E Supplementation May Increase All-Cause Mortality Edgar R. Miller et al. Annals of Internal Medicine 4 January 2005 | Volume 142 Issue 1 | Pages 37-46

(14) http://www.annals.org/cgi/content/full/142/1/I-40
SUMMARIES FOR PATIENTS Vitamin E Supplements May Be Harmful. Annals of Internal Medicine 4 January 2005 | Volume 142 Issue 1 | Page I-40

(15) http://ana-jana.org/reprints/VitaminEEditorialbyMarkHouston, MD.pdf JANA Vol. 8 No. 1, 2005, "Meta-Analysis, Metaphysics and Mythology" Scientific and Clinical Perspective on the Controversies Regarding Vitamin E for the Prevention and Treatment of Disease in Humans by Mark Houston, MD

(16) Nesaretnam K, Ambra R, Selvaduray KR, et al. (2004). Tocotrienol-rich fraction from palm oil and gene expression in human breast cancer cells. ANNALS OF THE NEW YORK ACADEMY OF SCIENCES 1031: 143-157.

(17) Conte C, Floridi A, Aisa C, et al. (2004). Gamma-Tocotrienol metabolism and antiproliferative effect in prostate cancer cells. ANNALS OF THE NEW YORK ACADEMY OF SCIENCES 1031: 391-394.

(18) Hasselwander O, Kramer K, Hoppe PP, et al. (2002). Effects of feeding various tocotrienol sources on plasma lipids and aortic atherosclerotic lesions in cholesterol-fed rabbits. FOOD RESEARCH INTERNATIONAL 35 (2-3): 245-251

(19) http://www.acgrace.com/index.php?option=com_virtuemart&Itemid=5
UNIQUE E® Tocotrienols—60 Softgels $39.50, AC Grace Co.

(20) Kappus H, Diplock AT. Tolerance and safety of vitamin E: a toxicological position report. Free Radic Biol Med 1992;13:55—'D074.

(21) Vitamins E and C are safe across a broad range of intakes. Hathcock JN, Azzi A, Blumberg J, Bray T, Dickinson A, Frei B, Jialal I, Johnston CS, Kelly FJ, Kraemer K, Packer L, Parthasarathy S, Sies H, Traber MG. Am J Clin Nutr. 2005 Apr;81(4):736-45.

(22) http://www.ncbi.nlm.nih.gov/pubmed/10480444
Clin Biochem. 1999 Jul;32(5):309-19. Tocotrienol: a review of its therapeutic potential.Theriault A, Chao JT, Wang Q, Gapor A, Adeli K.

(23) http://www.ncbi.nlm.nih.gov/pubmed/15753140 Ann N Y Acad Sci. 2004 Dec;1031:127-42. Tocotrienol: the natural vitamin E to defend the nervous system? Sen CK, Khanna S, Roy S.

(24) http://ajpheart.physiology.org/cgi/content/full/289/1/H361 Am J Physiol Heart Circ Physiol 289: H361-H367, 2005. Cardioprotection with palm tocotrienol: antioxidant activity of tocotrienol is linked with its ability to stabilize proteasomes. Samarjit Das et al.

(25) http://www.drpasswater.com/nutrition_library/bierenbaum.html
Reversing Arteriosclerosis with Tocotrienols: An interview with Marvin Bierenbaum, M.D. and Tom Watkins, Ph.D. by Richard A. Passwater, Ph.D.

(26) Passwater, R.A. (1992) Reversing atherosclerosis: An interview with Dr. Anthony Verlangieri. Whole Foods 15(9):27-30.

(27) Verlangieri, A.J. and Bush, M.K. (1992) Effects of d-alpha-tocopherol supplementation on experimentally induced primate atherosclerosis. J. Amer. Coll. Nutr. 11:131-138.

(28) Hodis, H.N.; Mack, W.J.; LaBree, L.; Cashin-Hemphill, L.; Sevanian, A.; Johnson, R. and Azen, S.P. (1995) Serial coronary angiographic evidence that antioxidant vitamin intake reduces progression of coronary artery atherosclerosis. JAMA 273(23):1849-1854.

(29) Kooyenga, D.K.; Geller,M.; Watkins, T.R. and Bierenbaum, M.L. (July 29, 1997) Antioxidant-induced regression of carotid stenosis

over three-years. Proceedings of the 16th International Congress of Nutrition. Montreal.

(30) Watkins, T.; Lenz, P.; Gapor, A.; Struck, M.: Tomeo, A. and Bierenbaum, M. (1993) Gamma—tocotrienol as a hypocholesterolemic and antioxidant agent in rats fed atherogenic diets. Lipids 28(12):1113-1118.

(31) Suzuki, Y.J.; Tsuchiya, M.; Wassall, S.R.; Choo, Y.M.; Govil, G.; Kagan, V.E. and Packer, L. (1993) Structural and dynamic membrane properties of alpha-tocopherol and alpha-tocotrienol: implication to the molecular mechanism of their antioxidant potency. Biochem. 32:10692-10699.

(32) Tomeo, A.C.; Geller, M.; Watkins, T.R.; Gapor, A. and Bierenbaum, M.L. (1995) Antioxidant effects of tocotrienols in patients with hyperlipidemia and carotid stenosis. Lipids 30(12):1179-1183.

(33) http://www.douglaslabs.com/pdf/nutrinews/Vitamin%20E%20NN%20(01-08).pdf Vitamin E: A New Perspective. NutriNews from Douglas Laboratories January/February 2008. Andreas M. Papas, Ph.D.

(34) http://stroke.ahajournals.org/cgi/content/full/36/10/e144 Stroke. 2005;36:e144. Neuroprotective Properties of the Natural Vitamin E—Tocotrienol Savita Khanna, PhD; Sashwati Roy, et al. T

(35) http://www.jacn.org/cgi/content/abstract/11/2/131
J Am Col of Nut, Vol 11, Issue 2 131-138, 1992. Effects of d-alpha-tocopherol supplementation on experimentally induced primate atherosclerosis. A. J. Verlangieri and M. J. Bush

(36) http://www.ncbi.nlm.nih.gov/pubmed/8622332 Lancet. 1996 Mar 23;347(9004):781-6. Randomised controlled trial of vitamin E in patients with coronary disease: Cambridge Heart Antioxidant Study (CHAOS)Stephens NG, Parsons A et al.

(37) http://jn.nutrition.org/cgi/content/full/131/10/2606
Journal of Nutrition. 2001;131:2606-2618. Novel Tocotrienols of Rice

Bran Inhibit Atherosclerotic Lesions in C57BL/6 ApoE-Deficient Mice. Asaf A. Qureshi et. al.

(38) http://jn.nutrition.org/cgi/content/abstract/130/10/2420
Palm Tocotrienols Protect ApoE +/—Mice from Diet-Induced Atheroma Formation Tracy M. Black et al. J. Nutr. October 1, 2000 vol. 130 no. 10 2420-2426

(39) http://atvb.ahajournals.org/cgi/content/full/19/6/1470 Arteriosclerosis, Thrombosis, and Vascular Biology. 1999;19:1470-1475.) Dietary ß-Carotene and—Tocopherol Combination Does Not Inhibit Atherogenesis in an ApoE-Deficient Mouse Model. Aviv Shaish et al.

(40) http://www.benbest.com/nutrceut/VitaminE.html
Vitamin E (Tocopherols and Tocotrienols) by Ben Best

(41) http://content.nejm.org/cgi/content/short/328/20/1450
NEJM Volume 328:1450-1456 May 20, 1993 Number 20. Vitamin E Consumption and the Risk of Coronary Heart Disease in Men. Eric B. Rimm et al.

(42) http://content.nejm.org/cgi/content/short/328/20/1444
NEJM Volume 328:1444-1449 May 20, 1993 Number 20 Vitamin E Consumption and the Risk of Coronary Disease in Women. Meir J. Stampfer, Charles H. Hennekens, JoAnn E. Manson, Graham A. Colditz, Bernard Rosner, and Walter C. Willett

(43) http://www.ncbi.nlm.nih.gov/pubmed/11072938
Lancet. 2000 Oct 7;356(9237):1213-8. Secondary prevention with antioxidants of cardiovascular disease in endstage renal disease (SPACE): randomised placebo-controlled trial. Boaz M, Smetana S, Weinstein T, Matas Z, Gafter U, Iaina A, Knecht A, Weissgarten Y, Brunner D, Fainaru M, Green MS.

(44) http://www.doctoryourself.com/biblio_shute.html
Wilfrid Shute, M.D and Evan Shute, M.D.Partial Bibliography of Papers and Books, website by Andrew Saul, PhD

(45) http://jn.nutrition.org/content/17/4/371.full.pdf
HERBERT MCLEAN EVANS (1882-1971) A Biographical Sketch by I. D. RAACKE. Journal of nutrition 1963;79:l-8. 20.

(46) http://jn.nutrition.org/content/17/4/371.full.pdf
THE PREVENTIVE EFFECT OF WHEAT GERM OILS AND OF a-TOCOPHEROL IN NUTRITIONAL MUSCULAR DYSTROPHY OF YOUNG RATS 1 MARIANNE GOETTSCH AND JOHANA EITZMANN. J. Nutrition, 1939 vol. 17, p. 371.

(47) http://jn.nutrition.org/content/22/5/463.full.pdf a-TOCOPHEROL REQUIREMENT OF THE RAT FOR REPRODUCTION IN THE FEMALE AND PREVENTION OF MUSCULAR DYSTROPHY IN THE YOUNG, MARIANNE GOETTSCH AND ALWIN M. PAPPENHEIMER JOURNAL OF OF NUTRITION 1941 P.463.

(48) VITAMIN E, Your Key To a Healthy Heart by Herbert Bailey. N. Y. Arc Books; 10th Printing edition (1971).

(49) http://www.ncbi.nlm.nih.gov/pubmed/16166580

(50) Stroke. 2005 Oct;36(10):2258-64. Neuroprotective properties of the natural vitamin E alpha-tocotrienol. Khanna S et al.

(51) Watkins TR, Bierenbaum ML, Giampaolo A. Tocotrienols: Biological and Health Effects. In Antioxidant Status, Diet, Nutrition and Health, Papas AM editor, CRC Press, Boca Raton, 1998;479-96)

(52) Ascorbate: The Science of Vitamin C, Dr. Steve Hickey & Dr. Hilary Roberts, LULU (May 20, 2004)

CHAPTER 44

Vitamin B6, Pyridoxine for Trigger Finger and Carpal Tunnel

Jim is a 46 year old retired New York policeman who uses power tools to repair his house. His problem is chronic pain at the base of the thumb and wrist. The pain worsens with use of the hand, making it difficult to use the power tools. Certain repetitive hand movements cause pain such as turning a key in a lock, unscrewing the lid of a jar, and opening the car door. Jim also has "trigger finger" involving the thumb joint. He reports tingling and numbness in the hands most noticeable at night just before sleep. Jim's hand pain worsened lately, so he went to a hand surgeon who gave him a steroid injection at the base of the thumb and applied a hand/wrist splint. These measures were ineffective, and his pain continued. The surgeon suggested operation. Jim came into the office to ask if anything else could be done to avoid surgery.

Vitamin B6, Pyridoxine for Trigger Finger

As it turns out, there is a simple and effective vitamin therapy for Jim's Trigger Finger hand condition.(1-9) This vitamin is Pyridoxine, vitamin B6. Jim was given a bottle of B6, pyridoxine phosphate (the activated form) and 3 weeks later, an amazed Jim returned to report that his pain and swelling is gone, and his trigger finger had also resolved. He no longer needs the operation.

John Ellis MD, The Doctor Who Looked At Hands

I first learned of Vitamin B6 for carpal tunnel from Dr Jonathan Wright's newsletter mentioning Dr. John Ellis, a Texas physician in the 1960's who discovered that vitamin B6 eliminates carpal tunnel syndrome, trigger finger, and other hand conditions. Examine the backs of your hands. Have you ever noticed the backs of your hands are puffy and swollen, making the tendons obscured? Are your hands so swollen that you can't touch your palms with the tips of your fingers? That's the positive "Ellis sign," indicating extra B6 could be helpful. Usual dosage is 20 milligrams three times daily of the activated P-5-P form of Vitamin B6. Old copies of Dr. Ellis' book "The Doctor Who Looked at Hands" originally written in 1966, are still available.(10)

Vitamin B6 Toxicity

Unlike other water soluble B vitamin which are safe at high doses, vitamin B6 (pyridoxine) can be toxic, causing sensory neuropathy at dosages above 300 mg per day.(11-15) The biologically active form of pyridoxine P-5-P (pyridoxal-5-phosphate) has no reported toxicity. Therefore, P-5-P is the preferred form of vitamin B6. Make sure your B Vitamin Complex uses the P-5-P version rather than plain old pyridoxine.

Warning—B6 Pyridoxine Toxicity
At high doses above 300 mg per day, Vitamin B6 (pyridoxine) can be toxic, causing sensory neuropathy.

For references and links, see my web site: www.bioidenticalhormones101.com

References for Chapter 44. Vitamin B6, Pyridoxine for Trigger Finger and Carpal Tunnel Syndrome

(1) http://www.pnas.org/content/79/23/7494.full.pdf
Response of vitamin B-6 deficiency and the carpal tunnel syndrome to pyridoxine. Proc. NatL Acad. Sci. USA Vol. 79, pp. 7494-7498, December 1982 Medical Sciences, (neuropathy/nutrition/vitamin supplementation/diet) by John Ellis et al.

(2) http://www.ncbi.nlm.nih.gov/pubmed/2921840
Klin Wochenschr. 1989 Jan 4;67(1):38-41. Carpal tunnel syndrome and vitamin B6. Laso Guzmán et al.

(3) http://www.ncbi.nlm.nih.gov/pubmed/877413
Res Commun Chem Pathol Pharmacol. 1977 Jun;17(2):283-93. Deficiency of vitamin B6 in women taking contraceptive formulations. Kishi H, Kishi T, Williams RH, Watanabe T, Folkers K, Stahl ML.

(4) http://www.ncbi.nlm.nih.gov/pubmed/7288513
J Nutr Sci Vitaminol (Tokyo). 1981;27(3):193-7. Distribution of vitamin B6 deficiency in university students. Shizukuishi S, Nishii S, Folkers K.

(5) http://www.ncbi.nlm.nih.gov/pubmed/3823219
Plast Reconstr Surg. 1987 Mar;79(3):456-62. Carpal tunnel syndrome and vitamin B6. Kasdan ML, Janes C.

(6) http://www.ncbi.nlm.nih.gov/pubmed/11506323
Ann Plast Surg. 2001 Aug;47(2):153-60. Experimental model of pyridoxine (B6) deficiency-induced neuropathy. Dellon AL et al.

(7) http://www.thorne.com/altmedrev/.fulltext/6/1/87.pdf
Pyridoxine & Pyridoxal 5'Phosphate. Alternative Medicine Review Thorne. Volume 6, Number 1 x 2001.

(8) http://www.ncbi.nlm.nih.gov/pmc/articles/PMC2572855
J Am Coll Nutr. 2008 June; 27(3): 421-427. Vitamin B6 Is Associated with Depressive Symptomatology in Massachusetts Elders Cristina Merete, MS, Luis M. Falcon, PhD, and Katherine L. Tucker, PhD

(9) http://www.garynull.com/documents/arthritis/carpal_tunnel_syndrome.htm Vitamin B6 Therapy The Case of Tunis Johnson, Gary Null B5 Arthritis, The Case of Ellen Cardwell, The Case of Joseph DeChamp, The Cases of Sarah and Gerald Black, The Research of John Marion Ellis, M.D.

(10) The Doctor Who Looked At Hands, by John M Ellis, ARC Books (1971)

(11) http://www.ncbi.nlm.nih.gov/pmc/articles/PMC1798481 Ann Rheum Dis. 2006 December; 65(12): 1666-1667. Pyridoxine toxicity courtesy of your local health food store by C D Silva and D P D'Cruz

(12) http://www.ncbi.nlm.nih.gov/pubmed/3041185 Med J Aust. 1987 Jun 15;146(12):640-2. Pyridoxine neuropathy. Waterston JA, Gilligan BS.

(13) http://www.ncbi.nlm.nih.gov/pubmed/2993949
Neurology. 1985 Oct;35(10):1466-8. Sensory neuropathy with low-dose pyridoxine.Parry GJ et al.

(14) http://www.ncbi.nlm.nih.gov/pubmed/6308447 N Engl J Med. 1983 Aug 25;309(8):445-8. Sensory neuropathy from pyridoxine abuse. A new megavitamin syndrome. Schaumburg H et al.

(15) http://www.orthomolecular.org/library/jom/2003/pdf/2003-v18n02-p065.pdf Indices of Pyridoxine Levels on Symptoms Associated with Toxicity: A Retrospective Study
Aliya N. Chaudary et al.

CHAPTER 46

Wheatgrass, the Path to Health

A while ago, a colleague and good friend confided in me and related a story about his patient with breast cancer who declined treatment with surgery and chemotherapy, and instead spent two weeks at a wellness retreat specializing in wheatgrass juice and a "live food", vegetarian diet. Three months later, the patient reported that the mass in her breast had regressed and was so small she couldn't feel it any more. The patient was also taking Iodine supplements. (See the chapter on Iodine and Breast Cancer.)

After three months, follow up MRI scans showed dramatic improvement, and the radiologist announced, "*the chemotherapy was working*"!! This story intrigued me, as it suggested a biologically active agent in the wheatgrass juice with a beneficial effect on breast cancer. Over the years, I had seen wheatgrass juice sold at various juice bars, and have even tried it a few times without thinking much of it. However, this story motivated me to look further.

Eydie Mae Hunsberger—Breast Cancer Survivor

I discovered a book from the 1970's entitled "How I Conquered Cancer Naturally" by Eydie Mae Hunsberger.(9) This is a true story of a woman in the 1970's who had recurrent axillary lymph node enlargement following lumpectomy for breast cancer. She declined chemotherapy and instead visited Ann Wigmore in Boston where she learned about wheatgrass juice and a live food diet, to which she attributed her recovery and remission from what appeared to be fatal breast cancer. (5-7) Here is a quote from Eydie Mae Hunsberger from page 131 of her book:

"*Here I am a cancer patient not long ago given an eighty per cent chance to live one year. I'm supposed to be sick and dying. And now I am seemingly free from all symptoms, except my lumps, and they are diminishing all the time . . . just as long as I continue to eat live foods, and drink my wheatgrass juice. How incredible, here at our fingertips for so long, an answer to cancer! No One will believe us. It's too simple. It's too easy. This phantom cancer has been such a hopeless subject for so long, no one will believe us. I don't care whether anyone believes us or not. I am going to tell the whole world."* (9)

Wheatgrass, Natures Finest Medicine by Steve Meyerowitz

I also discovered another anecdotal case of recovery from breast cancer with wheatgrass juice in Steve Meyerowitz's book, Wheatgrass, Natures Finest Medicine. (8) Two more anecdotal cases of breast cancer with remission attributed to wheatgrass juice were found in the book, "How and When To Be Your Own Doctor" written by Dr. Isabelle A. Moser with her husband Steve Solomon and published in 1997.(14) Another striking case report in the 2005 medical literature concerns a case of peritoneal cancer, a form of cancer which is rapidly fatal. This 89 year old patient refused chemotherapy and instead used wheat grass therapy with complete remission of the cancer four years after treatment.(15,16) The beneficial anti-cancer effects of wheatgrass are thought to be due to abscisic acid, a plant hormone which delays germination.(10-12)

Hemoglobin and Chlorophyll—Similar Chemical Structure

The intense green color of wheatgrass juice is due to the chlorophyll content. The molecular structure of chlorophyll is virtually identical to hemoglobin, the oxygen carrying red pigment of our blood. The major difference between chlorophyll and hemoglobin is the central metal atom. In hemoglobin the central atom is Iron (Fe), and in chlorophyll it is Magnesium (Mg). This similarity in chemical structure is thought to explain the beneficial effect of wheatgrass juice in cases of chronic anemia such as thalassemia. A report from India showed reduction of transfusion requirements in children with thalassemia who received wheatgrass juice therapy.(13)

Anemia from Chemotherapy

According to Bar-Sela at Rambam Medical Center, wheatgrass juice prevents bone marrow toxicity from chemotherapy without diminishing the effects of the chemo. This study was done in terminal breast cancer patients who noted improvement in blood count after wheatgrass therapy.(18)

Inflammatory Conditions

Wheatgrass juice has a long history of use as antimicrobial, anti-inflammatory and to promote wound healing. A 2002 report showed that Wheatgrass juice appeared safe and effective as a treatment for Ulcerative Colitis, an inflammatory condition of the colon. (21) Chris Reynolds, an Australian Practitioner, has also reported success with Crohn's disease, an inflammatory condition of the small bowel.(25-30) A 1988 review article by Chernomorsky & Segelman reported anti-inflammatory, wound healing and odor reducing capabilities of chlorophyllin (a component of wheatgrass). (23) Chlorophyllin has bacteriostatic properties aiding in wound healing, and stimulates the production of hemoglobin and erythrocytes in anemic animals. It has been used to treat various kinds of skin lesions, burns and ulcers where it acts as a wound healing agent, stimulating granulation tissue and epithelialization. Research from the 1940's describes improved healing for osteomyelitis, deep suppurative or draining wounds, diabetic ulcers, Vincent's stomatitis and pyorrhea.

According to Benjamin Gruskin, M.D., wheatgrass juice clears up foul smelling odors, neutralizes strep infections, heals wounds, hastens skin grafting, cures chronic sinusitis, overcomes chronic inner-ear inflammation and infection, reduces varicose veins and heals leg ulcers, eliminates impetigo and other scabby eruptions, heal rectal sores, successfully treat inflammation of the uterine cervix, gets rid of parasitic vaginal infections, reduces typhoid fever, and cures advanced pyorrhea in many cases.(32)

Dr. Chris Reynolds, a wheatgrass practitioner from Australia recommends wheatgrass for treatment of various conditions: Acne, Alopecia, Anal fissure, Crohn's Disease, Eczema, Hematoma (bruising), Molluscum contagiosum, Multiple sclerosis, Skin and skin-related conditions, Sports and soft tissue injuries, Wound healing. (25-32)

My Own Experience with WheatGrass:

I was intrigued by the benefits of Wheatgrass, and motivated to try it. I called a local producer who grows trays of wheatgrass and delivers the trays directly to your home. This grower plants the seeds and grows the trays which he irrigates with ocean water. The ocean water irrigation gives the wheatgrass bioavailable minerals from the sea. Once the trays were delivered to my home, I prepared the wheatgrass juice daily. Using a pair of scissors, the wheatgrass is cut and placed into an Omega Juicer. This home prepared fresh juice is much sweeter and palatable than the juice bar variety. I noticed more energy, clarity of mind, improvement in mood, and a general anti-inflammatory effect. I noticed that aches and pains seemed to disappear and old areas of hidden inflammation or infection seemed to resolve. There is something to this wheatgrass juice that is very beneficial.

Which Wheatgrass Products to Select?

There are many companies offering wheatgrass juice products. A few are listed in the Steve Meyerowitz Wheatgrass book and offered on his web site. Even though I had live wheatgrass trays, I decided to try the frozen and the freeze dried products. I ordered the frozen wheatgrass juice from Dynamic Greens.(49) The product arrived promptly to my house as frozen cubes of wheatgrass juice. Preparing a glass of wheatgrass was easy. Simply pop the green cubes into a glass, add water, wait a few minutes for the cubes to melt, and it's ready to drink. I found the taste to be pleasant and quite enjoyable. In his book, Meyerowitz speaks highly of various freeze-dried wheat grass powder products.(52-59) I decided to try this as well. The dried power mixed easily with water and had a pleasant taste. I can recommend it. I must apologize for not including many other good products, but time constraints have limited this list.

Which Wheatgrass Products is the Best?

There is no question in my mind that the maximal health benefit is gained by preparing your own fresh juice at home from live wheatgrass.

However, for those of us looking for a more convenient way to go, there is still considerable nutritional benefit from the frozen juice or the freeze dried juice. For anyone traveling, the freeze dried powder is a good travel solution. Note: I have no financial interest in any of the products or books mentioned above.

A Fertile Ground for New Research

There must be some unknown healing "wheat grass juice factor" beneficial for the immune system, involved in cell signaling, and inhibiting cancer. Could this factor be abscisic acid, chlorophyll, Vitamin K2, or some other unknown plant compound? Wheatgrass is a natural substance which cannot be patented so if we depend on drug company research, we may never find the "Wheat Juice Factor". This is where public funding with NIH research grants for basic science in the University setting can play an important role. Clearly, this is an area ripe for new discoveries which can lead to great medical benefits.

Disclaimer: This article in no way advocates wheatgrass as a replacement or substitute for mainstream medical advice or treatment for any medical condition or disease. Please consult your personal physician regarding questions about medical conditions, medications, nutritional supplements, or diet. **Disclosure:** I have no financial interest in any of the above wheatgrass companies or products.

For references and links, see web site: www.bioidenticalhormones101.com

References for Chapter 45. Wheatgrass, the Path to Health

(1) http://www.sproutman.com/ Sproutman—Steve Meyerowitz.

(2) http://sproutman.com/pdf/Grass The Medicine beneath our Feet.pdf Grass The Medicine beneath our Feet by Steve Meyerowitz

(3) http://sproutman.com/pdf/Freeze-Dried-Wheatgrass.pdf Freeze-Dried-Wheatgrass by Steve Meyerowitz

(4) http://sproutman.com/pdf/DOGS-PROVE-WHEATGRASS-WORKS.pdf DOGS-PROVE-WHEATGRASS-WORKS by Steve Meyerowitz.

(5) http://annwigmore.com/ Ann Wigmore web site

(6) http://www.hippocratesinst.org/ The Hippocrates Health Institute based on Ann Wigmore, Drs. Brian and Anna Maria Clement. Hippocrates Health Institute, West Palm Beach, FL

(7) http://books.google.com/books?id=9hgzJA7mPdwC&printsec=frontcover The Wheatgrass Book by Ann Wigmore.

(8) http://www.amazon.com/Wheatgrass-Natures-Finest-Revitalize-Meyerowitz/dp/B000E48LIU/ref=acc_glance_ktch_ai_-2_6_img Wheatgrass—Nature's Finest Medicine by Steve Meyerowitz.

(9) http://www.amazon.com/How-I-Conquered-Cancer-Naturally/dp/0895295180 How I Conquered Cancer Naturally by Eydie Mae Hunsberger, Avery; 2nd edition (March 1, 1992)

(10) http://www.biologie.uni-hamburg.de/b-online/e31/31e.htm Botany Online, by Peter v. Sengbusch Abscissic Acid Chemical Structure.

(11) http://www.fao.org/agris/search/display.do?f=./1982/v802/US8045841.xml;US8045841 Chiu-Nan Lai et al: The inhibitions of in vitro metabolic activation of carcinogens by wheat sprout extracts. Nutrition & Cancer, 1978,1(1) Fall: 27—30.

(12) CN Lai (1979) Chlorophyll: The active factor in wheat sprout extract inhibiting the metabolic activation of carcinogens in vitro. Nutrition and Cancer, 1 (3):19-21

(13) http://medind.nic.in/ibv/t04/i7/ibvt04i7p716.pdf http://cellfeast.com/why-wheatgrass-juice/wheatgrass-references-and-resources Wheat Grass Juice Reduces Transfusion Requirement in Patients with Thalassemia Major: A Pilot Study (Opens as pdf) R.K. Marwaha et al. India.

(14) http://www.healingcancernaturally.com/terminal-breastcure-wheatgrass.html Case report of two cases of terminal breast cancer cured with wheat grass. Excerpted from the book "HOW AND WHEN TO BE YOUR OWN DOCTOR" written by Dr. Isabelle A. Moser with her husband Steve Solomon and published in 1997.

(15) http://www.ncbi.nlm.nih.gov/pubmed/15750376
J Altern Complement Med. 2005 Feb;11(1):161-5. Bovine cartilage, coenzyme Q10, and wheat grass therapy for primary peritoneal cancer. Forgionne GA.

(16) http://www.cancerlynx.com/peritonealcase.html Case report of peritoneal cancer cured with wheatgrass. The results suggest that the primary peritoneal cancer is in remission for the studied patient more than 1 year after her surgery.

(17) http://www.thieme-connect.com/ejournals/abstract/plantamedica/doi/10.1055/s-2007-987320 Planta Med 2007; 73. Antiproliferative and apoptotic effects of wheatgrass (Triticum aestivum L.) extracts on chronic myeloid leukemia (CML) cell line. A Karadag et al.

(18) http://www.ncbi.nlm.nih.gov/pubmed/17571966
Nutr Cancer. 2007;58(1):43-8. Wheat grass juice may improve hematological toxicity related to chemotherapy in breast cancer patients: a pilot study.Bar-Sela G, Tsalic M, Fried G, Goldberg H. Division of Oncology, Rambam Medical Center and Faculty of Medicine, Technion-Israel Institute of Technology, Haifa 31096, Israel.

(19) Effect of Wheat Grass Juice in Supportive Care of Terminally Ill Cancer Patients—A Tertiary Cancer Centre Experience from India. Journal of Clinical Oncology 2006 ASCO Meeting Proceedings Part I. Vol 24, No. 18s (June 20 Supplement), 2006: 8634. Dey S et al.

(20) http://cancerpreventionresearch.aacrjournals.org/cgi/content/short/1/7_MeetingAbstracts/B139?rss=1
Cancer Prevention Research 1 (7 Supplement), B139, November

1, 2008. Effect of wheat grass juice in supportive care of terminally ill solid organ cancer patients: Experience from eastern India, Soma Mukhopadhyay et al, Kolkata, India

(21) http://www.ncbi.nlm.nih.gov/pubmed/11989836
Scand J Gastroenterol. 2002 Apr;37(4):444-9. Wheat grass juice in the treatment of active distal ulceative colitis: a randomized double-blind placebo-controlled trial. Ben-Arye et al. The Technion, Israel Institute of Technology, Haifa.

(22) http://www3.interscience.wiley.com/journal/112474006/abstract
Evaluation of the antioxidant activity of wheatgrass (Triticum aestivum L.) as a function of growth under different conditions Sunil D. Kulkarni 1, Jai. C. Tilak 2, R. Acharya 3, Nilima S. Rajurkar 1, T. P. A. Devasagayam 2, A. V. R. Reddy 3 * 1Department of Chemistry, University of Pune, Pune 411 007, India

(23) http://www.ncbi.nlm.nih.gov/pubmed/3050624
N J Med. 1988 Aug;85(8):669-73. Chernomorsky & Segelman. 1988. Review Article: Biological activities of chlorophyll derivatives

(24) http://www.wheatgrassprofessional.info/references.htm
A Selection of 27 Summaries From Medical and Scientific Journal Articles Supportive of Clinical Effectiveness of Wheatgrass

(25) http://www.drwheatgrass.com.au/LiteratureRetrieve.aspx?ID=29583.
Wound healing? Think growth factors. by Dr. Chris Reynolds. M.B.,B.S

(26) http://www.drwheatgrass.com.au/conditions/alopecia/case_2
ALOPECIA AREATA CASE

(27) http://www.drwheatgrass.com/info/newsletters/default.htm Dr. Chris' Wheatgrass

(28) http://www.wheatgrassprofessional.info/default.htm Wheatgrass For Inflammation Chris Reynolds

(29) http://www.tonicattack.com/documents/Wheatgrass for Crohns and IBS.pdf Wheatgrass and IBS/Crohns disease—by Dr. Chris Reynolds M.B.,B.S April, 2004—Crohn's Disease & The Return of Wheatgrass Healing Crohn's Disease

(30) http://ezinearticles.com/?Wheatgrass-For-Anal-Fissure—A-Medical-Breakthrough&id=118762 Wheatgrass For Anal Fissure—A Medical Breakthrough By Dr. Chris Reynolds

(31) http://74.125.47.132/search?q=cache:M0shTL1aA-wJ:www.tonicattack.com/documents/Wheatgrass for Crohns and IBS.pdf+Wheatgrass+Chris+Reynolds&cd=20&hl=en&ct=clnk&gl=us
In the AmericanJournal of Surgery (1940), Benjamin Gruskin, M.D. recommends chlorophyll for its antiseptic benefits.

(32) http://www.time.com/time/magazine/article/0,9171,764228,00.html
Chlorophyll for Colds Monday, Jul. 22, 1940 Professor Benjamin Gruskin of Philadelphia's Temple University

(33) http://www.xs4all.nl/~stgvisie/AMALGAM/NL/SUPPLEMENTEN/org chlorophyl.htm
ORGANIC CHLOROPHYLL FIGHTS INFECTIONS! By Dr. John Heinerman

(34) http://www.trc.dost.gov.ph/snapshots/snap the history of wheatgrass.pdf THE HISTORY OF WHEATGRASS—by KK Fowlkes

(35) http://www.authorstream.com/presentation/docgene-50235-Ten-Reasons-Why-Wheatgrass-10-Love-King-Alkaline-Foods-SUPPORTS-Science-Technology-ppt-powerpoint/ Ten Reasons Why Wheatgrass—Power Point slides.

(36) http://www.wheatgrass.com/book/chapter4.php
Cereal Grass—What's in it for you! Chapter 4: Chlorophyll as Therapy H.E. Kirschner, M.D.

(37) http://www.wheatgrass.com/book/titlepage.php
Cereal Grass—What's in it for you! CEREAL GRASS. WHAT'S IN IT FOR YOU! The Importance of Wheat Grass, Barley Grass and Other Green Vegetables in the Human Diet Edited by Ronald L. Seibold, M.S. PINES International, Inc. Lawrence, Kansas, online book.

(38) http://www.efph.purdue.edu/media/publication/NR_Ferruzzi_Blakeslee_2007.pdf Review Article Digestion, absorption, and cancer preventative activity of dietary chlorophyll derivatives, Mario G. Ferruzzia et al Brown University December 2006

(39) http://www.ncbi.nlm.nih.gov/pubmed/10495448
Teratog Carcinog Mutagen. 1999;19(5):313-22. Effect of dietary chlorophyll derivatives on mutagenesis and tumor cell growth. Chernomorsky S, Segelman A, Poretz RD.

(40) http://www.nutritionj.com/content/3/1/19/ USA Nutrition Journal 2004, 3, Review Nutrition and cancer: A review of the evidence for an anti-cancer diet. Michael S Donaldson et al.

(41) http://www.efph.purdue.edu/media/publication/NR_Ferruzzi_Blakeslee_2007.pdf Review Article Digestion, absorption, and cancer preventative activity of dietary chlorophyll derivatives Mario G. Ferruzzia,4, Joshua Blakesleeb

(42) Diaz GD, Li Q, Dashwood RH. Caspase-8 and apoptosis-inducing factor mediate a cytochrome c-independent pathway of apoptosis in human colon cancer cells induced by the dietary phytochemical chlorophyllin. Cancer Res 2003;63(6):1254—61.

(43) Chan JY, Tang PM, Hon PM, Au SW, Tsui SK, Waye MM, et al. Pheophorbide a, a major antitumor component purified from Scutellaria barbata, induces apoptosis in human hepatocellular carcinoma cells. Planta Med 2006;72(1):28—33.

(44) http://www.ncbi.nlm.nih.gov/pubmed/16142413 Chiu LC, Kong CK, Ooi VE. The chlorophyllin-induced cell cycle arrest and apoptosis in

human breast cancer MCF-7 cells is associated with ERK deactivation and cyclin D1 depletion. Int J Mol Med 2005;16(4):735—40.

(45) http://www.pnas.org/content/98/8/4782.full
A postgermination developmental arrest checkpoint is mediated by abscisic acid and requires the ABI5 transcription factor in Arabidopsis Luis Lopez-Molina, Sébastien Mongrand, and Nam-Hai Chua. PNAS April 10, 2001 vol. 98 no. 8 4782-4787

(46) http://www.google.com/patents?id=j7SZAAAAEBAJ
Patent for ABA as cancer preventive

(47) http://www.freshpatents.com/Abscisic-acid-against-cancer-dt20061228ptan20060292215.php?type=description
Patent by Dr. Livingston U.S. Pat. No. 3,958,025 (1976), col 8, line 50, that a hormone immuologically identical to HCG denominated microbic chorionic gonadotropin, produced from progenitor cryptocides, might be opposed or neutralized by a growth retardant in vitro. Such a growth inhibitor was identified as ABA. (Absciscic Acid)

(48) http://www.sproutman.com/ Sproutman Steve Meyerowitz

(49) http://www.dynamicgreens.com/ Dynamic Greens Wheatgrass 16128 9th Line Stouffville, ON L4A 7X4 Canada 1-877-910-0467 flash frozen wheatgrass juice shipped to you frozen overnight.

(50) http://wheatgrass.com/ PINES Wheat Grass Conveniently offered in tablets and powders first company in continuous operation in the U.S.A. to offer dehydrated wheat grass and barley grass to the public, starting in 1976.

(51) http://www.dyna-green.com/wheatgrass/wheatgrass-powder.html Freeze-dried wheat grass juice, like Dyna-Green. Dynamic Nutraceuticals Scott Smith P.O. Box 940 Sebastopol, CA 95473 Phone: 1-877-Dyna Green E-mail: dynamicn@earthlink.net

(52) http://www.wheatgrassexpress.com/ Freeze Dried Wheatgrass Juice Powder

(53) http://www.wholelifegreens.com/about.htm Vermont. Donna (Bergonzi) Boyle her brother Michael the Master Grower and Greenhouse Manager at Hippocrates Health Institute in West Palm Beach, FL 802-583-4769 or 802-793-2197 or e-mail DONNA AT info@wholelifegreens.com.

(54) http://bestjuiceextractorreviews.com/ Listing of Juicers. making your own decision about finding the right Breville, Omega, Braun, Champion, Jack Lalanne, Green Star juice extractor

(55) https://www.phporder.com/ProductPage.aspx?ItemID=60&ID=highpowersupplements The world's finest wheatgrass grown from the ancient Egyptian Kamut seed. The sweet taste of oat grass juice. The mineral rich juice from mature alfalfa leaves. Organic Kamut Blend

(56) http://www.phporder.com/WeightLossPlan.aspx?ID=highpowersupplements Weight Loss Battle Plan

(57) http://www.phporder.com/ScoopOfGreensInfo.aspx?ID=highpowersupplements Scoop Of Greens. for Diabetes and Weight Loss.

(58) http://img.exigo.com/public/1333/websites/41/images/wheatgrassca.pdf Wheatgrass Juice—Nature's Powerful Medicine. Organic Kamut Blend, containing one of the few still-wild wheatgrass strains available to consumers.

(59) http://www.google.com/patents?id=9tl7AAAAEBAJ Patent: Tablets of abscisic acid and a carrier are used to treat a vitamin deficiency of abscisic acid in man, animal and the avian species. Patent number: 3958025 Filing date: Jul 5, 1974 Issue date: May 18, 1976 Inventor: Virginia W-C Livingston.

(60) http://www.google.com/patents?id=j7SZAAAAEBAJ Abscisic acid against cancer US Patent 20060292215. Filing date: Jun 21, 2006 Inventor: Gonzalo Romero M.

SECTION TWELVE: IS YOUR FOOD MAKING YOU SICK?

CHAPTER 46

Selling Sickness in the Lobby, Fast Food in Hospitals

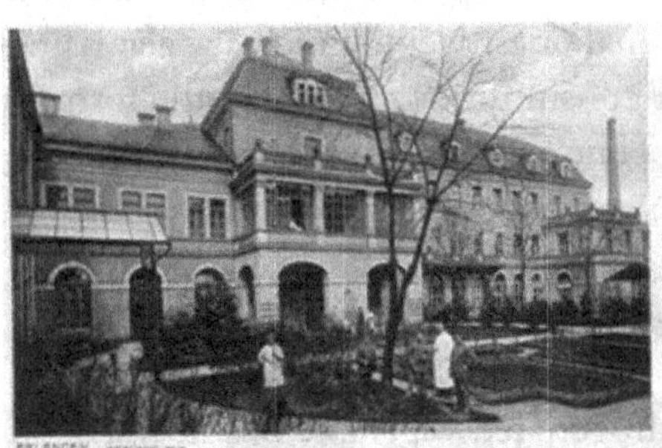

Old hospital building, Germany 1914, courtesy of Wikimedia commons.

Dr. Peter Cram reported in JAMA (Journal of the American Medical Association) that forty per cent of hospitals have fast food in the lobby.(3) While you might consider this an outrage, the hospital probably considers it business as usual. Your hospital banned cigarette smoking long ago,(47) yet still sends the message that fast food is healthy for you. In reality, fast food is unhealthy and leads to chronic diseases and new revenue for the hospital. For the hospital accounting department, looking at the bottom line, this is a good thing. Financial consideration, rather than the health of the community, is the deciding factor. Untrained in medical nutrition, hospital accountants may not understand that fast food causes obesity, metabolic syndrome, insulin resistant diabetes, hypertension and accelerated cardiovascular disease. (1-7)

Fast Food Causes Chronic Disease

Michael Pollen, a journalist and author of "In Defense of Food", and "Food Rules" says in a New York Times Editorial:

"*Fast food causes chronic disease, and there's lots of money to be made selling fast food, and then treating the diseases that fast food causes. One of the leading products of the American food industry has become patients for the American health care industry*". (8)

Fast Food, Obesity and Chronic Disease—What is the Evidence?

You might ask, what is the evidence that fast food causes obesity and chronic disease? For starters, a 2004 study published in Lancet found that eating Fast Food causes weight gain and insulin resistance. (29-30) The authors say, "*fast foods contain large amounts of partially hydrogenated oils, and this class of fatty acids can cause insulin resistance and increase risk of type 2 diabetes.*" Fast food also contains large amounts of highly refined starchy food and added sugars linked to increase risk for diabetes and obesity. The national obesity epidemic has been rising at parallel rates with refined sugar consumption, mostly in the form of high fructose corn syrup (HFCS). The average American consumes 70 pounds a year of refined sugar.

Health Risks of Sugar Consumption—HFCS

Ignoring for the moment the hydrogenated vegetable oils in fast food which are an enormous health risk, let's focus on the sweeteners, the high fructose corn syrup used in fast food and soft drinks. The evidence linking massive amounts of sugar consumption to chronic disease is overwhelming. (9-27) High Fructose Corn Syrup is our preferred sweetener, refined from government subsidized corn and used for processed foods. HFCS is cheaper and sweeter than regular table sugar (sucrose), and it prolongs shelf life. High Fructose corn syrup is a **4.5 BILLION** dollar industry, with our annual sugar consumption at **73.5 lbs per person**. Now, that's a lot of sugar!

Refined Sugar—Sucrose—This is an Addictive Drug

Some scientists say that refined table sugar (sucrose) is not food, and should be reclassified as a drug capable of producing craving, withdrawal effects and addiction.(44) A 2002 Princeton study showed addictive behaviors in rats given intermittent high sugar intake.(46) A 2008 report in NeuroScience examines the evidence for addiction associated with intermittent excess sugar intake.(45) The scientific evidence of sugar addiction is summarized nicely by Kathleen DesMaisons, Ph.D., author of "The Sugar Addict's Total Recovery Program", and "Potatoes

Not Prozac". Her program, called Radiant Recovery, is dedicated to helping people overcome sugar addition. (43)

HFCS—Comparing Fructose to Glucose

Chemically speaking, HFCS is a mixture of 55% fructose and 45% glucose, a ratio intended to mimic common table sugar, called sucrose. Sucrose is a simple molecule made of one fructose and one glucose molecule, so the corn industry can say that sucrose and HFCS are the same stuff. Of course this is partially true, but there is a difference. Firstly, HFCS has 10% more fructose than table sugar. Secondly the fructose in HFCS is absorbed into the bloodstream more rapidly, since the body must first cleave apart sucrose with enzymatic digestion, after which, the liberated fructose can be absorbed into the bloodstream. Once absorbed, fructose and glucose are metabolized quite differently.

IV Glucose is OK, IV Fructose is NOT OK.

Intravenous glucose is commonly given to patients in the hospital to sustain life. There is no IV fructose in the bag, because IV fructose is dangerous to your health. (48)

Warning—Fructose
Intravenous (IV) fructose is dangerous to your health and never given as an IV medication. On the other hand, IV glucose is routinely given in the hospital as a safe nutrient.

Health Risks of Fructose in Fast Food Sodas

In small amounts, fructose has always been a healthy part of human diet in fruits and vegetables. However, large amounts of fructose pose a serious health risk. Unlike glucose, fructose cannot be used by the body. Instead, it must be processed in the liver where it is uncontrollably converted into fat particles, triglycerides and atherogenic lipids. This causes insulin resistant diabetes, hypertension and cardiovascular disease. Thus, fructose is considered more dangerous and harmful than plain old glucose. Fructose also causes abnormal lipid panels in obese kids, who may then be given statin drugs. Wouldn't it make more sense to cut out the fructose instead?(9-27)

One in Five Teens have High Cholesterol

A recent CDC report raises alarms about increasing teen obesity and high cholesterol found in 20% of kids.(27) The CDC report went on to recommend that doctors adhere to guidelines calling for statin drugs for kids with high cholesterol.

Doctor, Surely You Must Be Joking?—Statins for Kids?

In 1998, the American Academy of Pediatrics convened a Committee on Nutrition to discuss "Cholesterol in Childhood" which published guidelines for treating kids with statin drugs for high cholesterol. (28) The guidelines were revised in 2008 by Dr. Stephen R. Daniels, causing a national uproar.(29) Apparently, Daniels and co-authors had undisclosed ties to Merck, maker of statin drug Mevacor™. (30) The problem with cholesterol guidelines for kids is absence of any medical data showing benefit from statin drugs in this age group. Alternatively, we have plenty of evidence that statin drugs cause harmful adverse side effects, especially considering a child starting a statin drug is committed to 40 years of drug treatment. Articles such as, "Storm Over Statins", promptly appeared in the media and medical literature raising opposition and creating backlash against the guidelines for statin drugs for kids.(33-35) In view of what we know about Fast Food causing teen obesity and abnormal lipid panels, it would seem the height of absurdity to give kids statin drugs, rather than address the fast food and soda pop diets.(38-40)

Fecal Contamination of Soda Fountains

Another problem with fast food in the lobby, is fecal contamination of soda fountains, reported in the Jan 2010 issue of the International Journal of Food Microbiology.(41-42) Take Action! Make a copy this article and give it to your local congressman, or hospital board member.

For references and links, see my web site: www.bioidenticalhormones101.com

References for Chapter 46. Selling Sickness in the Lobby, Fast Food in Hospitals

(1) http://pediatrics.aappublications.org/cgi/content/full/118/6/2290?vm=t PEDIATRICS Vol. 118 No. 6 December 2006 Marketing Fast Food: Impact of Fast Food Restaurants in Children's Hospitals, Hannah B. Sahud, MD et al.

(2) http://www.jabfm.org/cgi/content/full/19/5/526 Prevalence and Type of Brand Name Fast Food at Academic-affiliated Hospitals. J Am Board of Fam Med 19:526-527 (2006) Lenard I. Lesser, MD

(3) http://jama.ama-assn.org/cgi/content/full/287/22/2945 Vol. 287 No. 22, June 12, 2002 JAMA by Peter Cram, MD Fast Food Franchises in Hospitals

(4) http://www.yaleruddcenter.org/resources/upload/docs/what/industry/FoodTobacco.pdf The Perils of Ignoring History: Big Tobacco Played Dirty and Millions Died. How Similar Is Big Food? KELLY D. BROWNELL and KENNETH E. WARNER

(5) www.thesun.co.uk/sol/homepage/woman/health/health/2805543/Row-over-fast-food-in-hospitals.html Row over Fatty Grub in Hospitals, The Sun UK. By EMMA MORTON, 13 Jan 2010.

(6) www.dailymail.co.uk/news/article-1242815/NHS-pays-patients-lose-weight—opening-fast-food-branches-IN-hospitals.html Daily Mail, UK, NHS pays patients to lose weight—while opening fast food branches IN hospitals
By Sara Nelson 13th January 2010

(7) www.cmaj.ca/cgi/content/full/179/3/213 CMAJ July 29, 2008; 179 (3). Frying up hospital cafeteria food, Yoni Freedhoff and Rob Stevenson

(8) www.nytimes.com/2009/09/10/opinion/10pollan.html Big Food vs. Big Insurance By MICHAEL POLLAN September 9, 2009 NY Times.

(9) http://www.ncbi.nlm.nih.gov/pubmed/19956074 Curr Opin Lipidol. 2009 Dec 2. Soft drink consumption and obesity: it is all about fructose. Bray GA.

(10) http://www.ajcn.org/cgi/content/full/79/4/537 American Journal of Clinical Nutrition, Vol. 79, No. 4, 537-543, April 2004. Consumption of high-fructose corn syrup in beverages may play a role in the epidemic of obesity. George A Bray et al.

(11) http://www.cdc.gov/mmwr/preview/mmwrhtml/mm5902a1.htm Morbidity and Mortality Weekly Report (MMWR). Prevalence of Abnormal Lipid Levels Among Youths, United States, 1999-2006. January 22, 2010/59(02);29-33

(12) http://www.ncbi.nlm.nih.gov/pmc/articles/PMC2673878/?tool=pubmed J Clin Invest. 2009 May 1; 119(5): 1322-1334. 2009 April 20. Consuming fructose-sweetened, not glucose-sweetened, beverages increases visceral adiposity and lipids and decreases insulin sensitivity in overweight/obese humans by Kimber L. Stanhope et al.

(13) http://www.nutritionandmetabolism.com/content/2/1/5#B27 Fructose, insulin resistance, and metabolic dyslipidemia Heather Basciano, Lisa Federico and Khosrow Adeli. Nutrition & Metabolism 2005, 2:5

(14) http://ddr.nal.usda.gov/dspace/bitstream/10113/22238/1/IND44124650.pdf Br J Nutr. 2008 Nov;100(5):947-52. Consumption of fructose-sweetened beverages for 10 weeks increases postprandial triacylglycerol and apolipoprotein-B concentrations in overweight and obese women. Swarbrick MM et al.

(15) http://hyper.ahajournals.org/cgi/reprint/10/5/512 Hypertension, Vol 10, 512-516, Fructose-induced insulin resistance and hypertension in rats IS Hwang, H Ho, BB Hoffman and GM Reaven

(16) http://jama.ama-assn.org/cgi/content/full/292/8/927
JAMA. 2004;292:927-934, Sugar-Sweetened Beverages, Weight Gain, and Incidence of Type 2 Diabetes in Young and Middle-Aged Women by Matthias B. Schulze et al.

(17) http://www.kitchentablemedicine.com/high-fructose-corn-syrup-sugar/
Corn Syrup, Is it Really Just Like Sugar? January 30, 2009 by Kitchen Table Medicine

(18) http://www.westonaprice.org/The-Double-Danger-of-High-Fructose-Corn-Syrup.html The Double Danger of High Fructose Corn Syrup Written by Bill Sanda 2004-Feb-19

(19) http://www.lef.org/magazine/mag2008/dec2008_Metabolic-Dangers-of-High-Fructose-Corn-Syrup_02.htm LE Magazine December 2008 Metabolic Danger of High-Fructose Corn Syrup By Dana Flavin, MS, MD, PHD

(20) http://www.timesonline.co.uk/tol/news/uk/health/article6954603.ece
December 13, 2009 Child diabetes blamed on food sweetener, Times Online.

(21) http://www.sfgate.com/cgi-bin/blogs/sfmoms/detail?entry_id=55267
Corn syrup removed from SFUSD chocolate milk, SF Gate.

(22) http://www.trit.us/modernfood/highfructose.html#author
http://www.evadeandsurvive.com/syrup The Double Dangers of High Fructose Corn Syrup By Bill Sanda, BS, MBA

(23) http://www.slate.com/id/2216796/ Dark Sugar The decline and fall of high-fructose corn syrup. By Daniel Engber. April 28, 2009

(24) http://www.slashfood.com/2010/01/15/michael-pollan-on-food-rules/
Michael Pollen, Food Rules.

(25) http://www.nih.gov/news/pr/dec2004/nhlbi-30.htm
Eating at Fast-food Restaurants More than Twice Per Week is Associated

with More Weight Gain and Insulin Resistance in Otherwise Healthy Young Adults. NIH Gov News.

(26) http://www.ncbi.nlm.nih.gov/pubmed/15639678 Fast-food Habits, Weight Gain, and Insulin Resistance (The CARDIA Study): 15-Year Prospective Analysis". Mark Pereira et al. Lancet. 2005 Jan 1-7;365(9453):36-42.

(27) http://www.cdc.gov/mmwr/preview/mmwrhtml/mm5902a1.htm Prevalence of Abnormal Lipid Levels Among Youths—United States, 1999—2006 Weekly January 22, 2010/59(02);29-33 MM Weekly Report (MMWR) CDC

(28) http://pediatrics.aappublications.org/cgi/content/full/101/1/141 PEDIATRICS Vol. 101 No. 1 January 1998, pp. 141-147 Cholesterol in Childhood Committee on Nutrition

(29) http://pediatrics.aappublications.org/cgi/content/abstract/122/1/198 PEDIATRICS Vol. 122 No. 1 July 2008, pp. 198-208. Lipid Screening and Cardiovascular Health in Childhood, Stephen R. Daniels, MD, PhD, Frank R. Greer, MD and the Committee on Nutrition

(30) http://www.cspinet.org/integrity/watch/200807211.html Pediatrics Fails to Disclose Industry Ties in Lipid Guide for Kids.

(31) http://www.cnn.com/2010/HEALTH/01/22/teens.cholesterol/ CDC: 1 in 5 teens has cholesterol problems. Now what? By Sarah Klein, January 22, 2010 CNN News

(32) http://pediatrics.aappublications.org/cgi/content/full/122/4/904 PEDIATRICS Vol. 122 No. 4 October 2008, pp. 904-905 LETTER TO THE EDITOR An Assessment of the New Lipid Screening Guidelines Michael J. Steiner, MD Wallace D. Brown, MD

(33) http://nejm.highwire.org/cgi/content/full/359/13/1309 Volume 359:1309-1312 September 25, 2008 Number 13 NEJM Storm over Statins—The Controversy Surrounding Pharmacologic Treatment of

Children, Sarah de Ferranti, M.D., M.P.H., and David S. Ludwig, M.D., Ph.D.

(34) http://junkfoodscience.blogspot.com/2008/07/is-it-for-real-cholesterol-screening-in.html July 08, 2008 Is it for real? Cholesterol screening in toddlers and statins from elementary school age?

(35) http://www.nytimes.com/2008/07/08/health/08well.html?_r=2&ref=health&oref=slogin 8-Year-Olds on Statins? A New Plan Quickly Bites Back, by Tara Parker-Pope Jul 8, 2008 NYTimes

(36) http://www.reuters.com/article/idUSTRE60K54I20100122 One-fifth of U.S. teens have unhealthy cholesterol.Reuters News.

(37) http://abcnews.go.com/Health/WellnessNews/test-teens-high-cholesterol/story?id=9628671 Should We Test Teens for High Cholesterol? American Teens May Be at Risk for Problems Once Associated Only With Middle Age By JOHN GEVERJan. 22, 2010 MedPage Today Senior Editor

(38) http://www.npr.org/blogs/health/2010/01/high_cholesterol.html For Kids With High Cholesterol, Change Diet, Exercise Before Drugs January 22, 2010 By Nadja Popovich

(39) http://thespeckledbanana.blogspot.com/2010/01/more-business-for-big-pharma.html Saturday, January 23, 2010 More Business for Big Pharma.

(40) http://www.huffingtonpost.com/dr-michael-j-breus/statins-for-kids_b_116379.html Statins for Kids?Dr. Michael J. Breus 10-Day Boot Camp for a Healthier Lifestyle. Huffington Post.

(41) http://www.cnn.com/2010/HEALTH/01/08/soda.fountain.bacteria/index.html Soda fountains contained fecal bacteria, study found By Madison Park, CNN January 8, 2010 6:35 p.m. EST

(42) http://www.ncbi.nlm.nih.gov/pubmed/19926155 Int J Food Microbiol. 2010 Jan 31;137(1):61-6. Beverages obtained from soda fountain machines in the U.S. contain microorganisms, including coliform bacteria. Amy S. White, Renee D. Godard, Carolyn Belling Department of Biology, Hollins University,

(43) http://www.radiantrecovery.com/newsensitive6.htm
The scientific evidence of sugar addiction, Kathleen DesMaisons, Ph.D. is the best selling author of Potatoes Not Prozac, The Sugar Addict's Total Recovery Program, Your Last Diet, Little Sugar Addicts and Your Body Speaks.

(44) http://www.lurj.org/article.php/vol1n1/sugar.xml
The Reclassification of Sugar as a Drug—Marie-Hélène Lyle: The Reclassification of Sugar as a Drug. Lethbridge Undergraduate Research Journal. 2006. Volume 1 N 1.

(45) http://www.ncbi.nlm.nih.gov/pmc/articles/PMC2235907/ Neurosci Biobehav Rev. 2008; 32(1): 20-39. Published online 2007 May 18. Evidence for sugar addiction: Behavioral and neurochemical effects of intermittent, excessive sugar intake—Nicole M. Avena, Pedro Rada, and Bartley G. Hoebel*

(46) http://www.ncbi.nlm.nih.gov/pubmed/12055324 Obes Res. 2002 Jun;10(6):478-88. Evidence that intermittent, excessive sugar intake causes endogenous opioid dependence. Colantuoni C et al.

(47) http://jama.ama-assn.org/content/274/6/488.abstract Smoking Bans in US Hospitals Results of a National Survey. JAMA. 1995;274(6):488-491. Daniel R. Longo, ScD; Ross C. Brownson, PhD; Robin L. Kruse, PhD

(48) http://www.ncbi.nlm.nih.gov/pubmed/4118217 Lancet. 1972 Dec 23;2(7791):1354-7.Dangers of intravenous fructose.Woods HF, Alberti KG.

CHAPTER 47

The Grocery Store as Mine Field, Avoiding the Dangers

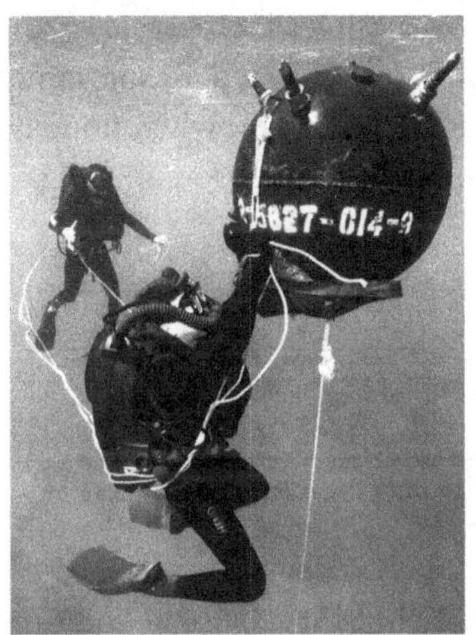

A U.S. Navy diver attaches charge to a training mine, during exercises, courtesy of Wikimedia Commons.

Is Your Supermarket a Minefield?

Recently, I went shopping with my 11 year old nephew, and was shocked and unprepared for the experience. Like other kids his age, he preferred diet sodas containing aspartame and Brominated Vegetable Oil (BVO). He also preferred processed foods high in MSG (mono sodium glutamate). I found myself protesting his choices, explaining the dangers of food additives, and removing these items from the shopping cart as fast I could. These food additives are harmful to health, and represent a minefield at the Supermarket waiting for the unsuspecting consumer.

Aspartame's Dubious Honor—Diet Sodas are a Mine Field

Since the 1981 approval as a food additive, aspartame has the dubious honor of the most complaints reported to the FDA's Adverse Reaction Monitoring System, accounting for 75 per cent of all complaints.(9) Aspartame is a chemical sweetener in diet sodas such as Diet Coke and Diet Pepsi with names such as Nutrasweet™, Equal™, etc. Little packets of aspartame are placed on the tables at restaurants for use as a coffee sweetener instead of sugar. The aspartame industry has sponsored 74 aspartame safety studies, all showing aspartame consumption is safe. When studies are done privately, with no connection to the aspartame industry or the FDA, 89 of 90 aspartame safety studies identified problems with aspartame use.(1) A disturbing 2007 study by Soffritti at the Ramazzini Institute in Italy showed aspartame to be a multipotential carcinogen.(2)

Avoiding the Aspartame Mine Field

Many people drink diet sodas with the mistaken belief that diet sodas will help them lose weight. A recent study shows this is a fallacy, finding a 41% increased risk of being overweight for every can or bottle of diet soft drink consumed daily.(8) The sweetener aspartame activates receptors in the brain to expect sugar (glucose), when none is forthcoming, the aspartame user merely increases junk food and sugar intake.

Warning
MSG, Monosodium Glutamate, and Aspartame are neurotoxins.

MSG—Chinese Restaurant Syndrome

Forty years ago, my earliest experience with MSG (Mono Sodium Glutamate) during medical school was a headache after eating at a Chinese restaurant. The MSG causes the Chinese Restaurant Syndrome.(3) Since my old medical school days, MSG has been added to thousands of products at the supermarket, and virtually all forms of fast food. Much of this MSG is hidden and does not appear on the label.

MSG and the Obesity Epidemic

MSG stands for mono sodium glutamate, and Glutamate is an excitatory neurotransmitter in the brain. Upregulation (stimulation) of the Glutamate pathway leads to neuron cell damage and cell death. MSG is associated with lesions in the hypothalamus (11), directly causes obesity (4), and a host of somatic and neurological symptoms. Laboratory mice studies show that MSG is a direct cause of obesity. Is our obesity epidemic caused by increased MSG consumption in the population?

Hidden Sources of MSG—It's Not On the Label.

Virtually all Fast Foods contain large amounts of MSG, and many processed foods now contain MSG. In other words, the processed food contains MSG in some form, yet the name MSG does not appear on the label.

Aspartame and MSG—Fibromyalgia Double Whammy

Both Aspartame and MSG are excitatory neurotoxins.(6) When aspartame and MSG are consumed together, as commonly found with fast food and diet sodas in the same meal, there can be a double whammy effect. A 2001 report describes four patients with fibromyalgia syndrome unresponsive to medical treatment.(7) These four patients noted complete resolution of chronic pain upon removing aspartame and MSG from the diet.(7) In addition, a lengthy list of medical and neurological symptoms are associated with MSG and aspartame. One syndrome includes slurred speech which looks like a TIA (transient ischemic attack). This usually resolves after elimination of MSG and aspartame from the diet. A 1981 study by Dhindsa showed that MSG administered to lab rats caused marked hypothyroidism with striking histology changes in the thyroid gland.(10) A study presented at the 2011 American Stroke Association Conference showed daily diet soda consumption had a **61 percent higher risk of stroke.**(57)

BVO—Brominated Vegetable Oil

Bromine (BVO) is a toxic substance added to sodas such as Mountain Dew, Gatorade, Powerade, Pineapple and Orange Fanta, Sun Drop, Squirt and Fresca. Bromine directly competes with Iodine in the body causing thyroid problems and Iodine deficiency states. BVO has been banned in India.

What About the FDA?

The FDA is an agency of our government, and like all other agencies, is infiltrated and corrupted by corporate lobbyists. Rather than an agency for the people, the FDA is an agency of the large corporations that manufacture food additives. The safety studies are manipulated to get FDA approval. And that's why the FDA cannot protect the American public from harmful food additives at our supermarket.

In Conclusion—Avoid the Minefield at the Supermarket

We have merely scratched the surface of harmful food additives to avoid at the Supermarket, concentrating on the excitatory neurotoxins Aspartame and MSG. There are other minefields at the grocery store to be avoided such as chemicalized food additives, flavorings, coloring, and trans-fats. Genetically Modified Food (GMO) should be avoided as hazardous to health.

For references and links, see my web site: www.bioidenticalhormones101.com

References for Chapter 47. The Grocery Store as Mine Field, Avoiding the Dangers

(1) http://www.westonaprice.org/modernfood/aspartame.html Aspartame: Diet-astrous Results By Rebecca Ephraim, RD, CCN, Weston Price.org

(2) http://www.ehponline.org/members/2007/10271/10271.pdf Soffritti M, Belpoggi F, Tibaldi E, Esposti DD, Lauriola M, 2007 Life-Span Exposure to Low Doses of Aspartame Beginning during Prenatal Life Increases Cancer Effects in Rats. Environ Health Perspect 115(9)

(3) http://www.sciencemag.org/cgi/content/abstract/163/3869/826 Science 21 February 1969:Vol. 163. no. 3869, pp. 826-828. Monosodium L-Glutamate: Its Pharmacology and Role in the Chinese Restaurant Syndrome. Herbert H. Schaumburg et al.

(4) http://www.nature.com/oby/journal/v16/n8/abs/oby2008274a.html Obesity (2008) 16 8, 1875-1880. doi: 10.1038/oby.2008.274 Association of Monosodium Glutamate Intake With Overweight in Chinese Adults: The INTERMAP Study

(5) http://www.holisticmed.com/aspartame/recent.html Aspartame and MSG Cause Painful Fibromyalgia Symptoms. Ann Pharmacother

2001 Jun;35(6):702-6 Relief of fibromyalgia symptoms following discontinuation of dietary excitotoxins. Smith JD et al.

(6) http://www.theannals.com/cgi/content/abstract/35/6/702 Aspartame and MSG Cause Painful Fibromyalgia Symptoms. Ann Pharmacother 2001 Jun;35(6):702-6. Relief of fibromyalgia symptoms following discontinuation of dietary excitotoxins. Smith JD et al.

(7) http://www.webmd.com/diet/news/20050613/drink-more-diet-soda-gain-more-weight Drink More Diet Soda, Gain More Weight? Overweight Risk Soars 41% With Each Daily Can of Diet Soft Drink By Daniel J. DeNoon WebMD Health News. Reviewed by Charlotte E. Grayson Mathis

(8) http://www.fda.gov/ohrms/DOCKETS/dailys/03/Jan03/012203/02P-0317_emc-000196.txt FDA Docket # 02P-0317. Recall Aspartame as a Neurotoxic Drug.

(9) http://www.ncbi.nlm.nih.gov/pubmed/7246043 Acta Anat (Basel). 1981;109(2):97-102. Histological changes in the thyroid gland induced by monosodium glutamate in mice. Dhindsa KS, Omran RG, Bhup R.

(10) http://www.ncbi.nlm.nih.gov/pubmed/827619
J Toxicol Environ Health. 1976 Nov;2(2):471-80. Hypothalamic morphology following ingestion of aspartame or MSG in the neonatal rodent and primate: a preliminary report. Reynolds WA, Butler V, Lemkey-Johnston N.

(11) http://fooddemocracy.wordpress.com/2008/01/18/the-dirty-dozen-12-foodsfood-additives-to-avoid-and-why/ The dirty dozen—12 foods/food additives to avoid and why January 18, 2008. Food Democracy

(12) http://www.supereco.com/glossary/high-fructose-corn-syrup/news/
High fructose corn syrup News (1-10 of 11) Cheat sheet: 20 worst food additives

(13) http://www.sweetpoison.com/food-additives-to-avoid.html Food Additives to Avoid

(14) http://articles.mercola.com/sites/articles/archive/2008/06/24/12-food-additives-to-avoid.aspx?source=nl 12 Food Additives to Avoid, Dr Mercola.

(15) http://www.momlogic.com/2008/06/10_food_preservatives_to_avoid.php 10 Preservatives to Avoid

(16) http://www.drrisley.com/html/excitotoxins.html A review of Dr. Russell Blaylock's book, "Excitotoxins: The taste that kills."

(17) http://kamdhenunews.blogspot.com/2009/06/chapter-15-dirty-dozen.html "The Dirty Dozen" details 12 foods/toxins which can pose serious health problems.

(18) http://www.huffingtonpost.com/dr-mj-wegmann/13-foods-to-avoid_b_184908.html Dr. M.J. Wegmann.Posted April 8, 2009 Foods To Avoid. Huffington Post.

(19) http://www.associatedcontent.com/article/398593/harmful_additives_in_everyday_food.html Harmful Additives in Everyday Food: What You Should Know

(20) http://thenaturalhealthplace.com/Articles/FoodAdditives.html Monosodium Glutamate (MSG)—Artificial Sweeteners (Aspartame)

(21) http://www.wereyouwondering.com/possible-and-suspected-carcinogens-found-in-food/ 24 Potentially Harmful Food Additives

(22) http://www.msgexposed.com/ MSG Exposed

(23) http://www.live-the-organic-life.com/food-additives.html Guide to Food Additives

(24) http://www.healthyeatingadvisor.com/food-additives.html Food Additives—Protect Your Family From Cancer-Causing Chemicals

(25) http://www.supereco.com/glossary/propylene-glycol/news/ Here's some ammunition: Super Eco's list of the Top 20 food additives to avoid.

(26) http://www.sandiegoreader.com/news/1999/jul/29/what-brominated-vegetable-oil-and-why-do-soda-comp/ What is brominated vegetable oil and why do soda companies put it in their drink? By Matthew Alice, Thursday, July 29, 1999

(27) http://www.msgexposed.com/page/2/ MSG—What is MSG and the Hidden Ingredients it lurks in March 5th, 2009

(28) http://www.ncbi.nlm.nih.gov/pubmed/9582101
Obesity induced by neonatal monosodium glutamate treatment in spontaneously hypertensive rats: an animal model of multiple risk factors. Iwase M, Yamamoto M, Iino K, Ichikawa K, Shinohara N, Yoshinari Fujishima. Hypertens Res. 1998 Mar

(29) http://www.ncbi.nlm.nih.gov/pubmed/729669 Hypothalamic lesion induced by injection of monosodium glutamate in suckling period and subsequent development of obesity. Tanaka K, Shimada M, Nakao K, Kusunoki Exp Neurol. 1978 Oct

(30) http://www.ncbi.nlm.nih.gov/pubmed/6541212 A. Frieder, B, and Grimm, VE. Prenatal monosodium glutamate (MSG) treatment given through the mother's diet causes behavioral deficits in rat offspring. Intern J Neurosci. 23:117-126,1984. Excitotoxins—The Taste That Kills' By Dr. Russell L Blaylock, MD, Health Press, December 1, 1996.

(31) http://www.ncbi.nlm.nih.gov/pubmed/1106764. Bunyan J, Elspeth A, Murrell A, Shah PP. The induction of obesity in rodents by means of monosodium glutamate. British Journal of Nutrition 35(1976): 25-39.

(32) http://www.ncbi.nlm.nih.gov/pubmed/7290289
Kanarek RB, Marks-Kaufman R. Increased carbohydrate consumption induced by neonatal administration of monosodium glutamate to rats. Neurobehavioral Toxicology Teratology 3(1981): 343-350

(33) http://www.ncbi.nlm.nih.gov/pubmed/565061 Nikoletseas MM. Obesity in exercising, hypophagic rats treated with monosodium glutamate. Physiology & Behavior 19(1977): 767-773.

(34) http://www.nature.com/oby/journal/v16/n8/abs/oby2008274a.html Obesity (2008) 16 8, 1875-1880. Association of Monosodium Glutamate Intake With Overweight in Chinese Adults: The INTERMAP Study

(35) http://www.ncbi.nlm.nih.gov/pubmed/5778021
Science. 1969 May 9;164(880):719-21.Brain lesions, obesity, and other disturbances in mice treated with monosodium glutamate. Olney JW.

(36) http://life-enthusiast.com/index/Articles/Blaylock/Toxic_Additives_in_Your_Food_and_Drink Toxic Additives in Your Food and Drink Not Just Another Scare by Russell L. Blaylock, M.D.

(37) http://w3.newsmax.com/newsletters/blaylock/issues/BlayOct07/blaylock_BlayOct07_40.pdf Food Additives:What You Eat Can Kill You by Russell L. Blaylock, M.D.

(38) http://www.youtube.com/watch?v=pvFRLIjOLOU
Aspartame—Nutrasweet video on You tube

(39) http://www.youtube.com/watch?v=9FeOtSNU900 Aspartame—the hidden poison for society—Viddeo on You Tube

(40) http://www.westonaprice.org/msg/msgobesity.html
The Obesity Epidemic: Should We Believe What We Read and Hear? By Jack L. Samuels. Weston Price.

(41) Reif-Lehrer, L. "A questionnaire study of the prevalence of Chinese restaurant syndrome." Fed. Proc. 36:1617-1623, 1977.

(42) Kenney, R. A. and Tidball, C. S. "Human susceptibility to oral monosodium L-glutamate." Am. J. Clin. Nutr. 25:140-146, 1972.

(43) Scopp, A. L. "MSG and hydrolyzed vegetable protein induced headache: a review and case studies." Headache. 31:107-110, 1991

(44) Allen, D. H. et al. "Monosodium L-glutamate-induced asthma." Journal of Allergy. 80: No 4, 530-537, 1987.

(45) http://www.aspartame.ca/epidemic-s3.pdf Aspartame Disease: AN FDA-Approved Epidemic, by H. J. Roberts, M.D.

(46) http://www.pubmedcentral.nih.gov/articlerender.fcgi?tool=pubmed&pubmedid=15061638 Tex Heart Inst J. 2004; 31(1): 105. Aspartame Disease—A Possible Cause for Concomitant Graves' Disease and Pulmonary Hypertension. H. J. Roberts, MD.

(47) http://www.ncbi.nlm.nih.gov/pubmed/8939194 J Neuropathol Exp Neurol. 1996 Nov;55(11):1115-23. Increasing brain tumor rates: is there a link to aspartame? Olney JW et al.

(48) http://www.ncbi.nlm.nih.gov/pubmed/12180494
Regul Toxicol Pharmacol. 2002 Apr;35(2 Pt 2):S1-93. Aspartame: review of safety. Butchko HH et al.

(49) http://www.westonaprice.org/modernfood/aspartame.html Aspartame: Diet-astrous Results By Rebecca Ephraim, RD, CCN Weston Price

(50) http://www.ramazzini.it/fondazione/blogDetail.asp?id=31 California Opens Proposition 65 File, Could Lead to aspartame State Suits re: Carcinogenic Properties by Stephen Fox.

(51) http://www.ncbi.nlm.nih.gov/pubmed/827619 J Toxicol Environ Health. 1976 Nov;2(2):471-80. Hypothalamic morphology following ingestion of aspartame or MSG in the neonatal rodent and primate: a preliminary report. Reynolds WA, Butler V, Lemkey-Johnston N.

(52) http://www.ncbi.nlm.nih.gov/pubmed/984473 Anat Rec. 1976 Oct;186(2):185-205. Monosodium glutamate induced lesions of the arcuate nucleus. I. Endocrine deficiency and ultrastructure of the median eminence.Holzwarth-McBride MA, Hurst EM, Knigge KM.

(53) http://www.ncbi.nlm.nih.gov/pubmed/1106764
British Journal of Nutrition (1976), 35:25-39 The induction of obesity in rodents by means of monosodium glutamate. J. Bunyana et al.

(54) http://www.scielo.br/scielo.php?pid=S0100-879X1997000500016&script=sci_arttext&tlng=en Braz J Med Biol Res, May 1997, Volume 30(5) 671-674. Monosodium glutamate (MSG)-obese rats develop glucose intolerance and insulin resistance to peripheral glucose uptake. A.E. Hirata et al.

(55) http://www.ncbi.nlm.nih.gov/pubmed/2047097 Oral Surg Oral Med Oral Pathol. 1991 May;71(5):560-4. Monosodium glutamate-related orofacial granulomatosis. Review and case report. Oliver AJ et al.

(56) http://www.ncbi.nlm.nih.gov/pubmed/3242382 Allergol Immunopathol (Madr). 1988 Nov-Dec;16(6):425-8. Monosodium glutamate and skin pathology in pediatric allergology. Botey J et al.

(57) http://www.newsroom.heart.org/index.php?s=43&item=1249 Diet soda may raise odds of vascular events. American Stroke Association Meeting Report: Abstracts P55 and 25. Study Highlights: Drinking diet soda daily is linked to a higher risk of stroke, heart attack and vascular-related deaths. American Stroke Association's International Stroke Conference 2011.

CHAPTER 48

Genetically Modified GMO Food, the Great Scandal

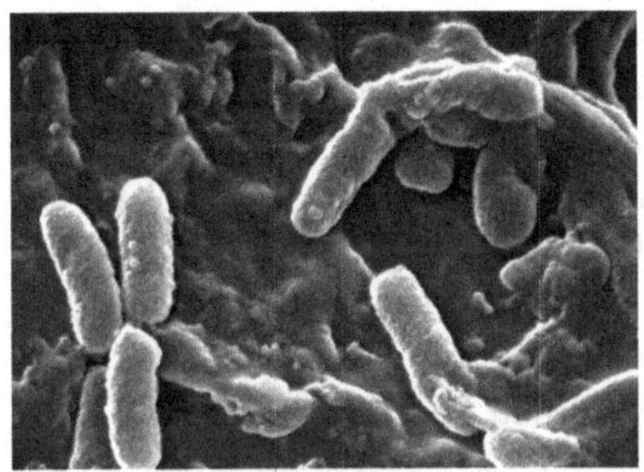

Bacteria froming rod-like shapes seen with SEM scanning electron microscope. GMOs, or Genetically Modified Organisms look like this, as well. Courtesy of Janice Haney Carr at the CDC (U.S. Center for Disease Control)

Jeffrey Smith writes about the dangers of Genetically Modified Food in his book, " Seeds of Deception". (18) This information about the health threat of genetically modified food may be new to you, since there has been a cover up with media censorship, and the suppression of key research scientists. Jeff Smith's book compiles 20 years of data on the health risks of genetically modified foods. This data includes studies in which GMO food is fed to laboratory animals resulting in thousands of sick, sterile and dead laboratory animals. Also included is data on human allergic reactions and toxicity from GMO foods. While American consumers remain oblivious, genetic modification has already spread to 70% of the supermarket food supply, mostly affecting corn, soy, cotton seed oil and canola oil. In spite of these obvious problems, the FDA does not require labeling or safety testing of genetically modified food. This is an outrage.(1-6)

L-Tryptophan, the First Genetically Engineered Food Supplement

Tryptophan is an amino acid in our diet, and a nutritional supplement. In 1984, a Japanese Company named Showa Denko manufactured Tryptophan the new GMO way, with genetically modified bacteria programmed to produce tryptophan. The programmed bacteria were "tweaked" so much, they also produced foreign proteins that were totally new and unknown, a form of undetected product contamination. These foreign proteins caused a new disease called EMS (Eosinophilia Myalgia Syndrome), leaving 37 people dead and thousands disabled. (45) On

November 11, 1989 the FDA (U.S. Food and Drug Administration) issued a nationwide warning to discontinue sales of L-tryptophan after 30 potential cases of EMS had been identified in New Mexico. (46) A lawsuit was eventually settled for 2 billion dollars which disclosed information that the company used bacterial strains 5, 4 and 3 which were genetically engineered causing the EMS disease outbreak between 1984 and 1989, caused by contaminants in the tryptophan product inherent to the technique of genetic modification. Tryptophan was banned temporarily until Non-GMO Tryptophan could be made available.(19)

Arpad Pusztai and Genetically Modified Potatoes

In 1995, a Hungarian Scientist working in Scotland by the name of Arpad Pusztai and his 20 member team was given the job of testing GMO food. Working in Scotland, the team created a potato that was genetically modified to produce a protein that was toxic to insects. Thus giving the potato a built-in insecticide. However, when lab rats were fed the genetically modified potatoes they developed health problems such as "*proliferative hyperplastic growth of the rat small intestine leading to crypt enlargement*". In testimony to Scottish Parliament, Dr Pusztai says, "*Rats fed GMO potatoes had interference in growth and development of some of their vital organs, had changes in gut structure and function and reduced immune responsiveness to injurious antigens. In contrast, the animals fed on diets containing the parent, non-GMO-potatoes or these potatoes supplemented with the gene product had no such effects.*"

When Arpad Pusztai went public on television interviews with his data, he was promptly fired and silenced after a stellar 35 year career. He was later vindicated, invited to speak before parliament, and published his study in Lancet, the most extensive animal feeding study on GMO foods. His work was credited with the banning of GMO food in Europe. (11-15) (36-37)

Transform Your GI Tract into a Toxic Factory

One common form of genetic modification for food plants is intended to confer insect resistance. This is commonly done by inserting a bacterial gene into the plant which codes for a protein toxic to insects, such as the Bt gene from the Bacillus Thuringiensis (BT). In 2004, Dr. Trudy Netherwood of Newcastle University studied the fate of these ingested BT genes after human ingestion of the GMO food. (40) However, before even starting the study, Dr. Netherwood found copies of the BT plant trans-genes already colonizing the gut bacteria of 3 of 7 human subjects. Apparently, these three human subjects had already consumed food contaminated with GMO products, just like all the rest of us trusting consumers.

We all have a few pounds of bacteria in our GI tract, called "friendly bacteria". After a round of antibiotics which kills off this "friendly bacteria" in our colon, we are often advised to consume probiotic capsules containing friendly bacteria to replenish our supply. Genes from the GMO food, such as the BT gene, are taken up by our "friendly bacteria", which in turn produce the toxic proteins inside of us. These proteins are not only the toxins and pesticides coded by the BT gene, but also unpredictable and unexpected proteins from the genetic manipulation. Thus, consuming GMO food transforms our own GI tract into a toxic factory. An even greater problem arises for genes coding for antibiotic resistance commonly spliced into plants during the GMO manufacturing process. These antibiotic resistance genes are then incorporated into our own gut bacteria. Thus we have created a new race of super antibiotic resistant bacteria waiting for a chance to cause an antibiotic resistant infection.(40-42)

To make matters worse, not only is the new genetic code from GMO food incorporated into friendly gut bacteria, it is also incorporated into the epithelial cells of the GI tract, and the liver. Dr. Netherwood's work was confirmed in a 2006 study by Dr. Sharma in Alberta Canada who found that transgenic DNA from Roundup Ready Canola Meal could be found in the gut epithelial tissues of pigs eating the GMO meal. (41)

Golden Rice and Grains of Hope—Vitamin A Gene Spliced into Rice

"Grains of Hope" was the cover story for the July 2000 issue of Time Magazine, highlighting genetically modified rice containing a gene for Vitamin A.(24) Back in the year 2000, I thought like everyone else this was a great thing. Rice lacks vitamin A, and impoverished people of third world countries subsist on rice, many going blind from vitamin A deficiency. On the surface, adding Vitamin A to rice would potentially prevent tens of thousands of cases of blindness. This was not to be. The Golden Rice was never approved for human consumption, and was labeled by critics as a hoax which caused birth defects and developmental anomalies.

Golden Rice Called a Hoax

"Phase II clinical trials on children have been conducted with unapproved experimental GM rice enhanced in pro-Vitamin A that has the potential to cause birth defects and developmental abnormalities . . . The 'golden rice' project was a useless application, a drain on public finance and a threat to health and biodiversity. It is being promoted in order to salvage a morally as well as financially bankrupt agricultural biotech industry, and is obstructing the essential shift to sustainable agriculture that can truly improve the health and nutrition especially of the poor in the Third World. This project should be terminated immediately before further damage is done . . . The 'golden rice' possesses all the usual defects of first generation transgenic plants plus multiple copies of the CaMV promoter (Cauliflower Mosaic Virus) which we have strongly recommended withdrawing from use on the basis of scientific evidence indicating this promoter to be especially unsafe. A growing number of scientists (318 scientists from 39 countries to-date) are calling for a global moratorium on the environmental releases of GMOs until and unless they can be shown to be safe." quoted from Mae-Wan Ho and Joe Cummins.(25-27)

Dr. Vandana Shiva calls Golden Rice a **HOAX,** which will not increase vitamin A consumption, and instead serves as a Trojan Horse for the corporate take-over of food production. She says:

"*while the complicated technology transfer package of "Golden Rice" will not solve vitamin A problems in India, it is a very effective strategy for corporate takeover of rice production, using the public sector as a Trojan horse.*" (38) (38A)

Genetic Pollution and Contamination of the Environment

Genetic engineering creates "genetic pollution", an uncontrolled spread of altered genetic information throughout the environment. Once released, genetic pollution cannot be recalled and is irreversible. The genetic contamination amplifies throughout the environment and soon becomes dominant. This is another disturbing aspect of genetic engineering. Unlike chemical pollution which does not replicate and gradually degrades in the environment, the genetic pollution replicates and amplifies throughout the plant and animal kingdom, creating far-reaching unpredictable consequences on the genetic diversity, and the number of species and varieties of organisms. We must stop genetic pollution of the planet.

Warning: Avoid GMO Food
GMO food should be avoided, as it is a health risk and causes genetic pollution of the environment.

Monsanto and Piracy by Science

Pirate Flag of Jack Rackam, courtesy of Wikimedia commons

By far, the largest player in the GMO game is a corporation called Monsanto. One of their GMO products is "Round-Up Ready" Soybeans. These are genetically modified soybeans which can tolerate large amounts of the herbicide Round-Up (also sold by Monsanto). Monsanto, with its long history of falsifying scientific studies, simply cannot be trusted. Monsanto's GMO manipulation of our food supply is a threat to our environment and the planet's bio-diversity. In addition, by owning patents on GMO foods, and seed, corporations like Monsanto could eventually own and control the global food supply, and with it, all life on the planet. Clearly, this is a misuse and abuse of science, and represents piracy of the highest order.

Many Countries Have Banned GMO Food

This information is changing daily. It is recommended that you do your own internet search to obtain information on which countries currently allow GMO, and which countries are banning GMO. Mexico rejected GMO corn on October 2006. The following countries have banned or restricted the import, distribution, sale, field trials and planting of GMO's: Algeria, Egypt, Sri Lanka, Thailand, Japan, Philippines, The European Union, Norway, Austria, Germany United Kingdom, Italy, Greece, France, Luxembourg, Portugal, Brazil, Saudi Arabia, American Samoa, Cook Islands, Fiji, Kiribati, Federated States of Micronesia, Marshall Islands, Nauru, Papua New Guinea, Samoa, Solomon Islands, Tonga, Tuvalu, Vanuatu, New Zealand. In North America, Genetically Modified foods are in widespread use throughout the U.S. Maryland has banned GMO fish, and North Dakota and Montana have filed bans on GE wheat. The Municipalities of Burlington, Vermont declared a moratorium on GE food. Boulder, Colorado has banned GE crops, and the City and County of San Francisco urged the federal government to ban GE food.

Medical Associations Asked For Moratorium On GMO Food

In 2002, the British Medical Association asked for a Moratorium on GMO Food, and on May 8, 2009, the American Academy of Environmental Medicine statement asked for a moratorium on GMO food, independent safety testing and labeling of GM foods, and urged the public to avoid GMO food.

We Need a Moratorium on GMO Food

Even though genetic modification of food is inherently unsafe, FDA regulations require no safety testing or labeling. In many animal feeding studies, consuming GMO food renders the animals diseased, sterile or dead. GMO feeding studies with human subjects reveal diseases such as EMS (Eosinophilia Myalgia), as well as allergic and toxic reactions to the ingested genetically modified foods. (45-46) Current biotech methods are crude and create totally new and unexpected genes and proteins which serve as toxins, allergens and cause diseases in humans and animals. The animal and human studies which show harmful effects of GMO foods have been suppressed, and the scientists fired and persecuted, such as the case of Arpad Pusztai.(36-37)

Mandatory Labeling of GMO Foods

Already 70% of food in stores is bioengineered, but not labeled as such. Labeling of genetically modified food (currently NOT DONE) should be mandated. Consumers have the right to know and need to know which products contain genetically modified foods.

GMO Modification Creates A New Drug

Genetic engineering of plants used as human food, in fact, creates a new drug. Genetically modified plants, grains, foods are not substantially equivalent to anything and are in fact new drugs, and as such, require the same scrutiny as any other new drug. FDA procedures already in place mandate process called an IND application, which is an application for an (IND) Investigational New Drug. This involves extensive animal and human safety studies. Any genetically modified food should be regulated by the FDA as a new drug.

Supreme Court Ruling Should be Overturned

It was a gross error for the Supreme Court to grant a patent for a living organism in 1980 (Diamond vs. Chakrabarty) for oil eating bacteria, which was then extended to all plant and animal life. (47) This ruling needs to be re-examined and overturned. This 1980 Supreme Court Decision (Diamond vs. Chakrabarty) is a misinterpretation of the patent laws passed by Congress. Therefore it is imperative that Congress clarify the patent laws by performing a review of previous patent legislation such as the 1930 Plant Patent Act and 1970 Plant Variety Protection Act. Congress must then pass patent law revisions and/or new patent laws which mandates that living organisms **cannot be patented**.

GMO Manufacturers Must be Held Liable for Genetic Pollution of the Environment

Similar to the way chemical companies are held accountable and liable for chemical pollution of the environment, manufacturers of genetically modified plants and animals must be held accountable and liable for genetic pollution of the environment. Genetic pollution from GMO causes far reaching irreversible damage to the environment, as well as economic loss for farmers. The environmental protection agency and the civil courts must play a role here.

Civil Litigation for GMO Food

On August 2004, Aventis settled a class-action lawsuit and paid farmers 110 million dollars for genetic contamination of farmer's fields with the Aventis Starlink™ Corn. A separate settlement paid 9 million dollars to consumers who had health problems from consuming the genetically modified Starlink corn. The courts considered the GMO Starlink™ Corn a "public nuisance", and this ruling was enough to cause Aventis to abandon its next GMO product, the Liberty Link™ Soybean. I predict that class action liability litigation against GMO Foods will increase, and become the next great bonanza for lawyers.

Federal Court Strikes Down USDA Approval for GMO Food as Illegal

Federal Court rules in three cases that GMO foods were illegally approved by USDA, violating the endangered species act and environmental policy act. Past approvals were ruled illegal.

1) In Hawaii, a federal district judge in Hawaii ruled in August 2006 that the USDA violated the Endangered Species Act as well as the National Environmental Policy Act in allowing drug-producing GM crops to be cultivated throughout Hawaii, without even an impact study. The USDA illegally approved GMO release into the wild without an environmental impact study on effect of horizontal gene transfer on endangered plant species.

2) February 2007, federal judge Harold Kennedy ruled that the USDA must halt approval of all new field trials until more rigorous environmental reviews are conducted. USDA's past GMO approvals was ruled illegal.

3) Feb 2007, a Federal Court ruled that Monsanto's Roundup Ready alfalfa had been approved for commercial release illegally, because there had been no Environment Impact Statement.

Using Science for Piracy and Robbery:

Patents for Living Organisms Based on Erroneous Supreme Court Ruling

A patent means that the patent holder has ownership rights and the right to collect royalties. Patents on living organisms were illegal until 1980 when an unprecedented US Supreme Court decision (Diamond vs. Chakrabarty) allowed a patent for genetically modified bacteria used for "eating" oil spills. (47) Lawyers and judges are not trained in science and have limited understanding, so it is not surprising that this Supreme Court ruling was a mistake and a failure to understand the science. This unprecedented ruling is a disaster and should be overturned as soon as possible. Perhaps a better approach would be for Congress to pass new patent laws which clearly state unequivocally and with no exceptions, that living organisms cannot be patented.

GMO Patents Revoke Our Inalienable Right to Life

The signers of the Declaration of Independence deemed it a ***"self evident truth"*** that all men are ***"endowed by their Creator with certain unalienable Rights". (48)*** These rights are life, liberty, and the pursuit of happiness, and these rights cannot be taken away, violated, or transferred. They are the most fundamental set of human rights, as the basic necessity of our human survival. Food is life, so therefore, included in these inalienable rights is the right to sustain life by planting and harvesting crops for food. In order to fully exercise these inalienable rights, and as a basic necessity for survival, the individual has the inalienable right to the free and open use of the natural plant and animal world, also known as farming. GMO Patents which grant corporate ownership of seed stock and living organisms revokes these inalienable human rights to life, and grants ownership to Monsanto. This is unethical, immoral and expressly prohibited by our Constitution. This ruling must be overturned. There can be no patent for Life because Life is not an invention of man; Life is an invention of the Creator given to man as an inalienable Right.

Do Not Buy GMO Foods, Consumer Sentiment Will Result in a Ban

As more and more people learn about the dangers posed by GMO food, the consumer avoidance pressures the food industry which then stops buying and stocking GMO products. Consumer avoidance has forced Gerber's Baby Food to remove GMO from their baby food products. Consumer avoidance in Europe forced most of Europe to ban GMO foods. In order to avoid buying GMO food, buy and consume Organic Food which is non-GMO. Avoid Soy, Corn, Cotton Seed and Canola products which are all GMO.

For references and links, see my web site: www.bioidenticalhormones101.com

References for Chapter 48. Genetically Modified GMO Food, the Great Scandal

(1) http://www.cqs.com/50harm.htm 50 Harmful Effects of Genetically Modified Foods By Nathan Batalion. 2000 Nathan B. Batalion, Published by Americans for Safe Food. Oneonta, N.Y.

(2) http://www.youtube.com/watch?v=a7rXIujvXGc Jeff Smith, Videos Interview at the A4M Meeting Feb, 2008. The effects of genetically modified foods.

(3) http://www.youtube.com/watch?v=94d-KVorSHM
The Health Dangers of Genetically Modified Foods PART 1-6, Jeff Smith Videos on You Tube—The Dangers of GMO FOODS, and the Cover-Up. This is a lecture by Jeffrey Smith, in which he summarizes

the contents of this book, Seeds of Deception. Introduction by Craig Winters, Campaign to Label GMO Foods.

(4) http://www.responsibletechnology.org/GMFree/Home/index.cfm Institute for Responsible Technology, Jeffrey Smith Web Site.

(5) http://www.actionbioscience.org/biotech/pusztai.html Genetically Modified Foods: Are They a Risk to Human/Animal Health?

(6) http://www.relfe.com/GMOs.html Genetically Engineered Organisms (GMOs): The Greatest Threat Ever to Humans and Animals

(7) http://www.westonaprice.org/federalupdate/aa2003/actionalert_072403.html July 24, 2003 Shopping List for GMO-Free Foods The Final Word, Weston Price.

(8) http://wideeyecinema.com/?p=105 The World According to Monsanto Video March 2008 by French journalist Marie-Monique Robin—A documentary.

(9) http://dandelionsalad.wordpress.com/2008/04/01/the-world-according-to-monsanto-a-documentary-that-americans-wont-ever-see-full-video/ The World According to Monsanto—A documentary that Americans won't ever see (video)

(10) http://fooddemocracy.wordpress.com/2008/04/14/video-the-world-according-to-monsanto/ Video: "The World According to Monsanto" April 14, 2008

(11) http://www.freenetpages.co.uk/hp/a.pusztai/ Árpád Pusztai's Homepage—GMO Potatoe

(12) Editorial (1999) 'Health risks of GM foods', The Lancet 353: 1811.

(13) http://www.ncbi.nlm.nih.gov/pubmed/10533866 Ewen, S.W.B. and Pusztai, A. (1999a) 'Effect of diets containing genetically modified potatoes expressing Galanthus nivalis lectin on rat small intestine', The Lancet 354: 1353-1354.

(14) Ewen, S.W.B. and Pusztai, A. (1999b) Authors' reply. The Lancet 354: 1726-1727.

(15) Pusztai A. and Bardocz S (2006). GMO in animal nutrition: potential benefits and risks. In: Biology of Nutrition in Growing Animals, eds. R. Mosenthin, J. Zentek and T. Zebrowska, Elsevier Limited, pp. 513-540.

(16) Schubbert R. et al. (1994) 'Ingested foreign (phage M13) DNA survives transiently in the gastrointestinal tract and enters the blood stream of mice', Molecules, Genes and Genetics 242: 495-504.

(17) Schubbert R. et al. (1998) 'On the fate of orally ingested foreign DNA in mice: chromosomal association and placental transmission in the fetus', Molecules, Genes and Genetics 259: 569-576.

(18) http://www.seedsofdeception.com/Public/Home/index.cfm Seeds of Deception, by Jeffrey M. Smith,

(19) http://www.seedsofdeception.com/Public/L-tryptophan/index.cfm Toxic L-tryptophan: Shedding Light on a Mysterious Epidemic by William E. Crist

(20) http://www.navdanya.org/publications/seeds-of-suicide.pdf Seeds of Suicide, The Ecological and Human Costs of Globalisation of Agriculture. Dr Vandana Shiva,

(21) http://www.pbs.org/frontlineworld/rough/2005/07/seeds_of_suicid.html Rough Cut, Seeds of Suicide, India's desperate farmers July 26, 2005

(22) http://www.vanityfair.com/politics/features/2008/05/monsanto200805 Monsanto's Harvest of Fear. Vanity Fair Article. by Donald L. Barlett and James B. Steele May 2008.

(23) http://www.greenleft.org.au/2008/754/38977 AUSTRALIA WA premier calls for GM product ban Annolies Truman 7 June 2008 Time

Magazine Cover Aug 7, 2000. Golden rice and co-creator Professor Ingo Potrykus on the cover of TIME magazine,

(24) http://online.sfsu.edu/~rone/GEessays/goldenricehoax.html THE "GOLDEN RICE" HOAX—When Public Relations replaces Science by Dr. Vandana Shiva "Golden Rice": A technology for creating Vitamin A deficiency.

(25) http://www.greenpeace.org/raw/content/international/press/reports/all-that-glitters-is-not-gold.pdf Greenpeace. 2005. All that Glitters is not Gold: The False Hope of Golden Rice

(26) http://www.i-sis.org.uk/rice.php The 'Golden Rice'—An Exercise in How Not to Do Science by Mae-Wan Ho, Institute of Science in Society, ISIS.

(27) http://www.ncbi.nlm.nih.gov/pubmed/10634784
Science. 2000 Jan 14;287(5451):303-5.Engineering the provitamin A (beta-carotene) biosynthetic pathway into (carotenoid-free) rice endosperm.Ye X, Al-Babili S, Klöti A, Zhang J, Lucca P, Beyer P, Potrykus I. Institute for Plant Sciences, Swiss Federal Institute of Technology

(28) http://www.time.com/time/magazine/article/0,9171,997586,00.html Grains of Hope Time MAgazine Monday, Feb. 05, 2001 By J. MADELEINE NASH A.

(29) http://www.agbioworld.org/biotech-info/articles/biotech-art/potrykus.html Experience from the Humanitarian Golden Rice Project: Extreme Precautionary Regulation Prevents Use of Green Biotechnology in Public Projects BioVision Alexandria 3-6 April 2004 By Ingo Potrykus Professor emeritus Plant Sciences, ETH Zuerich, Switzerland

(30) http://www.i-sis.org.uk/isisnews/sis37.php Redeeming Science from Corporate Corruption (SiS 37), We are faced with a corporate corruption of science in which every level of the corporate structure is complicit: the scientific establishment, journal editors and big government held to ransom by the biotech industry.

(31) http://www.seedsofdeception.com/DocumentFiles/138.pdf interview with Jeffrey Smith Documents made public from a lawsuit show that the overwhelming consensus among the FDA's own scientists was that GM crops were inherently unsafe and could create hard-to-detect, unpredicted toxins,allergens, new diseases.

(32) http://www.seedsofdeception.com/Public/GeneticRoulette/HealthRisksofGMFoodsSummaryDebate/index.cfm
The Health Risks of GM Foods: Summary and Debate.

(33) http://www.youtube.com/watch?v=94d-KVorSHM&feature=related— The Health Dangers of Genetically Modified Foods, with jeffrey M. Smith, author of "Seeds of Deception.

(34) http://www.globalresearch.ca/index.php?context=viewArticle&code=SMI20061119&articleId=3912 Monsanto Whistleblower Says Genetically Engineered Crops May Cause Disease.

(35) http://articles.mercola.com/sites/articles/archive/2007/08/01/genetically-modified-organisms-are-a-looming-threat.aspx Genetically Modified Foods—What to Know Before You Eat Them (from Mercola.com)

(36) http://www.somloquesembrem.org/img_editor/file/Brown-Journal-article%20-%20Arpad%20Pusztai.pdf Genetic Engineering—Genetechnology—Is It Salvation or Curse for the 21st Century? Arpad Pusztai, Ph.D., FRSE Aberdeen, Scotland UK

(37) http://www.gmfreeireland.org/potato/info/ArpadPusztai.pdf article by Arpad Pusztai, Proliferative hyperplastic growth of the rat small intestine leading to crypt enlargement and a part of the stomach enlargement was not a GNA lectin effect but was probably either due to some other component of the gene vector used for the genetic modification and/or the disruption caused by the incorporation of the vector in the plant genome

(38) http://userwww.sfsu.edu/~rone/GEessays/goldenricehoax.html THE "GOLDEN RICE" HOAX,When Public Relations replaces Science by Dr. Vandana Shiva, "Golden Rice": A technology for creating Vitamin A deficiency.

(38A) http://www.biotech-info.net/conway_greenpeace.pdf Response to the report by Dr. Vandana Shiva entitled "The Golden Rice Hoax" from Rockefeller Foundation

(39) http://www.foodsafetynetwork.ca/gmo/gmnewcastlereport.pdf Netherwood, T., Martin-Orue, S.M., O'Donnell,A.G., Gockling, S., Gilbert, H.J., and Mathers, J.C. "Transgenes in Genetically Modified Soya Survive Passage Through the Human Small Bowel but are Completely Degraded in the Colon."

(40) http://www.ncbi.nlm.nih.gov/pubmed/14730317 And also http://www.agbios.com/docroot/articles/06-272-005.pdf Nat Biotechnol. 2004 Feb;22(2):204-9. Assessing the survival of transgenic plant DNA in the human gastrointestinal tract. Netherwood T et al.

(41) http://www.ncbi.nlm.nih.gov/pubmed/16506822 Agric Food Chem. 2006 Mar 8;54(5):1699-709. Detection of transgenic and endogenous plant DNA in digesta and tissues of sheep and pigs fed Roundup Ready canola meal.Sharma R, Damgaard D, Alexander TW et al.

(42) http://www.mindfully.org/GE/2004/Transgenes-Human-Gut1feb04.htm The Fate of Transgenes in the Human Gut JOHN HERITAGE Nature Biotechnology v.22, n.2, 1feb2004

(43) http://www.botanischergarten.ch/debate/Newcastlereport.pdf Technical report on the Food Standards Agency project G010008. "Evaluating the risks associated with using GMOs in human foods"—University of Newcastle

(44) http://www.uspirg.org/uploads/h2/c7/h2c7fdGhH7uoszDFnGppnw/WeirdScience2003.pdf
The Brave New World of Genetic Engineering U.S. PIRG Education Fund October 2003

(45) http://www.ncbi.nlm.nih.gov/pubmed/9213377
Semin Arthritis Rheum. 1997 Jun;26(6):788-93.Eosinophilia myalgia syndrome.Blackburn WD Jr.

(46) http://www.cdc.gov/mmwr/preview/mmwrhtml/00001502.htm
Epidemiologic Notes and Reports Eosinophilia-Myalgia Syndrome and L-Tryptophan-Containing Products—New Mexico, Minnesota, Oregon, and New York, 1989. November 24, 1989/38(46);785-788 MMWR

(47) http://digital-law-online.info/cases/206PQ193.htm Diamond, Commissioner of Patents and Trademarks v. Chakrabarty United States Supreme Court June 16, 1980 447 U.S. 303, 206 USPQ 193

(48) http://www.ushistory.org/declaration/document/ Declaration of Independence. IN CONGRESS, JULY 4, 1776 The unanimous Declaration of the thirteen united States of America.

CHAPTER 49

Gluten Sensitivity, Is Your Food Making You Sick?

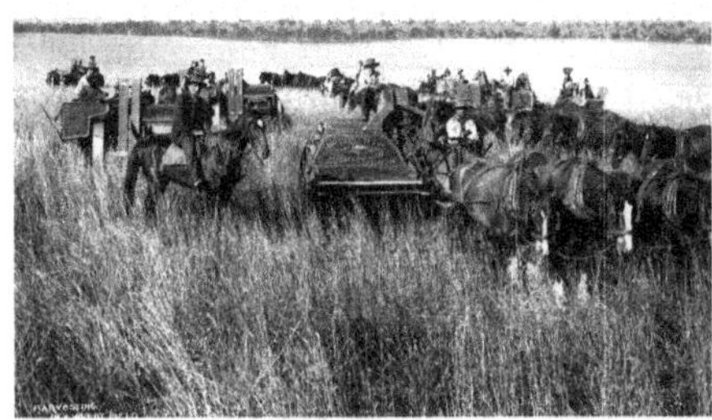

Harvesting in a wheat field, ca. 1900 Australia, courtesy of the Powerhouse Museum and wikimedia commons.

Jim suffered from frequent migraines which were severe and incapacitating. After seeing a number of neurologists and trying multiple medications with no improvement, Jim finally came to see me. His last neurologist found he had a low vitamin D level, and started Jim on 10,000 units per day of vitamin D3. Jim reported that his psoriatic skin lesions were markedly better. However, his migraines were unchanged.

Migraines and Food Allergies

A connection between gluten sensitivity and psoriasis is well known. (18-20) In addition, I mentioned to Jim that food allergies can cause migraines (7). Gluten is a wheat protein, and sensitivity to wheat gluten can cause migraine headaches (8,9). In fact, gluten sensitivity is associated with all sorts of neurological disorders: cerebellar ataxia, epilepsy, myoclonic ataxia, chronic neuropathies, and dementia, mainly in middle-aged adults.(10-13) I suggested to Jim it was likely that a gluten free diet would be helpful in reducing his migraines.(8-9)

Gluten Testing with Entero-Labs

Jim's lifestyle made it difficult for him to go Gluten free, so I suggested he try the EnteroLabs gluten test.(41) Sure enough, the test panel came back positive. Jim went on a gluten free diet, and 4 weeks later called me to report his migraines were much better. This article will discuss sensitivity to wheat gluten, a condition which is epidemic, yet mainly ignored or unknown by the medical system.(20)

What is wheat gluten sensitivity?

Gluten is a protein in wheat products, such as bread, pasta, wheat cereals etc. About 1% or more of the population reacts to wheat gluten with an immune response and an inflammatory disorder of the small intestine which may cause malabsorption of key minerals, amino acids and vitamins. (40) This has an inherited autoimmune component and genetic testing is available.(17) Other diagnostic testing involves looking for the antibodies called TTG (transglutaminase) in stool or blood samples.

Immune Response In the Wall of the Small Bowel-Malabsorption

The immune response involves production of various antibodies and immune cells which damages the small intestine, reducing its absorptive ability.(40) This is called malabsorption, and results in the inability to absorb key vitamins and minerals such as Iron, Calcium, folate and B12. These abnormalities will show up on the blood count as iron deficiency anemia, and B12/folate deficiency anemia.(22) Gluten sensitivity and celiac disease may cause malabsorption of calcium, and the DEXA bone density scan may show osteoporosis (21). The auto-immune response can circulate freely through the body, crossreacting with other organ systems, unpredictably.

Immune Response in the Skin and Hair Follicles

Another common place for the immune response to attack is the skin, with a characteristic skin lesion called Dermatiformis Herpetiformis (it resembles Herpes) with intense burning, itching and blistering skin rash which is usually symmetrically distributed on the elbows, knees and the buttocks. The rash usually starts as small blisters that erupt into small erosions. Dermatologists will make the diagnosis of gluten sensitivity by doing a skin biopsy showing characteristic findings. Immunofluorescence of normal skin next to the vesicle typically shows granular IgA deposits in the upper dermis. (27-29) If the scalp is involved, this is called Alopecia Areata with patchy hair loss caused by auto-antibodies reacting with the hair follicles.(25-26)

Vascular System

If the immune response attacks the vascular system, there may be increased venous thrombo-embolism, stroke (2)(3), and coronary artery disease, etc. Thus, gluten sensitivity is one of the major causes of migraine headaches since it may cause inflammation of cerebral arteries, or the brain itself. (9)

Neurological Problems

If the immune response attacks the brain or spinal cord, this may cause a neurological disorder (4, 10-16) such as ataxia (5), uncoordination, peripheral neuropathy (tingling with pins and needles)(6).

Going to the Endocrinologist

The patient with gluten sensitivity may end up at the endocrinologist's office with issues such as: Type 1 diabetes mellitus, autoimmune thyroid disease, Addison disease, osteomalacia, secondary hyperparathyroidism, vitamin D or iron deficiency, fertility problems, hypogonadism in men, and autoimmune hypopituitarism.(23) Autoimmune thyroid disease is especially common among people with gluten sensitivity, with elevated anti-thyroid antibodies (Hashimoto's Thyroiditis) which decrease after initiating a gluten free diet.(24) One can make a case for gluten sensitivity testing for all patients with autoimmune thyroid disease (Hashimoto's).

The Heart

The gluten sensitive patient may have heart involvement with cardiomyopathy, a serious and potentially lethal form of heart failure. In addition, the gluten sensitive individual may have heart rhythm abnormalities such as atrial fibrillation, reversible with a gluten free diet, if diagnosed early. Testing for gluten sensitivity should be done for such patients. (30-31)

Sarcoidosis

A unusual lung disease of unknown etiology called Sarcoidosis is linked to gluten sensitivity. Sarcoidosis is thought to be an auto-immune disease because the treatment is immune suppression with prednisone. These patients may benefit from a gluten free diet.(34)

Addison's Disease and Adrenal Failure

Complete failure of the adrenal glands to manufacture cortisol is called Addison's Disease and is associated with gluten sensitivity.(35) These patients may benefit from a gluten free diet.

Going on a Gluten Free Diet

Patients may go for decades with health problems, running through a succession of doctors, yet remain undiagnosed by the mainstream medical system. Treatment is usually curative with a Gluten Free Diet (GFD) which means avoiding all wheat products such as breads, pasta, wheat cereals, bakery goods etc.

Articles with related interest: See Celiac Disease, Gluten Intolerance, the Unsuspected Epidemic in the book, Natural Medicine 101.

Links and References

(1) http://charlotteceliacconnection.com/files/Green - NEJM - Celiac Disease.pdf Medical Progress, Celiac Disease, Peter H.R. Green, M.D., and Christophe Cellier, M.D., Ph.D. N Engl J Med 357;17 october 25, 2007

(2) http://www.ncbi.nlm.nih.gov/pubmed/15301836
Pediatr Neurol. 2004 Aug;31(2):139-42. Celiac disease and childhood stroke. Goodwin FC, Beattie RM, Millar J, Kirkham FJ.

(3) http://www.ncbi.nlm.nih.gov/pubmed/19144365 Rev Neurol (Paris). 2009 Nov;165(11):962-6. Epub 2009 Jan 13. [Celiac disease and ischemic stroke].[Article in French] El Moutawakil B et al.

(4) http://www.ncbi.nlm.nih.gov/pubmed/19845007 Mov Disord. 2009 Dec 15;24(16):2358-62. Neurological symptoms in patients with biopsy proven celiac disease. Bürk K, Farecki ML, Lamprecht G, Roth G, Decker P, Weller M, Rammensee HG, Oertel W.

(5) www.ncbi.nlm.nih.gov/pubmed/12566288 Brain. 2003 Mar;126(Pt 3):685-91. Gluten ataxia in perspective: epidemiology, genetic susceptibility and clinical characteristics. Hadjivassiliou M et al.

(6) http://www.etseq.urv.es/cdmedics/pdfs/Celiac%20disease%20from%20gut%20to%20brain.pdf Lancet Neurol 2010; 9: 318-30 Gluten sensitivity: from gut to brain. Marios Hadjivassiliou et al.

(7) http://www.ncbi.nlm.nih.gov/pubmed/87628 Lancet. 1979 May 5;1(8123):966-9. Food allergies and migraine.Grant EC.

(8) http://www.ncbi.nlm.nih.gov/pubmed/12650798 http://www.nature.com/ajg/journal/v98/n3/abs/ajg2003147a.html Am J Gastroenterol. 2003 Jul;98(7):1674; Association Between Migraine and Celiac Disease: Results From a Preliminary Case-Control and Therapeutic Study. Maurizio Gabrielli MD et al.

(9) http://www.sciencedaily.com/releases/2001/02/010213072604.htm American Academy of Neurology (2001, February 14); Gluten In The Diet May Be The Cause Of Recurring Headaches; Science Daily.

(10) http://www.celiacosmadrid.org/Gluten_sensitivity_from_gut_to_brain.pdf Lancet Neurol 2010; 9: 318-30 Gluten sensitivity: from gut to brain. Marios Hadjivassiliou, David S Sanders, Richard A Grünewald, Nicola Woodroofe, Sabrina Boscolo, Daniel Aeschlimann

(11) http://menwit.ru/The_gluten_syndrome__A_neurological_disease.pdf The gluten syndrome: A neurological disease . . . Rodney Philip Kinvig Ford * The Children's Gastroenterology and Allergy Clinic, P.O. Box 25-265, Christchurch 8144, New Zealand

(12) http://www.acnr.co.uk/pdfs/volume2issue6/v2i6reviewart2.pdf M Hadjivassiliou—acnr.co.uk ACNR 2003 Gluten and neurologic disorders

(13) http://pediatrics.aappublications.org/cgi/reprint/113/6/1672 http://pediatrics.aappublications.org/cgi/content/abstract/113/6/1672Range of Neurologic Disorders in Patients With Celiac Disease Nathanel Zelnik, MD etr al.

(14) http://www.etseq.urv.es/cdmedics/pdfs/Celiac%20disease%20from%20gut%20to%20brain.pdf Lancet Neurol 2010; 9: 318-30 Gluten sensitivity: from gut to brain Marios Hadjivassiliou, David S Sanders, Richard A Grünewald, Nicola Woodroofe, Sabrina Boscolo, Daniel Aeschlimann

(15) http://www.charlotte-celiac-connection.org/files/Narrative_Review_Celiac_Disease_Understanding_A_Complex.pdf Narrative Review: Celiac Disease: Understanding a Complex Autoimmune Disorder Armin Alaedini, PhD, and Peter H.R. Green, MD Ann Intern Med. 2005;142:289-298.

(16) http://ir.library.oregonstate.edu/xmlui/bitstream/handle/1957/17611/Thesis%20Electronic%20Copy%20Dougher.pdf?sequence=1 http://ir.library.oregonstate.edu/xmlui/handle/1957/17611 Living Gluten-Free: An Analysis of Illness and Coping Narratives. Authors: Dougher, Carly E. Citation URL: http://hdl.handle.net/1957/17611

(17) http://www.ncbi.nlm.nih.gov/pubmed/20947431
Trends Mol Med. 2010 Nov;16(11):537-50. Epub 2010 Oct12. A genetic perspective on coeliac disease. Trynka G, Wijmenga C, van Heel DA.

(18) http://www.wjgnet.com/1007-9327/13/2138.pdf
Celiac disease and skin: Psoriasis association. L Abenavoli, L Leggio, G Gasbarrini, G Addolorato. World J Gastroenterol 2007 April 14; 13(14): 2138-2139

(19) http://www.ncbi.nlm.nih.gov/pubmed/12949434
Digestion. 2003;68(1):9-12. Epub 2003 Aug 29. Rapid Regression of Psoriasis in a Coeliac Patient after Gluten-Free Diet. A Case Report and Review of the Literature Giovanni Addoloratoa, et al.

(20) Celiac Disease (Revised and Updated Edition) A Hidden Epidemic By Peter H.R. Green, M.D., Rory Jones William Morrow and Company, 2010

(21) http://www.ncbi.nlm.nih.gov/pubmed/15738367
Increased prevalence of celiac disease and need for routine screening among patients with osteoporosis. Stenson WF, Newberry R, Lorenz R, Baldus C, Civitelli R.

(22) http://bloodjournal.hematologylibrary.org/content/109/2/412.full and also: http://www.ncbi.nlm.nih.gov/pmc/articles/PMC1785098/ Blood. 2007 January 15; 109(2): 412-421. Hematologic manifestations of celiac disease. Thorvardur R. Halfdanarson et al.

(23) http://www.ncbi.nlm.nih.gov/pubmed/18463048
Endocr Pract. 2008 Apr;14(3):381-8. Celiac disease and the endocrinologist: a diagnostic opportunity. Fisher AH, Lomasky SJ, Fisher MJ, Oppenheim YL.

(24) http://www.ncbi.nlm.nih.gov/pubmed/11280546 Am J Gastroenterol. 2001 Mar;96(3):751-7. Prevalence of thyroid disorders in untreated adult celiac disease patients and effect of gluten withdrawal: an Italian multicenter study. Sategna-Guidetti C et al.

(25) http://www.ncbi.nlm.nih.gov/pubmed/8176253
J Invest Dermatol. 1994 May;102(5):721-4. Antibodies to hair follicles in alopecia areata. Tobin DJ, Orentreich N, Fenton DA, Bystryn JC.

(26) http://www.ncbi.nlm.nih.gov/pubmed/16338213 Autoimmun Rev. 2006 Jan;5(1):64-9. Epub 2005 Aug 8. Alopecia areata: a tissue specific autoimmune disease of the hair follicle.Gilhar A, Kalish RS.

(27) http://digestive.niddk.nih.gov/ddiseases/pubs/dh/Dermatitis Herpetiformis_CDAC_PP.pdf
Dermatitis HerPetiformis: Skin Manifestation of Celiac Disease. A skin biopsy is the first step in diagnosing DH. Direct immunofluorescence of clinically normal skin adjacent to a lesion shows granular IgA deposits in the upper dermis.

(28) http://www.ncbi.nlm.nih.gov/pubmed/19344979
Rose C, Armbruster FP, Ruppert J, Igl BW, Zillikens D and Shimanovich I Autoantibodies against epidermal transglutaminase are a sensitive diagnostic marker in patients with dermatitis herpetiformis on a normal or gluten-free diet. J Am Acad Dermatol 2009; 61:39-43 Zone JJ Skin manifestations of celiac disease.

(29) http://www.ncbi.nlm.nih.gov/pubmed/16521210 Abenavoli L, Proietti I, Leggio L, et al. Cutaneous manifestations in celiac disease. World Journal of Gastroenterology. 2006;12(6):843-852.

(30) http://www.ncbi.nlm.nih.gov/pubmed/10421311
Curione M, Barbato M, De Biase L, Viola F, Lo Russo L, Cardi E. Prevalence of Coeliac Disease in Idiopathic Dilated Cardiomyopathy. The Lancet 1999; 354: 222-223.

(31) http://www.mayoclinicproceedings.com/content/80/5/674.full.pdf
Cardiomyopathy Associated With Celiac Disease. Mayo Clin Proc. 2005;80(5):674-676
CASE REPORT NISHEETH K. GOEL et al.

(32) http://www.biomath.info/Protocols/PGY2/docs/ChangMatt.pdf Risk of Coronary Artery Disease in Celiac Disease Patients

(33) http://www.ncbi.nlm.nih.gov/pmc/articles/PMC1955032/ Heart. 2007 September; 93(9): 1111-1115. Vascular disease in a population-based cohort of individuals hospitalised with coeliac disease J F Ludvigsson, U de Faire, A Ekbom, and S M Montgomery

(34) http://www.ncbi.nlm.nih.gov/pubmed/18496982 Sarcoidosis Vasc Diffuse Lung Dis. 2007 Sep;24(2):121-6. Coeliac disease and risk

of sarcoidosis. Ludvigsson JF, Wahlstrom J, Grunewald J, Ekbom A, Montgomery SM.

(35) http://www.ncbi.nlm.nih.gov/pubmed/17595243
J Clin Endocrinol Metab. 2007 Sep;92(9):3595-8. Epub 2007 Jun 26. Risk of primary adrenal insufficiency in patients with celiac disease. Elfström P, Montgomery SM, Kämpe O, Ekbom A, Ludvigsson JF.

(36) http://charlotteceliacconnection.com/files/Green - NEJM - Celiac Disease.pdf Medical Progress, Celiac Disease, Peter H.R. Green, M.D., and Christophe Cellier, M.D., Ph.D. n engl j med 357;17 october 25, 2007

(37) http://www.charlotte-celiac-connection.org/files/The Many Faces Of Celiac Disease.pdf The Many Faces of Celiac Disease: Clinical Presentation of Celiac Disease in the Adult Population. Peter H. R., Green. Gasteroenterology Vol. 128, No. 4 April Supplement 2005. Celiac Disease Center at Columbia University, Columbia University Medical Center, New York.

(38) http://www.direct-ms.org/pdf/ImmunologyOther/SollidCeliac.pdfAnnu. Rev. Immunol. 2000. 18:53-81. MOLECULAR BASIS OF CELIAC DISEASE Ludvig M. Sollid Institute of Immunology, Rikshospitalet

(39) http://findarticles.com/p/articles/mi m0ISW/is 2002 Dec/ai 94538644/pg 2 Gluten intolerance: A Paradigm of an Epidemic. Townsend Letter for Doctors and Patients, Dec, 2002 by Stacy Astor Shaul.

(40) http://www.scientificamerican.com/article.cfm?id=celiac-disease-insights
Celiac Disease Insights: Clues to Solving Autoimmunity by Alessio Fasano, July 27, 2009 Scientific American

(41) http://www.enterolab.com/ Kenneth Fine MD, 10875 Plano Rd.Suite 123 Dallas, TX 75238 PH: 972-686-6869

Section Thirteen: Mind Body Connection and Spirituality

CHAPTER 50

Signature in a Cell, Aging, Disease and Death

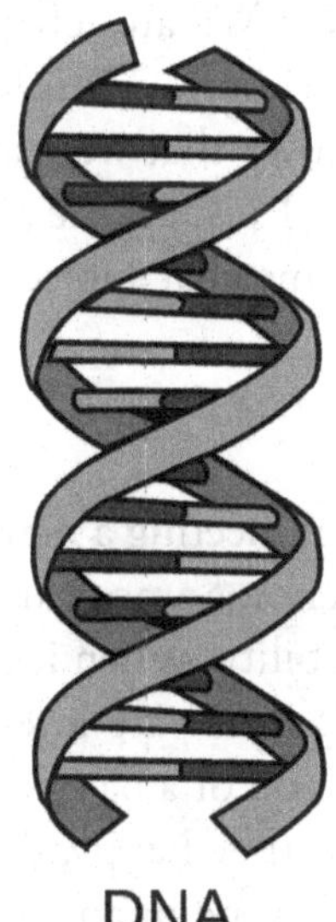

DNA double helix, courtesy of Wikimedia commons

Intelligent Design—Metaphysical Speculation or Science?

The central argument of Stephen Meyer's book, "Signature in a Cell", is that coded instruction sets in cellular DNA, just like computer code, require intelligence for their origin.(1) Meyer calls this the best inference from the evidence, a valid argument used in science. I think this argument is a valid one. One can make the inference that the origin of information indicates intelligence. Meyer's argument remains science because it stops short of the next step, which is to make the metaphysical inference that the "intelligent agent" that originates the information in nature is God, the creator of the universe. This metaphysical inference is the old "Watchmaker Argument" by William Paley written in 1826.(2) So, in order to avoid this for the moment, let's not make this metaphysical inference.

Observing Origination of New Code

We can observe a coded instruction set originate when a computer programmer writes new code for a computer program. The human computer programmer is said to be "an intelligent agent". We can actually sit behind the man as he does his work, observing new computer software being written. What about computer software in nature? Unfortunately none of us current day humans will ever directly observe the origin of the first information in DNA, at the dawn of life billions of years ago.

What is Intelligence?

So once we agree that the best inference is that coded instructions in DNA originated from intelligence, then what? We are left with the problem of defining "intelligence". We think we know what intelligence is, yet once we look at the definition, we discover that we really don't have a good scientific definition of intelligence. I suspect the reason for this is that our recognition of intelligence is somewhat subjective.

Reading Other People's Intelligence

For example, one of the first things we do when meeting a new person, is to try assessing that person's level of intelligence. Some of us have an innate ability to do this. Some of us lack this ability. When it comes to reading other people, in addition to intelligence, we are interested in other qualities in the new person. Are they a good or a bad person, are they trustworthy, truthful, capable of love, are they happy, depressed, confident, fearful? Is this new person a threat to me in any way? Will they be a potential ally or a foe?

Intelligence is in the Subjective Realm

We can also try to assess the intelligence of animals, such as our cats and dogs that we are familiar with around the house. We can also get the feeling that there is artificial intelligence in some forms of computer software such as chess programs that exhibit a form of artificial intelligence. Again, we do not have any instruments to measure intelligence in an objective way. IQ testing doesn't seem to be a very good tool. Our knowledge of intelligence seems to remain in the subjective realm. Science is concerned with the objective realm, and doesn't do very well with the subjective realm.

The Implications of A Non-Human Intelligent Agent.

Let's assume that we all agree that this is a valid inference, that the coded instruction set in DNA is evidence of the work of an intelligent agent.

Is the Intelligent Agent Friend or Foe?

This brings us back to popular movies like Space Odyssey or Contact in which extra-terrestrial intelligence is the subject of the movie. When primitive man came across tracks or markings indicating an intelligent agent, the intelligent agent was either another primitive human, or else an animal. Either way, the highest priority consideration is whether the intelligent agent is a threat or a friend. This is true for ANY new found intelligent agent in the wild, and must be applied to our new found intelligent agent, the originator of the information in coded DNA.

If a Foe, is the Foe Dangerous to Me?

The first thing we would ask is, "what is the level of this intelligence relative to mine or other humans?" Molecular biologists have concluded that the complexity and elegance of the coded instruction set in DNA is far in excess of anything humans could produce. This is a frightening realization, because, if this intelligent agent is a threat rather than a friend, then we are at a serious disadvantage. A foe with more intelligence means a foe with better technology and better weapons.

Aging, Disease and Death

Fortunately for us, it seems that the intelligent agent, if there was malevolent one, has left the scene. And if the agent was a threat, then the only malevolent features being left behind for us are the coded instruction sets for pre-programmed aging, disease and death. I would remiss if I ended this discussion on such a pessimistic and depressing note. There is another take on things.

Gratitude for Life.

There is another more optimistic viewpoint based on our understanding of the coded instruction sets in our DNA. This is the miracle of life, our own individual life that began as two microscopic specks of matter containing paired instruction sets in the DNA. The underlying intelligence required for the origin of this instruction set is something the ancients understood well. Whether we use the most powerful instruments to examine the galaxies in space or the smallest particles of the atom, or whether we use the naked eye and the five senses to examine our immediate natural world, we are confronted with the obvious conclusion that the world is permeated with intelligence. This intelligence makes all life possible, including our individual life. This realization leads to a sense of gratitude to the Creator, and a sense of wonder and awe. Yes, we are faced with the eventual prospect of aging, disease and death. But until that time comes, we will celebrate life.

References for Chapter 50. Signature In A Cell, Aging Disease and Death

(42) Signature in the Cell: DNA and the Evidence for Intelligent Design by Stephen C. Meyer, HarperOne (June 23, 2009)

(43) http://books.google.com/books/about/Natural_theology_or.html?id=cvAQAAAAYAAJ Natural theology: or Evidences of the existence and attributes of the Deity, collected from the appearances of nature, by William Paley,1826,Lincoln-Rembrandt Pub.; 12 edition (August 1986)

CHAPTER 51

Finding God in Mr. Foley's I.V.

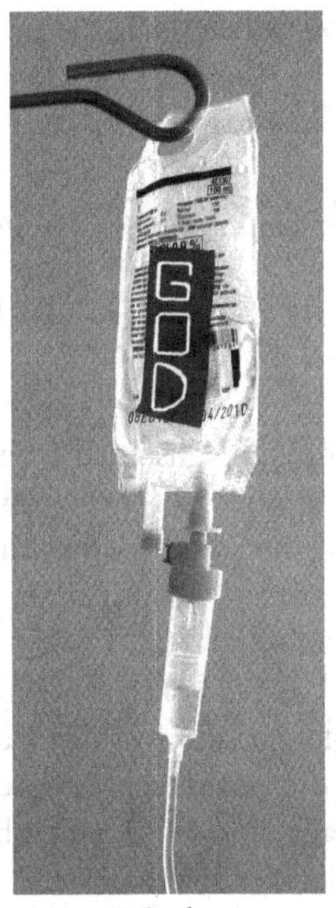

Intravenous (IV) bag courtesy of Wikimedia commons

As I walked through the snow covered parking lot into the hospital building, the place was strangely vacant. The hospital was a lonely place during the break between Christmas and New Year's. The house staff had vanished for the holiday, and as the medical student on call, I was left behind to care for the sick and dying on the sixth floor medical ward at the University of Illinois Hospital.

My patient for the week, Mr. Foley, was dying. His failing liver would last for a few more days at the most. What had caused his failing liver? I don't recall and it doesn't matter. Perhaps it was alcohol toxicity, perhaps something else. I entered the room with a fresh bag of saline for his IV line and found him sitting up in bed. His jaundiced eyes gazed out the window past the parking lot to the ice covered tree branches.

His yellow, green skin was thin and fragile from chronic wasting. At the bedside, his tray of hospital food was untouched. The room had been cleaned by the hospital staff, yet still emanated a distinctive aroma of ammonia, bile, and fecal residue. The whole ward smelled like that. Foley knew he was dying. And I knew that he knew, yet he seemed in good spirits. As I examined his two arms for a suitable vein to restart his failed I.V. line, Foley struck up a conversation.

"*Doc, he said, do you believe in God?*"

I confessed to Mr. Foley that I had my doubts about it. After four years of studying science in college and a year of medical school, I had drifted into agnosticism. Science could not demonstrate the existence of God, and since I could not see, touch or feel God in this material world of science, how could I be sure of God's existence?

"*No, Doc, you are wrong*", *said Mr. Foley. "There is a God, I know it.*"

I looked into his sad, yellow eyes and asked back, "*How do you know*"?

Mr. Foley's emaciated face revealed a sincerity and wisdom that I had rarely seen. He said. "*It is obvious. I just know that's all.*"

The IV needle found its vein easily, and the light glistened from the droplets of saline as they dripped into the chamber under the bag, and then into Mr. Foley. My task completed, I returned to the nursing station for my next assignment.

That small conversation about God with Mr. Foley marked the beginning of a drastic change in how I looked at the world. I learned a very important thing from Mr. Foley. He did not merely believe that God existed, he knew it. That was 35 years ago, and I still remember as if it was yesterday. Mr. Foley died ten days later of liver failure.

Section Fourteen: The Future of Medicine

CHAPTER 52

Cannabis, Miracle Drug of the 21st Century

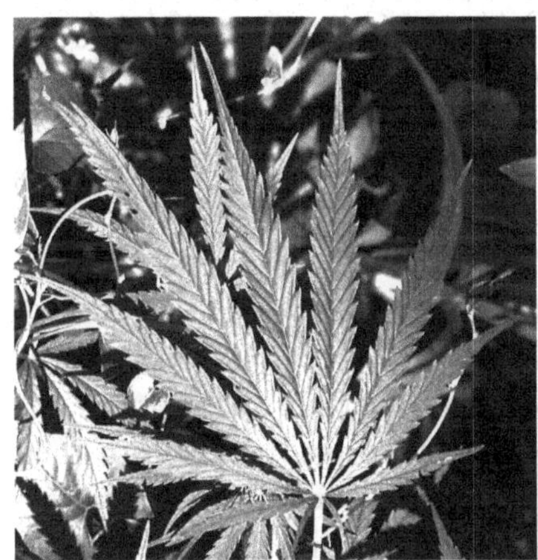

Cannabis plant photograph, courtesy of the United States Fish and Wildlife Service.

Although cannabis (marijuana) was a medicinal plant for thousands of years, its use was suppressed and banned throughout most of the 20th century. Banned in England, Canada and the US in the 1930's, medical cannabis represents the first casualty in the war against natural medicine waged by the pharmaceutical industry. While banned in the US, there have been major scientific breakthroughs in Israel, Spain, Italy and Brazil over the last two decades. These breakthroughs have made cannabis "the wonder drug of the 21st century".

The Father of Medical Cannabis Research

The greatest cannabis researcher is unquestionably Raphael Mechoulam from Israel.(76) In 1964, Mechoulam discovered the active ingredient in cannabis, THC (Tetra-Hydro-Cannabinol). (2) In 1992, he discovered the first endogenous endo-cannabinoid, Anandamide, a sanskrit word translated as "bliss".(78) Endo-Cannabinoids are marijuana-like compounds made by our own brain, and circulate normally in your body.

A Treasure Trove Waiting for Discovery

When asked why he devoted his entire lifetime studying the biochemistry of cannabis, Dr. Raphael Mechoulam said the following:

"The three major illicit drugs derived from plants were then (at the beginning of my career), and still are, opium, coca and cannabis. Morphine had been isolated from opium early in the 19th century and structure elucidated in the 1920s by Robert Robinson. Cocaine was isolated from coca leaves in the middle of the 19th century and structure described by Richard Willstatter in the last decade of the 19th century. I believe that the cannabinoids represented a medicinal treasure trove which waits to be discovered."(79-82)

Just Like the Opiate Receptor Story

In a story very similar to the discovery of opiate receptors in the brain, cannabinoid receptors have been discovered along with their endogenous cannabinoids, representing the largest neurotransmitter system in the brain and immune system. This neurotransmitter system went undetected for decades because it involves an unheard of concept, retrograde transmission, or reversed flow of information from the post synapse to the pre-synapse.

A List of the Medical Uses of Cannabinoid Drugs:
Relieves Chronic Pain Reduces need for narcotics in chronic pain or Narcotics Addiction Anti-Cancer Activity Relieves Post Traumatic Stress Disorder, Phobias Relieves Nausea and Vomiting associated with Chemotherapy Improves Appetite in Wasting Syndromes Relieves Migraine Headache Relieves Glaucoma Relieves Bladder incontinence Used as Anti-convulsant Used as Anti-depressant Used as Atypical anti-psychotic Used for Bi-Polar Syndrome Used for Multiple Sclerosis, ALS

The Cannabinoid Receptor Story

In the 1970s, Morphine was isolated from the poppy plant and found to bind to opiate receptors in the brain. Scientists eventually discovered that people make their own opioids, called enkephalins and endorphins. Morphine simply hijacks the receptors for the brain's opioids. It seemed likely that something similar was happening with THC and the cannabinoid receptors in the brain and the immune system. The health implications of the endo-cannabinoid system are staggering. Cannabinoids act as a bioregulatory mechanism for most life processes

Timeline for Cannabinoids and Receptor System
2,000 BC to 1,800 AD Medicinal Cannabis used in Ancient China, Egypt, India, ancient Greeks. **800 AD to 1,800 AD** Medical Cannabis was used extensively in the medieval Islamic World. **1800-1900** Medical Cannabis commonly used entire world as primary pain reliever until the invention of aspirin. **1925** England bans cannabis with Dangerous Drugs Act, and non-medicinal cannabis made illegal in Britain. **1927** Canada bans all forms of cannabis. **1937** Even though there are 28 cannabis pharmaceuticals on the American market, Cannabis banned in US with federal law, the 1937 Marijuana Tax Act. **1964** THC, tetra hydro cannabinol, the psycho-active component of cannabis, isolated by Raphael Mechoulam at Weizmann Institute in Israel. **1970** Marijuana fully outlawed in US by Controlled Substances Act of 1970. **1975** Munson shows anti cancer effects of cannabis in Lewis Lung Tumors. **1980-2000** Cannabis research banned in US (de facto). **1985** FDA approves Marinol drug, a pure THC drug. **1992** First endo-cannabinoid isolated by Hanuš and Devane in Raphael Mechoulam's lab at the Hebrew University in Jerusalem. This new substance is named Anandamide. **1992** endo-cannabinoid CB1 receptors cloned and found in brain

1993 endo-cannabinoid CB2 receptors cloned and found in the immune system.
1998 Di Marzo's in Naples Italy group found that cannabinoids (anandamide) inhibit breast cancer cell proliferation.
1999 Marinol (THC) was rescheduled from Schedule II to III of the Controlled Substances Act,
2000 Guzman's group in Spain found that cannabinoids inhibit the growth of C6 glioma cells.
2005 Sativex approved in Canada. Sativex is a whole cannabis plant extract, mouth spray approved for multiple sclerosis patients to alleviate neuropathic pain and muscle spasticity.
2006 Cannabindiol found useful as anti-psychotic drug São Paulo, Brasil.
2007 Sean D. McAllister—Cannabidiol inhibits aggressive breast cancer cells.
2008 Acomplia, Rimonabant (also known as SR141716) first CB1 receptor blocker suspended from the UK market because of adverse effects of suicidality, depression. This agent blocks the endo-cannabidiol receptors.
2009 Two components of cannabis plant identified. THC which is psychoactive, and the non-psychoactive Cannabidiol "CBD" represents up to 40% of extracts of the medical cannabis plant. Cannabidiol relieves convulsion, inflammation, anxiety, nausea, and inhibits cancer cell growth. Cannabidiol as effective as atypical antipsychotics in treating schizophrenia.
2010—10 million people have been arrested for marijuana possession since 1967. In the US, 13 states have approved medical use of cannabis.

Safety of Marijuana:

There has never been a documented human fatality from marijuana. The respiratory depression from opiates does not happen with cannabinoids. The active ingredient in cannabis is Cannabidiol, a Schedule I drug in the USA, despite having no psychoactive effects and no known abuse potential. Cannabidiol kills cancer cells, relieves pain, serves as an anti-depressant, and has numerous other medical uses. In the US, 13 states that have passed laws legalizing medicinal cannabis. You can join the movement to legalize the medicinal use of cannabis by calling, emailing or writing your congressman today.

Warning and Disclaimer:

Marijuana is an illegal drug in many US states and other countries. It is illegal to grow or possess the marijuana plant, also known as the hemp plant. Even when used as a prescribed medicine, marijuana use may result in arrest, fines or imprisonment. Only use marijuana as a drug if it has been legally prescribed by a licensed physician in a state or country that has legalized the use of medical marijuana.

For references and links, see web site: www.bioidenticalhormones101.com

References for Chapter 52. Cannabinoids, Miracle Drug of the 21st Century

(1) http://www.altmd.com/Videos/Cancer-Cure—Cannabis-Cannabinoids Video filmed in 2006, Dr. Robert Melamede, Professor of Biology at the University of Colorado, explains how the body's Endo-Cannabinoid system kills cancer cells and inhibits tumor growth.

(2) http://pubs.acs.org/doi/abs/10.1021/ja01062a046 Isolation, Structure, and Partial Synthesis of an Active Constituent of Hashish. Y. Gaoni, R. Mechoulam J. Am. Chem. Soc., 1964, 86 (8), pp 1646-1647.April 1964

(3) http://www.ncbi.nlm.nih.gov/pubmed/616322
Cancer Biochem Biophys. 1977;2(2):51-4. In vivo effects of cannabinoids on macromolecular biosynthesis in Lewis lung carcinomas. Friedman MA.

(4) http://americanmarijuana.org/Guzman-Cancer.pdf
http://www.nature.com/nrc/journal/v3/n10/abs/nrc1188.html
Nature Reviews Cancer 3, 745-755 (October 2003) Cannabinoids: Potential AntiCancer Agents by Manuel Guzmán.

(5) http://www.cannabis-med.org/english/journal/en_2006_02_1.pdf
Cannabinoids: potential antitumoral agents? Manuel Guzmán Madrid, Spain, 2006

(6) http://www.brainlife.org/reprint/2008/sarfaraz_s080115.pdf Cancer Res 2008;68(2):339-42. Cannabinoids for Cancer Treatment: Progress and Promise. Sami Sarfaraz et al University of Wisconsin, Madison, Wisconsin

(7) http://www.geocities.com/cannabinoidscience/Cancer.html Cannabinoids as Anti-Cancer Agents.

(8) http://www.ncbi.nlm.nih.gov/pubmed/16250836 Mini Rev Med Chem. 2005 Oct;5(10):941-52. Cannabinoids and cancer. Kogan NM. Hebrew University, Pharmacy School, Department of Medicinal Chemistry and Natural Products, Israel.

(9) http://mct.aacrjournals.org/cgi/content/full/6/11/2921 see also http://safeaccess.ca/research/cbd_breast_cancer.pdf Molecular Cancer Therapeutics 6, 2921, November 1, 2007. Research Articles: Therapeutics, Targets, and Development.Cannabidiol as a novel inhibitor of Id-1 gene expression in aggressive breast cancer cells. Sean D. McAllister et al.

(10) http://news.bbc.co.uk/1/hi/health/7098340.stm Cannabis compound 'halts cancer' BBC News Nov 2007. http://erc.endocrinology-journals.org/cgi/content/abstract/15/2/391 Endocrine-Related Cancer 15 (2) 391—408. Endocannabinoids in endocrine and related tumours Maurizio Bifulco et al; Napoli, Italy

(11) http://jnci.oxfordjournals.org/cgi/content/abstract/djm268v1 Journal of the National Cancer Institute December 25, 2007. Inhibition of Cancer Cell Invasion by Cannabinoids via Increased Expression of Tissue Inhibitor of Matrix Metalloproteinases-1. Robert Ramer et al.

(12) http://www.ncbi.nlm.nih.gov/pubmed/19047095 Clin Cancer Res. 2008 Dec 1;14(23):7691-700. Cannabinoid receptor activation induces apoptosis through tumor necrosis factor alpha-mediated ceramide de novo synthesis in colon cancer cells. Cianchi F et al. University of Florence, Florence, Italy.

(13) http://www.spandidos-publications.com/or/article.jsp?article id=or_17_4_813 Endocannabinoids as emerging suppressors of angiogenesis and tumor invasion (Review) MAURIZIO BIFULCO et al. Napoli, Italy August 7, 2006

(14) http://www.pubmedcentral.nih.gov/articlerender.fcgi?tool=pubmed&pubmedid=9653194 Proc Natl Acad Sci U S A. 1998 July 7; 95(14): 8375-8380. PMCID: PMC20983 The endogenous cannabinoid anandamide inhibits human breast cancer cell proliferation. Luciano De Petrocellis and Vincenzo Di Marzo et al. Naples, Italy;

(15) http://jpet.aspetjournals.org/cgi/content/full/318/3/1375 Antitumor Activity of Plant Cannabinoids with Emphasis on the Effect of Cannabidiol on Human Breast Carcinoma. JPET 318:1375-1387, 2006 Vincenzo Di Marzo et al. Napoli, Italy

(16) http://www.thenhf.com/articles/articles_659/articles_659.htm Hemp Oil and Cancer By Mark Sircus Ac., OMD February 23, see also www.phoenixtears.ca

(17) http://pr.cannazine.co.uk/20090205875/cannabis-news/cannabis-cancer-and-hemp-medicine.html Cannabis, Cancer and Hemp Medicine by Rick Simpson

(18) http://www.phoenixtearsmovie.com/ Rick Simpson, video, anti cancer effects of hemp cannabis

(19) http://video.google.com/videoplay?docid=-7331006790306000271 run from the cure-rick simpson entire movie

(20) http://www.huffingtonpost.com/2009/02/26/holder-vows-to-end-raids_n_170119.html Obama's Attorney General, Holder, Vows To End Raids On Medical Marijuana Clubs

(21) http://www.informapharmascience.com/doi/abs/10.1517/13543780802691951 Expert Opinion on Investigational Drugs February 2009, Vol. 18, No. 2, Pages 125-133 Cannabinoids

against pain. Efficacy and strategies to reduce psychoactivity: a clinical perspective Matthias Karst† MD PhD & Sonja Wippermann

(22) http://www.medboardwatch.com/wb/pages/therapeutic-effects.php Russo and Grotenhermen report: Review of Therapeutic Effects of cannabis. Relieves Nausea and vomiting, anorexia, and weight loss associated with chemotherapy or HIV/AIDS. Relieves spasticity, neurogenic pain, asthma, glaucoma.

(23) http://www.ncbi.nlm.nih.gov/pubmed/11106791 Chem Phys Lipids. 2000 Nov;108(1-2):191-209. Endocannabinoids and fatty acid amides in cancer, inflammation and related disorders.De Petrocellis L, Melck D, Bisogno T, Di Marzo V. Istituto di Cibernetica, Consiglio Nazionale delle Ricerche, Via Toiano 6, 80072 Arco Felice, Napoli, Italy.

(24) http://www.jackherer.com/chapters.html The emperor wears no clothes, Jack Herer.

(25) http://www.suntimes.com/news/huntley/1456881,CST-EDT-hunt03.article Legalizing marijuana makes sense, cents March 3, 2009 BY STEVE HUNTLEY Chicago Sun TImes.

(26) http://www.associatedcontent.com/article/1524315/california_state_assembly_considering.html?cat=8 California State Assembly Considering Marijuana Legalization. March 03, 2009 by P. Trembeth. Could Widespread Marijuana Legalization Be Just Around the Corner? AP News

(27) http://newmexicoindependent.com/20182/feds-make-medical-marijuana-de-facto-legal Obama Administration makes medical marijuana de facto legal. By Marjorie Childress 3/2/09 9:28 AM U.S.

(28) http://www.scielo.br/pdf/bjmbr/v39n4/6164.pdf see also http://www.scielo.br/scielo.php?pid=S0100-879X2006000400001&script=sci_arttext Braz J Med Biol Res, April 2006, Volume 39(4) 421-429 (Review) Cannabidiol, a Cannabis sativa constituent, as an antipsychotic drug.A.W. Zuardi et al.

(29) http://finola.com/CBDreview2008.pdf Cannabidiol: from an inactive cannabinoid to a drug with wide spectrum of action Antonio Waldo Zuardi, Brazil

(30) http://videos.med.wisc.edu/videoInfo.php?videoid=1107 Cannabis and Cannabinoids in the 21st Century: Medical Marijuana. David Bearman, MD

(31) http://americanmarijuana.org/ The American Medical Marijuana Association

(32) http://www.nature.com/bjp/journal/v146/n7/pdf/0706415a.pdf see also http://www.nature.com/bjp/journal/v146/n7/full/0706415a.html Plant cannabinoids: a neglected pharmacological treasure trove. Raphael Mechoulam. British Journal of Pharmacology (2005) 146, 913-915

(33) http://www.jleukbio.org/cgi/content/full/82/6/1390 Journal of Leukocyte Biology. 2007;82:1390-1392.) Endocannabinoids, cannabinoid receptors and inflammatory stress: an interview with Dr. Pál Pacher Helene F. Rosenberg1 Laboratory of Allergic Diseases, National Institute of Allergy and Infectious Disease, National Institutes of Health, Bethesda, Maryland, USA

(34) http://www.endocannabinoid.net/Mechoulam.aspx Excerpt from the journal, Addiction. Conversation with Raphael Mechoulam. Addiction. 2007; 102(6), 887-893.

(35) http://www.bioteach.ubc.ca/Journal/V02I01/Cannabis.pdf Half-Baked Science: A Primer on Medicinal Cannabis Ryan Philippe

(36) http://edrv.endojournals.org/cgi/content/full/27/1/73 Endocrine Reviews 27 (1): 73-100, 2006. The Emerging Role of the Endocannabinoid System in Endocrine Regulation and Energy Balance. Uberto Pagotto, Giovanni Marsicano, Daniela Cota, Beat Lutz and Renato Pasquali

(37) http://cancerres.aacrjournals.org/cgi/content/full/66/13/6748 Cancer Research 66, 6748-6755, July 1, 2006. Cannabinoids Induce Apoptosis

of Pancreatic Tumor Cells via Endoplasmic Reticulum Stress-Related Genes. Arkaitz Carracedo1, Meritxell Gironella2, Mar Lorente1, Stephane Garcia2, Manuel Guzmán1, Guillermo Velasco1 and Juan L. Iovanna2

(38) http://www.fuoriluogo.it/medicalcannabis/documenti/bifulco2002.pdf Targeting the endocannabinoid system in cancer therapy: A call for further research MAURIZIO BIFULCO1 & VINCENZO DI MARZO
NATURE MEDICINE • VOLUME 8 • NUMBER 6 • JUNE 2002

(39) http://www.aapsj.org/articles/aapsj0802/aapsj080234/aapsj080234.pdf Cannabinoid Receptors and Endocannabinoids: Evidence for New Players, AAPSJ, April 28, 2006 Ken Mackie 1 and Nephi Stella 2 1 Departments of Anesthesiology and Physiology.

(40) http://pharmrev.aspetjournals.org/cgi/content/full/58/3/389 The Endocannabinoid System as an Emerging Target of Pharmacotherapy. Pharmacol Rev 58:389-462, 2006. Pál Pacher, Sándor Bátkai and George Kunos.

(41) http://www.scielo.br/scielo.php?script=sci_arttext&pid=S1516-44462006000200015&tlng=en&lng=en&nrm=iso Rev. Bras. Psiquiatr. vol.28 no.2 São Paulo June 2006. History of cannabis as a medicine: a review Antonio Waldo Zuardi

(42) http://www.illinoisnorml.org/index2.php?option=com_content&do_pdf=1&id=104 Cannabis' Potential Exciting Researchers in Treatment of ALS, Parkinson's Disease—URB597. Last Updated Friday, 15 June 2007

(43) http://jpet.aspetjournals.org/cgi/content/full/322/1/236 Journal of Pharmacology And Experimental Therapeutics Fast Forward. JPET 322:236-242, 2007. The Fatty Acid Amide Hydrolase Inhibitor URB597 (Cyclohexylcarbamic Acid 3'-Carbamoylbiphenyl-3-yl Ester) Reduces Neuropathic Pain after Oral Administration in Mice. Roberto Russo et al Naples, Italy

(44) http://www.pubmedcentral.nih.gov/articlerender.fcgi?tool=pubmed&pubmedid=16352709 Proc Natl Acad Sci U S A. 2005 December 20; 102(51): 18620-18625. The National Academy of Sciences. Neuroscience—Antidepressant-like activity and modulation of brain monoaminergic transmission by blockade of anandamide hydrolysis. G. Gobbi et al.

(45) http://www.sciencedaily.com/releases/2005/12/051213172852.htm New Antidepressant Drug Increases 'Brain's Own Cannabis. Science Daily 2005.

(46) http://www.doctordeluca.com/Library/WOD/BrainsOwnMJ-SA04-NoPix.pdf The Brain's Own Marijuana by Roger A. Nicoll and Bradley N. Alger Scientific American, December 2004, pages 69-75.

(47) http://cancerres.aacrjournals.org/cgi/content/abstract/64/16/5617 Cancer Research 64, 5617-5623, August 15, 2004, Cannabinoids Inhibit the Vascular Endothelial Growth Factor Pathway in Gliomas. Manuel Guzmán et al., Spain

(48) http://www.ncbi.nlm.nih.gov/pubmed/19047095 Clinical Cancer Research 14, 7691, December 1, 2008. Cannabinoid Receptor Activation Induces Apoptosis through Tumor Necrosis Factor-Mediated Ceramide De novo Synthesis in Colon Cancer Cells. Fabio Cianchi et al, Italy

(49) http://www.aapsj.org/view.asp?art=aapsj070364 Pertwee RG. The Therapeutic Potential of Drugs That Target Cannabinoid Receptors or Modulate the Tissue Levels or Actions of Endocannabinoids. AAPS Journal. 2005; 7(3): E625-E654.

(50) http://www.usdoj.gov/dea/ongoing/marinol.html MARINOL DEA Page

(51) http://www.marijuanalibrary.org/HT_Marinol_0794.html High Times, July 1994, pp. 18-21 Marinol: The Little Synthetic That Couldn't. By Elsa Scott

(52) http://www.iowatelecom.net/~sharkhaus/marinol_long.html Marinol vs. Marijuana: Politics, Science, and Popular Culture Kambiz. Akhavan

(53) http://www.endocannabinoid.net/ endocannabinoid system network

(54) http://www.icb.cnr.it/erg/ The Endocannabinoid Research Group (ERG) is a multi-disciplinary research group established in 1995 and based in the laboratories of several Institutes of the Italian National Research Council (CNR) and of Universities in the Naples and Salerno area.

(55) http://www.cannabinoidsociety.org/ The International Cannabinoid Research Society.

(56) http://www.ukcia.org/research/CannabidiolWonderDrug.html Cannabidiol: The Wonder Drug of the 21st Century?

(57) http://www.smart-publications.com/articles/MOM-mechoulam.php The New Science of Cannabinoid-Based Medicine: An Interview with Dr. Raphael Mechoulam By David Jay Brown

(58) http://www.endocannabinoid.net/Mechoulam.aspx Interview with Mechoulam.

(59) http://www.hempfood.com/IHA/iha01113.html Interview Professor Dr. Raphael Mechoulam, the discoverer of THC

(60) http://www.chipsbooks.com/cannabin.htm Cannabinoids as Therapeutics by Raphael Mechoulam, the book.

(61) http://www.youtube.com/watch?v=IgjLLHJdv3Q You Tube Video, Cannabinoid cancer treatment

(62) http://www.henriettesherbal.com/eclectic/kings/cannabis.html Cannabis Indica (U. S. P.)—Indian Cannabis. Indian hemp. ILLUSTRATION: Bentley and Trimen, Med. Plants, 231.

(63) http://www.youtube.com/watch?v=VHWuD8a3INs&NR=1 You Tube Video April 4, 2008—5th Clinical Conference on Cannabis Therapeutics in Pacific Grove, CA, Deputy Director of NORML Paul Armentano talks Cannabis (marijuana) and the Endo-Cannabinoid system

(64) http://YouTube.com/SurvivingALS Cannabis Therapeutics Conference hosted by Patients Out of Time

(65) http://www.abc.net.au/quantum/poison/marijuan/lester.htm Interview with Lester Grinspoon 1997.

(66) http://articles.latimes.com/2006/may/05/opinion/oe-grinspoon5 Puffing is The Best Medicine By Lester Grinspoon M.D. Los Angeles Times—May 5, 2006.

(67) http://www.iht.com/articles/2007/03/01/opinion/edgrinspoon.php Marijuana, the wonder drug of the 21st century. Lester Grinspoon The Boston Globe. March 1, 2007

(68) http://www.jimboland.com/2009/03/07/common-sense-compassion-overcome-marijuana-propaganda/ Common Sense and Compassion Overcome Marijuana Propaganda March 7th 2009

(69) http://www.lewrockwell.com/spl/legalize-marijuana-sense-cents.html Legalizing Marijuana Makes Sense, Cents by Steve Huntley

(70) http://www.neurology.org/cgi/content/abstract/68/7/515 Cannabis in painful HIV-associated sensory neuropathy A randomized placebo-controlled trial D. I. Abrams, MD et al

(71) http://www.cmcr.ucsd.edu/images/pdfs/Abrams_2007.pdf Abrams DI, Jay CA, Shade SB, Vizoso H, Reda H, Press S, Kelly ME, Rowbotham MC, Petersen KL. Cannabis in painful HIV-associated sensory neuropathy: A randomized placebo-controlled trial. Neurology 2007 68: 515-521.*

(72) http://www.safeaccessnow.org/downloads/medical_cannabis_research.pdf MEDICAL CANNABIS RESEARCH: WHAT DOES THE EVIDENCE SAY?

(73) http://query.nytimes.com/gst/fullpage.html?res=9C04E7D71E3FF936A25751C1A9679C8B63 After Two-Decade Halt, Marijuana Research Is Set By PHILIP J. HILTS. Dec 15, 2001. NY Times.

(74) http://bja.oxfordjournals.org/cgi/content/abstract/101/1/59 British Journal of Anaesthesia 2008 101(1):59-68; Therapeutic potential of cannabis in pain medicine. R. D. Hosking and J. P. Zajicek* Neurology Research Group, Peninsula Medical School, Plymouth, UK

(75) http://www.ccrmg.org/journal/06spr/index.html Spring 2006. O'Shaughnessy's. Journal of the California Cannabis Research Medical Group

(76) http://www.ccrmg.org/journal/06spr/aday.html A Day in the Life of a Cannabis Consultant. Philip A. Denney, M.D. Journal of the California Cannabis Research Medical Group.

(77) Cannabinoids As Therapeutic Agents by Raphael Mechoulam (Editor) Chapman and Hall/CRC; 1 edition (July 1, 1986)

(78) http://www.ncbi.nlm.nih.gov/pmc/articles/PMC1576036/ Br J Pharmacol. 2005 February; 144(4): 459-465.The expanding field of cannabimimetic and related lipid mediators by Heather B Bradshaw and J Michael Walker

(79) http://www.ncbi.nlm.nih.gov/pubmed/1470919 Science. 1992 Dec 18;258(5090):1946-9.Isolation and structure of a brain constituent that binds to the cannabinoid receptor.Devane WA, Hanus L, Breuer A, Pertwee RG, Stevenson LA, Griffin G, Gibson D, Mandelbaum A, Etinger A, Mechoulam R.

(80) http://matters.ecnp.nl/number11/interview2.shtml Interview with the winner of the first ECNP Lifetime Achievement Award:Raphael Mechoulam, Israel Maria Vrijmoed—de Vries, The Netherlands, editor

(81) http://www.druglibrary.net/olsen/HEMP/IHA/iha01113.html Interview with Professor Dr. Raphael Mechoulam, the discoverer of THC, (June 17 1994)

(82) http://www.medicalmarijuana411.com/2010/05/07/dr-raphael-mechoulam_part-one/ Dr. Raphael Mechoulam—Medical Marijuana 411.com Interview—Part One

(83) http://www.lmreview.com/articles/view/new-developments-in-cannabinoid-based-medicine-an-interview-with-dr-raphael-mechoulam/ New Developments in Cannabinoid-Based Medicine: An Interview with Dr. Raphael Mechoulam by Lara Pizzorno, MDiv, MA, LMT

CHAPTER 53

The Trophoblastic Theory of Cancer

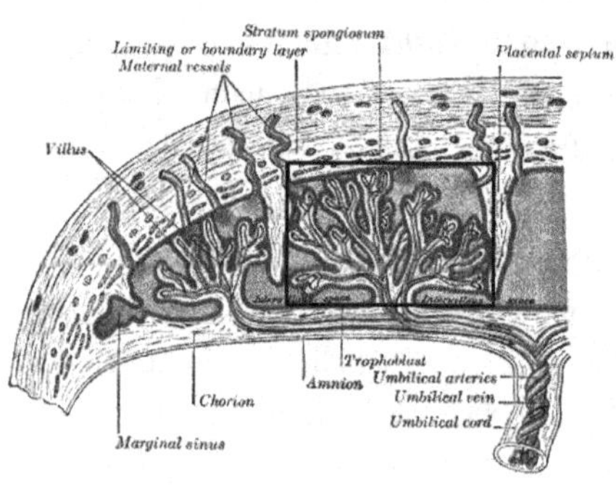

Placenta anatomic diagram from Gray's Anatomy published in 1918.

Have you ever wondered why cancer treatment has not changed much in over 70 years? Why is chemotherapy still the mainstay of conventional cancer treatment after all these years of disappointing results for the majority of cancer cell types? Perhaps we should be exploring alternatives. At a medical meeting I attended, Nicholas Gonzalez MD presented his views on the etiology of cancer and cancer treatment. Dr. Gonzalez is actively engaged in medical practice in Manhattan where he treats advanced cancer successfully with high dose oral pancreatic enzymes. (1-7) This treatment regimen is based on the Trophoblastic Theory of cancer. This theory was originally proposed by a Scottish embryologist named John Beard (1858-1924), and was resurrected by William Donald Kelley, DDS (1926-2005).(8-16)

John Beard and the Trophoblast Theory

John Beard (1858-1924), was a Scottish embryologist who used the light microscope to study developmental embryology as well as cancer pathology.(10-12) In 1905, Beard was the first to report that trophoblast cells act and behave in a manner identical to cancer cells, acting invasively, and inducing their own blood supply.(40-41) This observation has been confirmed with more recent research.(56) The trophoblast cell is a cell derived from the Placenta, a structure inside the uterus of a pregnant mother which serves as blood supply for the developing embryo.

What are Trophoblasts? Similarity with Cancer Cells

In the pregnant mother, trophoblasts are the infiltrative components of the developing embryo which form the placenta. These cells invade and infiltrate into the wall of the mother's uterus. This behavior is very similar to the way cancer cells infiltrate and invade surrounding tissues. These trophoblast cells are known to produce human chorionic gonadotropin (HCG). In fact, production of HCG is the basis for the widely used pregnancy test. If cancer cells and trophoblast cells are similar, one would expect cancer cells to also produce HCG. That is exactly what they do. This was reported in 1995 by Hernan Acevedo, PhD, and published in the journal, Cancer. (42-44) He found that every cancer produces HCG, same as the trophoblast cells of pregnancy. Since John Beard's day about one hundred years ago, modern biologists have found even more similarities between trophoblasts and malignant cancer cells. Dr. C. Ferretti in the October 2006 issue of Human Reproduction Update, states that both cancer and trophoblast cells share the same molecular circuitry for their proliferative, invasive and migratory capacities.(53)

CT Antigens Discovered

Another twist to the story is the recent discovery of a new class of human tumor antigens called CT (cancer/testis) antigens.(49-52) About 90 genes have been found having messenger RNA expression in both germ cells (testis) and cancer cells, and no expression in otherwise normal cells. This is further evidence linking the trophoblast cells, which are, in fact, germ cells (also called stem cells), with cancer cells. These recent advances in molecular biology have shown that John Beard was quite correct to point out the similarity between placental trophoblast cells and malignant cancer cells. Beard's forgotten predictions in the early 1900's seem to have an uncanny way of resurfacing 100 years later.

Pancreatic Enzymes on Day 56

On Day Fifty Six of embryonic development, John Beard observed through his microscope trophoblast cells suddenly transform from malignant, invasive cells into mature and well behaved cells. This day 56 transformation also coincides with the appearance of enzyme granules (also called zymogen granules) in the fetal pancreas. Obviously, since all nutrition comes from the maternal blood supply, the developing fetus in-utero has no need for pancreatic enzymes. These are used later after the fetus is born when the baby starts eating food. Beard theorized the appearance of pancreatic enzymes was no accident, and that the enzymes caused transformation of the trophoblast cells behavior from "malignant" to a "benign" cell type. This logic suggested the use of digestive enzymes to control cancer cells. A number of studies in both animal models and humans have actually confirmed the utility of pancreatic enzyme for cancer treatment.

About the same time as John Beard's early work, Madam Curie's (1867-1934) work treating cancer with radiation took the spotlight, and captured the imagination of the media and the public. John Beard's work on the Trophoblast Theory was dismissed by mainstream medical science and almost forgotten.

An excellent review of recent research confirming John Beard's work as well as the value of enzyme treatments for cancer is: "A Critique of the Kelley Nutritional-Metabolic Cancer Program" by Melina A. Roberts BSc. From the Townsend Letter for Doctors & Patients June 2003. (30) A leading biochemist, Ernst Krebs, wrote an important 1950 paper supporting the Trophoblast Theory of Cancer entitled "The Unitarian or Trophoblastic Thesus of Cancer" by Ernst T. Krebs, Jr., Ernst T. Krebs, Sr., and Howard H. Beard. (57)

William Donald Kelley Resurrects John Beard's Work

Years later in the 1960's, William Kelly discovered Beard's forgotten papers, and resurrected the treatment of cancer with pancreatic enzymes. Kelly had considerable success treating patients with this alternative cancer treatment approach. However, Kelly was a dentist, and bitterly opposed by mainstream medicine, and as expected, had difficulties with the authorities. Kelly was convicted of practicing medicine without a license in 1970, his dental license was suspended in 1976, and he passed away on Jan. 30, 2005 at the age of 79.

Nicholas Gonzalez' Research

In 1981, during the Kelly's early years, a medical student at Cornell Medical School by the name of Nicholas Gonzalez was given a summer project to interview William Donald Kelly and evaluate his results with cancer patients using the pancreatic enzyme treatment. Gonzalez did a retrospective review of 1300 patients who had been treated over a 20-year period with the Kelley protocol with enzymes, diet and nutritional support. Gonzalez was so impressed with the data, and the superior patient outcomes, that this summer project expanded into a book, and later adopted as his own life's work.

Continuing after Kelly, Nicholas Gonzalez MD carried on with his legacy at a Manhattan office, documenting remarkable success over the past decade or so. Selected case reports from the Gonzalez Manhattan office show dramatic clinical results not possible with conventional mainstream cancer treatment. This information is posted on the Dr Gonzalez web site.(1)

In 1999, Gonzalez published a 2 year pilot study of 10 patients with inoperable advanced pancreatic cancer treated with large doses of orally ingested pancreatic enzymes.(92) Results showed 80% survival after 1 year, 45% survival after 2 years and 36% survival after 3 years. (92) These results are far above the 25% one year, 10% two year, and 6 % three year survival reported in the National Cancer Data Base for inoperable pancreatic cancer. (93) Shortly after this, Gonzalez received a $1.4 million grant from the National Center for Complementary and Alternative Medicine at the National Institutes of Health for further study on enzyme therapy and pancreatic cancer. (94) The study was to be conducted at Columbia-Presbyterian Medical Center in New York under the supervision of the NCI and with approval from the FDA. This study ran into snags and is yet to be completed or published.

Otto Warburg

Otto Warburg made important contributions to the understanding of the metabolic activity of cancer. All cancers, as well as trophoblast cells have a high glucose utilization using the primitive glycolysis pathway. They tend not to use oxidative phosphorylation and thrive in a low oxygen environment. This is known as the Warburg Effect. Recent work has built on Warburg's ideas using inhibitors of glycolysis such as 3 bromopyruvate to kill cancer cells by stopping glycolysis. (77)(82) Others have used insulin induced hypoglycemia to starve cancer cells of their glucose substrate. (84-90) Avid glucose uptake is the basis of modern PET (positron emission tomography) imaging of the body which is capable of showing cancer deposits with radiolabeled 17-Flouro-deoxyglucose. This has prompted interest in compounds which inhibit glucose metabolism such as 2-De-Oxy-Glucose, which kills cancer cells.(73)

Aneuploidy—and Confined Placental Mosaicism

Recently there has been resurgence of interest in aneuploidy and cancer championed by Peter Duesberg in his 2007 article in Scientific American, "Chromosomal Chaos and Cancer". (95) Aneuploidy or abnormal and multiple sets of chromosomes is commonly found in cancer, and also found in the placenta. (65-70) Using ultrasound guided chorionic villous sampling, it has been discovered that between 2-5% of placental samples show aneuploid cells; this is called confined placental mosaicism, which apparently does not affect the developing embryo.

No Coexistence of Cancer with Circulating Enzymes of Pancreatitis

One last point I am compelled to mention. During my 30 year career as a radiologist much of my time was spent reading images of metastatic cancer on CAT scans. One of the things I noticed was that I never witnessed the presence of metastatic cancer in patients who had pancreatic enzymes circulating freely in the bloodstream from acute or chronic diffuse pancreatitis. Excluded of course was focal pancreatitis caused by an obstructed pancreatic duct due to a small pancreatic cancer. Thus I had independently confirmed the major tenet of John Beard and Ernst Krebs many years before I even heard of the trophoblastic theory of cancer.

Cancer of Small Bowel Relatively Rare

Another observation most experienced radiologists and surgeons will make is the relative rarity of neoplasm involving the small bowel compared to the relative common appearance (50 times more common) of neoplasm in the colon and the stomach. Ernst Krebs makes this same observation in his landmark 1950 paper on the Unified Trophoblast Theory of Cancer, and Krebs suggests that pancreatic enzymes released into the duodenum at the duct of Wirsung and Santorini are responsible for this 50 times reduction in small bowel cancer. (57) The age-adjusted death rate for cancer of the colon is 47 times higher than cancer of the small bowel, at 0.4 for small bowel and 18.8 for colon cancer per 100,000 men and women per year. (96)

NIH Grant Proposal to Study Cancer

The NIH (National Institute of Health) has spent literally trillions over four decades on failed cancer research. It is time to take a different approach with a few proposals to investigate the trophoblast theory of cancer. A widely used technique in molecular biology is the tracer study. The older tracer method involved the use of Carbon 14 radio-labeling. The newer method uses insertion of the green florescent protein (GFP) into the protein one wishes to study.

Carbon 14 Radio-Labeled Trypsin

The proposed study can be done by using Carbon 14 radio-labeling of key amino acids in the pancreatic enzyme, trypsin, and feeding these radio-labeled amino acids to the pigs used to harvest the trypsin for later use. Then administer the radio-labeled trypsin enzymes to an animal model of cancer looking for the distribution of the radio-label in the sacrificed animals. If there is an effect on the cancer cells, I would expect to find the radio-labeled enzymes at the surface of the cancer cells.

GFP Green Florescent Protein

Another more elegant approach would be to genetically modify the pancreatic trypsin enzyme in mice by adding a green florescent marker gene (GFP), a common technique used in molecular biology. If pancreatic enzymes control the trophoblast, then the experiments should confirm the presence of the florescent marker at the trophoblast cells after day 56 in the developing embryo. To study cancer, the green florescent gene (GFP) can be inserted into DNA of the animals (usually pigs) used to manufacture the pancreatic enzymes. These labeled enzymes can then be administered to mice pretreated with cancer cells. Knowledge about the rate of survival of the treated vs. control mice as well as the fate of the labeled enzymes would be useful. If the enzymes are having an effect on the cancer cells, then I would expect the florescent label or radio-label to be found at the tumor site.

Using the NIH to Find a Cure for Cancer

A few decades ago, Richard Nixon, declared a war against cancer and ramped up funding for NIH research which mostly went towards proving the idea that cancer was caused by a virus. This line of research expended massive amounts of money and ended a dismal failure. A new and more promising direction for cancer research would be to investigate the mysteries of the trophoblast which shares so many features in common with cancer cells. We now have the molecular tools that John Beard a century ago could only imagine. How do we get the NIH to pursue this? Use political pressure by contacting your congressman and asking them to push the NIH to fund the research.

Conclusion: Advances in molecular biology now make it fairly straightforward to validate and expand on the early work of Scottish embryologist John Beard, Ernst Krebs and Otto Warburg. The research costs for such a program would be minimal and the potential gains enormous.

For references and links, see my web site: www.bioidenticalhormones101.com

References for Chapter 53. The Trophoblastic Theory of Cancer

(1) http://www.dr-gonzalez.com/index.htm Nicholas J. Gonzalez, M.D. Web Site

(2) http://www.michaelspecter.com/ny/2001/2001_02_05_gonzalez.html Annals of medicine the outlaw doctor Cancer researchers used to call him a fraud. What's changed? february 5, 2001. Michael Specter. The New Yorker

(3) http://www.dr-gonzalez.com/totalhealth_7b_00.htm Dr Nicholas Gonzalez video presentation on John Beard's theories. A recording of Dr. Gonzalez's speech at Boulderfest 2008, sponsored by Crayhon Research, is available (for purchase) at the following link: http://www.newspringpress.com/lectures.html

(4) http://www.alternative-therapies.com/at/web_pdfs/isaacs.pdf EVALUATING ANECDOTES AND CASE REPORTS Linda L. Isaacs, MD. Alternative Therapies.

(5) http://www.prevention.com/cda/article/alternative-medicine-saved-our-lives/4b8b9f9ad6914110VgnVCM10000013281eac_____/health/healthy.living.centers/cancer/ Alternative Medicine Saved Our Lives How unconventional treatments paid off for 4 desperately ill womenTalk to these four women and their health care providers on our discussion forums September 4 through 30. Prevention Magazine.

(6) http://www.alternative-therapies.com/at/web_pdfs/gonzalez1.pdfTHE GONZALEZ THERAPY AND CANCER:A COLLECTION OF CASE REPORTS. Nicholas J. Gonzalez, MD; Linda L. Isaacs, MD. Alternative Therapies.

(7) http://www.dr-gonzalez.com/best_cases.htm On July 7, 1993, at the NCI I presented 25 histories of my "best cases": patients with diagnosed, biopsy-proven cancer who enjoyed either documented regression of disease or long-term survival on their nutritional protocol. Here are three of those 25 cases. Nicholas Gonzalez MD.

(8) http://www.alternative-doctor.com/cancer/kelley.htm
Dr. Kelley's Do-it-Yourself Book one answer to cancer Reviewed after 32 years 1967—1999 By Dr. William Donald Kelley, D.D.S., M.S. 1999 THIS IS THE ENTIRE BOOK ON ONE WEB PAGE!

(9) http://www.alternative-doctor.com/cancer/beard.htm
John Beard's Trophoblast Cell Theory

(10) Beard, J: "The Action of Trypsin . . ." Br Med J 4, 140-41, 1906.

(11) Beard, J: "The Enzyme Treatment of Cancer" London: Chatto and Windus, 1911.

(12) Cutfield, A: "Trypsin Treatment in Malignant Disease" Br Med J 5, 525, 1907.

(13) Wiggin, FH: "Case of Multiple Fibrosarcoma Of The Tongue, With Remarks on the Use of Trypsin and Amylopsin in the Treatment of Malignant Disease" JAMA 47, 2003-08. 1906.

(14) Gotze, H, Rotham SS: Enterohepatic Circulation of Digestive Enzymes As A Conservative Mechanism" Nature 257 (5527).

(15) Shively, FL: "Multiple Proteolytic Enzyme Therapy Of Cancer." Dayton, Johnson-Watson, 1969.

(16) Little, WL: "A Case Of Malignant Tumor, With Treatment." JAMA 50, 1724, 1908.

(17) Kelley, WD: "One Answer To Cancer" latest update—33,000 cancer cases over three decades. New Century Promotions 3711 Alta Loma Drive Bonita, CA 91902 800-768-8484 or 619-479-3829.

(18) http://www.medscape.com/medline/abstract/11561867?prt=true
Mixture of trypsin, chymotrypsin and papain reduces formation of metastases and extends survival time of C57Bl6 mice with syngeneic melanoma B16. Cancer Chemother Pharmacol. 2001; 47 Suppl:S16-22

(ISSN: 0344-5704) Wald M; Olejár T; Sebková V; Zadinová M; Boubelík M; Poucková P

(19) http://www.mucos.cz/eng/onko/con_onco_com.htm references for proteolytic enzymes

(20) Wald M, Olejár T, Poucková P, Zadinová M. Proteinases Reduce Metastatic Dissemination and Increase Survival Time in C57BI6 Mice with the Lewis Lung Carcinoma. Life Sciences 1998a; 63(17):237-243.

(21) Wald M, Olejár T, Poucková P, Zadinová M. The influence of proteinases on in vivo blastic transformation in rat species SD/Ipcv with spontaneous lymphoblastic leukemia. British Journal of Haematology 1998b;102 (1): 294.

(22) Wald M, Olejár T, Sebkova V, Zadinová M, Boubelík M, Pouckova P. Mixture of trypsin, chymotrypsin and papain reduces formation of metastases and extends survival time of C57BI6 mice with syngeneic melanoma B16. Cancer Chemother Pharmacol 2001;47(Suppl):S16-S22.

(23) Wald M, Poucková P, Hloušková D, Altnerová M, Olejár T. The influence of trypsin, chymotrypsin and papain on the growth of human pancreatic adenocarcinoma transplanted to nu/nu mice. The European Journal of Cancer 1999;35(4),No. 543:148.

(24) http://users.navi.net/~rsc/beard066.htm
MEDICAL RECORD Page 1020, [June 23, 1906] Correspondence TRYPSIN AND AMYLOPSIN IN CANCER.

(25) http://whale.to/cancer/kelley.html Dr. William Donald Kelley, D.D.S., M.S.

(26) http://www.cancerdecisions.com/070202.html Part Two of the Beard Paper Centenary

(27) http://www.outsmartyourcancer.com/pdf/ScientificArticleForSite.PDF.pdf The Scientific Basis Behind Alternative Cancer Treatments by Tanya

Harter Pierce, MA, MFCC This is the second article in a 3-part series on alternative cancer treatments.

(28) http://www.cancure.org/science_paper1.htm Trophoblasts: On the Cause of Birth And Its Relationship to Cancer Regression

(29) http://www.holisticjunction.com/articles/2404.html
The Cure for Cancer: Theory, History and Treatment by Owen R. Fonorow

(30) (http://www.townsendletter.com/June2003/kelleycritique0603.htm
A Critique of the Kelley Nutritional-Metabolic Cancer Program by Melina A. Roberts BSc. (Hons.) University of Waterloo, 3rd year at the Canadian College of Naturopathic Medicine. From the Townsend Letter for Doctors & Patients June 2003

(31) http://hungerforhealth.wordpress.com/2008/05/29/enzyme-therapy-for-cancer-prevention-and-treatment/ see also http://members.aol.com/pbchowka/gonzalez2002.html One Man, Alone Dr. Nicholas Gonzalez has compelling results and a landmark grant from the National Cancer Institute. Now he just needs to convince doctors to trust him with their patients. By Peter Barry Chowka with Kathi Head, N.D. Alternative Medicine Magazine. April 2002

(32) http://scholar.google.com/scholar?hl=en&lr=&q=related:jNPD1mSZmHcJ:scholar.google.com/

(33) http://www.cancure.org/trophoblastic_nature_of_cancer.htm The Trophoblastic Nature of Cancer and Pregnancy Cycle as the Basis for the Enzyme Treatment of Cancer by Roger Cathey

(34) http://www.alkalizeforhealth.net/Lstemcells.htm
Ralph W. Moss, Ph.D. Weekly CancerDecisions.com. Newsletter #81 04/26/03 Scientists Identify Stem Cells As Hidden Cause of Cancer

(35) Al-Hajj M, et al. From the cover: prospective identification of tumorigenic breast cancer cells. Proc Natl Acad Sci U S A. 2003 Apr 1;100(7):3983-8.

(36) http://www.med.umich.edu/opm/newspage/2003/tumorsc.htm
Steinberg D. Stem cell discoveries stir debate. The Scientist 2000;14:1. Accessed at
http://www.the-scientist.com/yr2000/nov/steinberg_p1_001113.html.

(37) Thomson JL, et al. Embryonic stem cell lines derived from human blastocysts. Science 1998;282:1145-7.

(38) Goshen R, et al. Hyaluronan, CD44 and its variant exons in human trophoblast invasion and placental angiogenesis. Mol Hum Reprod. 1996;2:685-91.

(39) U.S. Patent No. 5,843,780, "Primate embryonic stem cells"; accessible at www.uspto.gov.

(40) Beard J. Embryological aspects and etiology of carcinoma. Lancet 1902;1:1758.

(41) Beard J. The Enzyme Treatment of Cancer. London: Chatto & Windus, 1911.

(42) Acevedo HF, et al. Detection of membrane-associated human chorionic gonadotropin and its subunits on human cultured cancer cells of the nervous system. Cancer Detect Prev. 1997;21(4):295-303.

(43) Acevedo HF and Hartsock RJ. Metastatic phenotype correlates with high expression of membrane-associated complete beta-human chorionic gonadotropin in vivo. Cancer. 1996 Dec 1;78(11):2388-99.

(44) Acevedo HF, et al. Human chorionic gonadotropin-beta subunit gene expression in cultured human fetal and cancer cells of different types and origins. Cancer. 1995 Oct 15;76(8):1467-75.

(45) Regelson W. Have we found the "definitive cancer biomarker"? The diagnostic and therapeutic implications of human chorionic gonadotropin-beta expression as a key to malignancy. Cancer. 1995;76:1299-301.

(46) http://www.oasisadvancedwellness.com/health-articles/2008/06/suppression-of-alternative-cancer.html June 24, 2008 The Suppression of Alternative Cancer Treatments CancerDecisions Newsletter Archives For June 22, 2008 A GREAT OPPORTUNITY LOST Ralph Moss, Ph.D

(47) http://tsienlab.ucsd.edu/Publications/Tsien%201998%20Annu.%20Rev.%20Biochem%20-%20GFP.pdf THE GREEN FLUORESCENT PROTEIN by Roger Y. Tsien.

(48) http://www.cancerimmunity.org/v7p19/071019.htm
Cancer Immunity, Vol. 7, p. 19 (6 November 2007). Cancer is a somatic cell pregnancy. Lloyd J. Old. Ludwig Institute for Cancer Research, New York Branch at Memorial Sloan-Kettering Cancer Center, New York, NY, USA

(49) http://www.medscape.com/viewarticle/510222?rss
From Nature Reviews Cancer. Cancer/Testis Antigens, Gametogenesis and Cancer Posted 08/12/2005 Andrew J. G. Simpson; Otavia L. Caballero; Achim Jungbluth; Yao-Tseng Chen; Lloyd J. Old Nat Rev Cancer. 2005;5(8):615-625.

(50) http://www.ncbi.nlm.nih.gov/pubmed/11934257
Can J Physiol Pharmacol. 2002 Feb;80(2):142-9. Human placental trophoblast as an in vitro model for tumor progression. Lala PK, Lee BP, Xu G, Chakraborty C.

(51) http://cancerres.aacrjournals.org/cgi/content/abstract/67/19/9528
Immunology A Placenta-Specific Gene Ectopically Activated in Many Human Cancers Is Essentially Involved in Malignant Cell Processes. Michael Koslowski1, Ugur Sahin1, Rita Mitnacht-Kraus2, Gerhard Seitz3, Christoph Huber1 and Özlem Türeci2

(52) http://www.cancerci.com/content/5/1/4 see also http://www.biomedcentral.com/content/pdf/1475-2867-5-4.pdf Cancer/testis antigens and gametogenesis: a review and "brain-storming" session Martins Kalejs* and Jekaterina Erenpreisa Cancer Cell International 2005, 5:4

(53) http://humupd.oxfordjournals.org/cgi/reprint/dml048v1 Molecular circuits shared by placental and cancer cells, and their implications in the proliferative, invasive and migratory capacities of trophoblasts. C.Ferretti et al. Human Reproduction Update Advance Access published October 26, 2006

(54) http://www.stopcancer.com/enzymes_wobenzym.htm Wobenzym enzymes 1-(888) 484-8264 http:// www.wobenzym.com

(55) http://www.oasisadvancedwellness.com/health-articles/2008/06/suppression-of-alternative-cancer.html Tuesday, June 24, 2008 The Suppression of Alternative Cancer Treatments

(56) http://www.ncbi.nlm.nih.gov/pubmed/9458933
Review: analogies between trophoblastic and malignant cells. Mullen CA.Am J Reprod Immunol. 1998 Jan;39(1):41-9.

(57) http://www.cancergnosis.com/History/Trophablastic%20theory.pdf
THE UNITARIAN OR TROPHOBLASTIC THESIS OF CANCER by Ernst T. Krebs, Jr., Ernst T. Krebs, Sr., and Howard H. Beard (Reprinted From the Medical Record, 163:149-174, July 1950)

(58) http://users.navi.net/~rsc/thesis.htm On the Cause of Birth and Its Relation to Cancer Regression. Roger S. Cathey Updated July 12, 2003

(59) http://lib.bioinfo.pl/pmid:15141079/pmid/cit Mol Biol Cell. 2005 Apr;16 (4):1901-12 Hypoxia-inducible factor regulates alphavbeta3 integrin cell surface expression. Karen D Cowden Dahl, Sarah E Robertson, Valerie M Weaver, M Celeste Simon

(60) http://www.pubmedcentral.nih.gov/articlerender.fcgi?artid=1073670
Mol Biol Cell. 2005 April; 16(4): 1901-1912. Hypoxia-inducible Factor Regulates αvβ3 Integrin Cell Surface Expression. Karen D. Cowden Dahl,* Sarah E. Robertson,† Valerie M. Weaver,‡§ and M. Celeste Simon*

(61) http://www.pubmedcentral.nih.gov/articlerender.fcgi?tool=pmcentrez&artid=407853 Reprod Biol Endocrinol. 2004; 2: 15. Trophoblast

'pseudo-tumorigenesis': Significance and contributory factors. Rama Soundararajan1 and A Jagannadha Rao1,2

(62) http://www.redorbit.com/news/science/94009/trophoblast_differentiation_during_embryo_implantation_and_formation_of_the_maternalfetal/ see also http://www.pubmedcentral.nih.gov/articlerender.fcgi?tool=pubmed&pubmedid=15372095 J Clin Invest. 2004 September 15; 114(6): 744-754. American Society for Clinical Investigation. Trophoblast differentiation during embryo implantation and formation of the maternal-fetal interface Kristy Red-Horse et al.

(63) http://www.pubmedcentral.nih.gov/articlerender.fcgi?tool=pubmed&pubmedid=17288592 Reprod Biol Endocrinol. 2007; 5: 6. Control of human trophoblast function, Laura Lunghi,1 Maria E Ferretti,1 Silvia Medici,1 Carla Biondi,1 and Fortunato Vesce2

(64) http://www.ncbi.nlm.nih.gov/pubmed/16234296
Hum Reprod Update. 2006 Mar-Apr;12(2):137-44 The regulation of trophoblast differentiation by oxygen in the first trimester of pregnancy. James JL, Stone PR, Chamley LW.

(65) http://www.sciencemag.org/cgi/content/abstract/221/4611/665 Science 12 August 1983:Vol. 221. no. 4611, pp. 665-667. Chromosomal mosaicism confined to the placenta in human conceptions. DK Kalousek and FJ Dill

(66) http://www.ncbi.nlm.nih.gov/pubmed/16333823
Am J Med Genet A. 2006 Jan 1;140(1):24-30. Investigation of confined placental mosaicism (CPM) at multiple sites in post-delivery placentas derived through intracytoplasmic sperm injection (ICSI).Minor A, Harmer K, Peters N, Yuen BH, Ma S.

(67) http://www.ncbi.nlm.nih.gov/pubmed/16274964
Mech Dev. 2005 Dec;122(12):1266-81. Fate of tetraploid cells in 4n<—>2n chimeric mouse blastocysts.Mackay GE, West JD.

(68) http://www.pubmedcentral.nih.gov/picrender.fcgi?artid=1735725&blobtype=pdf Detection of cell free placental

DNA in maternal plasma: direct evidence from three cases of confined placental mosaicism. H Masuzaki, K Miura, K-i Yoshiura, S Yoshimura, N Niikawa, T Ishimaru J Med Genet 2004;41:289-292. doi: 10.1136/jmg.2003.015784

(69) http://www.ncbi.nlm.nih.gov/pubmed/11973523 J Gynecol Obstet Biol Reprod (Paris). 2002 Feb;31(1 Suppl):2S70-4.[Confined placental mosaicism: definition, consequences and outcome][Article in French] Viot G.

(70) http://www.ncbi.nlm.nih.gov/pubmed/8338621
Fetal Diagn Ther. 1993 Mar-Apr;8(2):102-8. Viable pregnancies after diagnosis of trisomy 16 by CVS: lethal aneuploidy compartmentalized to the trophoblast. Johnson MP, Childs MD, Robichaux AG 3rd, Isada NB, Pryde PG, Koppitch FC 3rd, Evans MI.

(71) http://www.whale.to/a/warburg.html The Prime Cause and Prevention of Cancer with two prefaces on prevention

(72) http://healingtools.tripod.com/primecause2.html
Revised lecture at the meeting of the Nobel-Laureates on June 30, 1966 at Lindau, Lake Constance, Germany by Otto Warburg. Director, Max Planck-Institute for Cell Physiology, Berlin-Dahlem

(73) http://www.nature.com/bjc/journal/v87/n7/abs/6600547a.html
Experimental Therapeutics British Journal of Cancer (2002) 87, 805-812. Evaluation of 2-deoxy-D-glucose as a chemotherapeutic agent: mechanism of cell death R L Aft, F W Zhang and D Gius

(74) http://lib.bioinfo.pl/pmid:17879147 J Bioenerg Biomembr. 2007 Sep 19; : 17879147 Warburg, me and Hexokinase 2: Multiple discoveries of key molecular events underlying one of cancers' most common phenotypes, the "Warburg Effect", i.e., elevated glycolysis in the presence of oxygen. [My paper] Peter Pedersen

(75) http://www.ncbi.nlm.nih.gov/pubmed/11578813
Ko YH, Pedersen PL, Geschwind JF (2001). "Glucose catabolism in the

rabbit VX2 tumor model for liver cancer: characterization and targeting hexokinase". Cancer Lett. 173 (1): 83-91. PMID 11578813.

(76) http://www.ncbi.nlm.nih.gov/pubmed/17879147 Pedersen PL (2007). "Warburg, me and Hexokinase 2: Multiple discoveries of key molecular events underlying one of cancers' most common phenotypes, the "Warburg Effect", i.e., elevated glycolysis in the presence of oxygen". doi:10.1007/s10863-007-9094-x. PMID 17879147.

(77) http://www.ncbi.nlm.nih.gov/pubmed/15465013 Ko YH, Smith BL, Wang Y, et al (2004). "Advanced cancers: eradication in all cases using 3-bromopyruvate therapy to deplete ATP". Biochem. Biophys. Res. Commun. 324 (1): 269-75.

(78) http://www.ncbi.nlm.nih.gov/pubmed/17404823 J Bioenerg Biomembr. 2007 Feb;39(1):1-12. The cancer cell's "power plants" as promising therapeutic targets: an overview. Pedersen PL.

(79) http://cancerres.aacrjournals.org/cgi/content/full/62/14/3909 Geschwind JF, Ko YH, Torbenson MS, Magee C, Pedersen PL (2002). "Novel therapy for liver cancer: direct intraarterial injection of a potent inhibitor of ATP production". Cancer Res. 62 (14): 3909-13.

(80) http://www.kosen21.org/upload_repository2/community/01230411451209597a.pdf full text REVIEW Glycolysis inhibition for anticancer treatment. H Pelicano1, DS Martin2,{, R-H Xu3 and P Huang1 Oncogene (2006) 25, 4633-4646

(81) http://www.hopkinskimmelcancercenter.org/news/details.cfm?documentid=673 OCTOBER 14, 2004. Audio file of Peter Pedersen, Ph.D., discussing the success in treating advanced liver cancers in rats. "ENERGY BLOCKER" KILLS BIG TUMORS IN RATS

(82) http://www.kjronline.org/abstract/view_articletext.asp?year=2007&page=216 FDG-PET for Evaluating the Antitumor

Effect of Intraarterial 3-Bromopyruvate Administration in a Rabbit VX2 Liver Tumor Model. Hee Sun Park, MD et al. Korean Journal of Radiology; 2007 June; 8(3):216-224

(83) http://acs.confex.com/acs/norm07/techprogram/P44814.HTM June 20, 2007. Glycolytic enzyme inhibitors as novel anti-cancer drugs. James C.K. La et al.

(84) http://www.iptq.com/ Insulin Potentiation Therapy (IPT)

(85) http://www.contemporarymedicine.net/pub06_insulin_chemotherapy.htm Insulin, Chemotherapy and the Mechanisms of Malignancy: The Design and the Demise of Cancer S.G. Ayre, D.P. Garcia y Bellon, D.P. Garcia Jr Medical Hypotheses (2000) 55(4), 330-334

(86) Ayre SG, Perez Garcia y Bellon D, Perez Garcia D Jr. Insulin potentiation therapy: a new concept in the management of chronic degenerative disease. Med Hypotheses 1986;20(2):199-210

(87) Ayre SG, Garcia y Bellon DP, Garcia DP Jr. Insulin, chemotherapy, and the mechanisms of malignancy: the design and the demise of cancer. Med Hypotheses 2000;55(4):330-4

(88) http://www.ncbi.nlm.nih.gov/pubmed/14655024 Lasalvia-Prisco E, Cucchi S, Vazquez J et al. Insulin-induced enhancement of antitumoral response to methotrexate in breast cancer patients. Cancer Chemother Pharmacol 2004;53(3):220-4

(89) http://www.ncbi.nlm.nih.gov/pubmed/14458502 Koroljow, S. Two cases of malignant tumors with metastases apparently treated successfully with hypoglycemic coma. Psychiatric Quarterly 1962; 36(1):261-270.

(90) http://www.ncbi.nlm.nih.gov/pubmed/14479168 Neufeld, O. Insulin therapy in terminal cancer: a preliminary report. J Amer Geriatric Soc 1962; 10(3):274-6.

(91) Warburg O. The metabolism of carcinoma cells. J Cancer Res 1925; 9:148-163.

(92) http://www.ncbi.nlm.nih.gov/pubmed/10368805 Nutr Cancer. 1999;33(2):117-24.Evaluation of pancreatic proteolytic enzyme treatment of adenocarcinoma of the pancreas, with nutrition and detoxification support. Gonzalez NJ, Isaacs LL.

(93) http://www.ncbi.nlm.nih.gov/pubmed/8635074 Cancer. 1995 Nov 1;76(9):1671-7. The National Cancer Data Base report on pancreatic cancer. Niederhuber JE, Brennan MF, Menck HR.

(94) http://www.ncbi.nlm.nih.gov/pmc/articles/PMC1071044/ West J Med. 2000 September; 173(3): 153-154. US cancer institute funds trial of complementary therapy Deborah Josefson

(95) http://www.nature.com/bjc/journal/v87/n7/abs/6600547a.html Chromosomal Chaos and Cancer By Peter Duesberg, Scientific American 296, May 52-59.

(96) http://seer.cancer.gov/statfacts/ National Cancer Institute, Cancer Stat Fact Sheets are a collection of statistical summaries for a number of common cancer types.

CHAPTER 54

Anti-Aging Breakthrough with Bioidentical Hormones

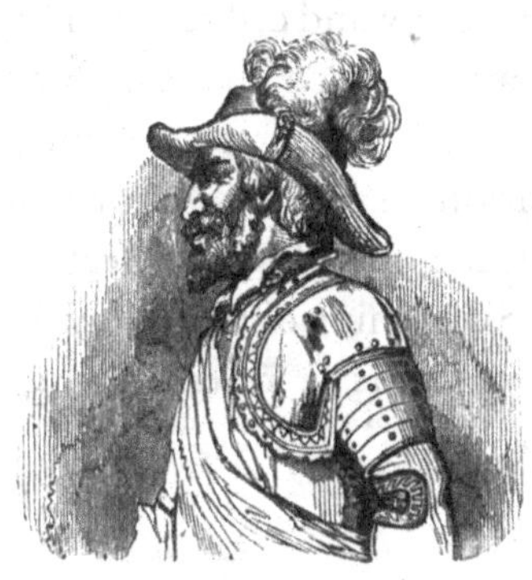

Ponce de Leon.

Kapitel VIII.

Florida.

Juan Ponce De Leon, famous explorer searched for the fountain of youth. Wood engraving 1858, courtesy of Library of Congress

Ponce de Leon was the famous explorer who searched for the fountain of youth, the magic waters that restored youth and vigor and reversed aging. Although Ponce de Leon failed to find the "fountain of youth", Ronald A. DePinho, a Harvard professor may have succeeded with his genetically modified mouse experiment which reversed aging in mice. This study was published in Nature.(1-2) The doctor used special mice that had been genetic engineered to age rapidly. The gene that controls aging had been "knocked out", so these mice had accelerated aging with shrinkage (atrophy) of the brain, spleen, loss of sense of smell, and loss of fertility with testicular atrophy.

Reversing Aging with the "The Ponce De Leon Effect"

The next step of the aging mouse experiment was to reverse aging and make the mice younger. This was done by giving back the missing gene that had been "knocked out" and see if that would reverse all these signs of aging in the mice. For this next step, the aged mice were treated with a drug (4-OHT) which dramatically reversed the signs of aging. The aged mice were surprisingly rejuvenated. Their shrunken brains, spleens and testes resumed normal size, and they regained their sense of smell. The infertile males once again became fertile, and fathered large litters. Is this the next anti-aging breakthrough? Can this type of treatment potentially restore organ function and reverse degenerative disease in the elderly?

What is a Telomere? Telomeres are the Biological Clock that Control Aging

De Pinho's mouse aging experiment was based on our knowledge of the telomere which serves as a biological clock for aging and cell replication. The telomere is a strand of DNA information which shortens with each cell replication. After about 50 cell replications or so, telomere shortening instructs the cell to stop replication in a process known as "cell senescence", or the Hayflick limit.(3) Cessation of cell replication directly causes aging, senescence and death. Shortening of the telomeres hastens aging, and lengthening the telomeres halts or reverses aging, producing the Ponce De Leon, "fountain of youth" effect.

Nobel Prize for Telomere Research

Much of our knowledge of telomeres and aging is credited to the work of Carol Grieder and her colleagues, awarded the 2009 Nobel Prize in Medicine for discovery and work on telomerase, the enzyme that lengthens telomeres.(4) In 1984, Greider discovered the enzyme telomerase and later she found that telomerase can prevent shortening of the telomeres, which prevents and reverse the aging process. Her findings were published in 1985 in the journal, Cell.(5) Activating the enzyme, telomerase, protects the telomeres from shortening and serves as an anti-aging treatment, slowing or reversing aging. On the contrary, knocking out or inhibiting telomerase activity allows telomeres to shorten and accelerate aging.

The Race to Activate Telomerase

How can we activate telomerase? The answer to this question can be found in an excellent 2002 review article by Cong entitled, "Human Telomerase and Its Regulation".(7) Among other things, the bioidentical hormones, 17 beta estradiol (estrogen) activates telomerase.

hTERT Gene and Estrogen Activation of Telomerase

The major mechanism for control and activation of telomerase is the hTERT promoter gene which stands for the human Telomerase Reverse

Transcriptase (hTERT) gene. When the hTERT gene is sequenced, and the code examined, one finds two estrogen receptor elements in this gene. This explains why 17-beta estradiol activates telomerase. The fact that there are estrogen receptors in the hTERT gene means that estrogen activates telomerase.(7) Estrogen blockers such as Tamoxifen™ block these receptors and turn off telomerase. Androgens were also found to turn on the hTERT gene and activate telomerase, and as expected, androgen blocker drugs inhibit telomerase.(7)

Doing Genetic Gymnastics To Use Tamoxifen™

Although much of the scientific research on telomerase activity has focused on estrogen (a bioidentical hormone) as the regulator and activator of telomerase activity, the DePinho Harvard group did something different. They genetically modified the mouse TERT gene so they could use a synthetic hormone called 4-OHT, which is actually Tamoxifen™. Normally, Tamoxifen™ is an estrogen receptor blocker and inhibitor of telomerase activity. The Depinho group did some genetic gymnastics and modified the genes of the mice so the Tamoxifen™ would activate the TERT gene, rather than inhibit it.

More on Tamoxifen™

Tamoxifen™, originally made by Astra-Zeneca, had global sales in 2001 of a billion dollars. This was a big seller, a blockbuster. As you might guess, Astra-Zeneca is a large pharmaceutical company with deep pockets for funding academic research.(8)(9) So, why did the Harvard group use a synthetic hormone called 4-OHT, to increase telomere length when research over the past decade shows that 17 Beta-Estradiol is the natural agent for this? Why not use 17-Beta Estradiol to produce the same anti-aging effects as the DePinho mouse telomere study?

Bioidentical Hormones are the Most Logical Choice

Whether you happen to be a human being or a mouse, then the most logical and effective way to increase telomerase activity, lengthen the telomeres and reverse aging is with the human bioidentical hormone, 17-Beta-Estradiol, also known as estrogen. In 1999, more than a decade ago, Kyo demonstrated that 17-Beta-Estradiol activates telomerase via direct and indirect effects on the hTERT promoter region.(10) In 2000 Silvia Misiti showed that telomerase activity and TERT gene expression is regulated by and dependent on 17 Beta Estradiol, which by the way, is a Bioidentical Hormone.(11) In 2008, Bayne showed that estrogen deficiency in mice leads to telomere shortening and rapid aging. (12) Another study in 2009 by Rodrigo T. Calado from the NIH (National Institute of Health) showed that 17-Beta-Estradiol was effective in increasing TERT gene expression and telomerase enzymatic activity. Quite contrary to DePinho's mouse aging model, the beneficial effect of 17-Beta Estradiol on telomerase function was abolished by Tamoxifen™, an estrogen blocker drug.(13)

A recent December 2010 study from Imanishi from Japan showed that 17-Beta-Estradiol (estrogen) augments telomerase activity, thereby accelerating recovery after injury and reducing the effects of aging (reducing senescence). If this isn't a description of anti-aging effects, I don't know what is.(14)(15)

Published in the journal Gut in 2004, Sato found that Estradiol prevents telomere shortening in normal human liver cells, as well as in a mouse model of chemically induced liver cirrhosis. Sato states that estradiol is the preferred treatment and superior to Dr. Depinho's genetic engineering proposals.(16)

An important study in Circulation 2006 found that 17-Beta Estradiol enhances recovery after heart attacks by augmenting incorporation of endothelial stem cells and inducing new collateral vessels in the ischemic myocardium. This beneficial effect is related to telomerase activation of the Endothelial Progenitor cells. (17)

Bioidentical Hormones Levels Decline After Age 50

Bioidentical hormones are the hormones normally found in the human body. After age 50, hormone levels decline in men and women, heralding the onset of degenerative changes also known as aging. It makes sense to replenish these hormones to normal levels which we now know activates telomere lengthening, and reverses senescence.

Why the Genetic Engineering Gymnastics?

In real life, Tamoxifen™ is anti-estrogen and acts to inhibit telomerase activity. So, you might be wondering why DePinho's group did some genetic engineering gymnastics to get the right receptors loaded onto the TERT gene, so that Tamoxifen could be used as the promoter drug, a drug that actually blocks the effect of 17-Beta Estradiol and is a TERT inhibitor in actual real life. It's all about Big Business and Big Pharma.

Pharmaceutical Industry and a Conflict of Interest

If you are wondering if telomere research at Harvard is tainted by Big Business and Big Pharma money, the answer is yes, of course. It's all disclosed in the public record.(18) The anti-aging mouse study author, Dr. DePinho received more than $83,000 dollars as a consultant to the Glaxo-Smith Klein drug company in 2009-2010.(18) Dr DePinho also co-founded Karyopharm, a privately held Oncology company which raised $20 Million in financing for its line of Novel Nuclear Transport Modulators. Dr DePinho is also one of the Directors at the Dana-Farber Cancer Institute which recently raised 1 Billion Dollars to fund its research activities (how much of this from Big Pharma?). So yes, of course, there is big money and big pharma involved in the halls of academic medicine, and this explains why a synthetic drug like 4-OHT (4 hydroxy tamoxifen) was used in the mouse telomere study instead of the more logical choice of 17 beta estradiol (estrogen).

The Race for Natural Substances That Activate Telomerase and Reverse Aging

Resveratrol, Silymarin and Gingko Biloba are natural substances found to activate telomerase with potential for anti-aging. (19-21) Calvin Harley of Geron Corporation, and John Anderson and William H Andrews of Sierra Sciences are leading the race to develop safe products as nutritional supplements to activate telomerase and reverse aging. Dr. Andrews says "***Telomerase activation technology promises to be the most significant advance in human health since germ theory.***"(22-23)

References For Chapter 54. Anti-Aging Breakthrough

(1) http://www.nature.com/news/2010/101128/full/news.2010.635.html Published online 28 November 2010 Nature—Telomerase reverses ageing process—Dramatic rejuvenation of prematurely aged mice hints at potential therapy.

(2) http://www.nature.com/nature/journal/vaop/ncurrent/full/nature09603.html Telomerase reactivation reverses tissue degeneration in aged telomerase-deficient mice Mariela Jaskelioff,Florian L. Muller,Ji-Hye Paik,Emily Thomas,Shan Jiang,Andrew C. Adams,Ergun Sahin,Maria Kost-Alimova,Alexei Protopopov,Juan Cadiñanos,James W. Horner,Eleftheria Maratos-Flier& Ronald A. DePinho Nature (2010) Published online 28 November 2010

(3) http://www4.utsouthwestern.edu/cellbio/shay-wright/publications/hayflick.nature.pdf Hayflick, his limit, and cellular ageing Jerry W. Shay and Woodring E.Wright Nature Reviews Mol Cell Bio 72 | OCTOBER 2000 | VOLUME 1

(4) http://www.nytimes.com/2009/10/06/science/06nobel.html New York Times—3 Americans Share Nobel for Medicine By NICHOLAS WADE October 5, 2009

(5) http://www.ncbi.nlm.nih.gov/pubmed/3907856 Cell. 1985 Dec;43(2 Pt 1):405-13. Identification of a specific telomere terminal transferase activity in Tetrahymena extracts. Greider CW, Blackburn EH.

(6) http://www.ncbi.nlm.nih.gov/pubmed/9335332 Cell. 1997 Oct 3;91(1):25-34. Telomere shortening and tumor formation by mouse cells lacking telomerase RNA. Blasco MA, Lee HW, Hande MP, Samper E, Lansdorp PM, DePinho RA, Greider CW. Cold Spring Harbor Laboratory, New York 11724, USA.

(7) http://www.ncbi.nlm.nih.gov/pmc/articles/PMC120798/ Microbiol Mol Biol Rev. 2002 September; 66(3): 407-425. Human Telomerase and Its Regulation. Yu-Sheng Cong,* Woodring E. Wright, and Jerry W. Shay

(8) http://www.news-medical.net/health/What-is-Tamoxifen.aspx Tamoxifen is an antagonist of the estrogen receptor in breast tissue. Global sales of tamoxifen in 2001 were $1,024 million.

(9) http://www.womenshealthtrack.vcu.edu/pdf/Osborne.pdf ALASTAIR J.J. WOOD, M.D., Editor Drug Therapy, Tamoxifen in the Treatment of Breast Cancer C. Kent Osborne, M.D., NEJM 1998 Volume 339 Number 22, 1609

(10) http://cancerres.aacrjournals.org/content/59/23/5917.full Estrogen Activates Telomerase. Satoru Kyo1, Masahiro Takakura, Taro Kanaya, Wang Zhuo, Kohtaro Fujimoto, Yukihito Nishio, Akira Orimo, and Masaki Inoue. Cancer Res December 1, 1999 59; 5917

(11) http://mcb.asm.org/cgi/content/full/20/11/3764 Molecular and Cellular Biology, June 2000, p. 3764-3771, Vol. 20, No. 11 Induction of hTERT Expression and Telomerase Activity by Estrogens in Human Ovary Epithelium Cells. Silvia Misiti, et al., Molecular Oncogenesis Laboratory, Regina Elena Cancer Institute, Rome, Italy.

(12) http://www.ncbi.nlm.nih.gov/pubmed/18936784 Cell Res. 2008 Nov;18(11):1141-50. Estrogen deficiency leads to telomerase inhibition, telomere shortening and reduced cell proliferation in the adrenal gland of mice. Bayne S, Jones ME, Li H, Pinto AR, Simpson ER, Liu JP. Department of Immunology, Central Eastern Clinical School, Monash University, Melbourne, Australia.

(13) http://bloodjournal.hematologylibrary.org/cgi/content/full/114/11/2236 Blood, 10 September 2009, Vol. 114, No. 11, pp. 2236-2243. Sex hormones, acting on the TERT gene, increase telomerase activity in human primary hematopoietic cells. Rodrigo T. Calado et al. National Institutes of Health, Bethesda, MD

(14) http://www.ncbi.nlm.nih.gov/pubmed/19965898 Ther Adv Cardiovasc Dis. 2010 Feb;4(1):55-69. Epub 2009 Dec 4. Endothelial progenitor cell senescence—is there a role for estrogen? Imanishi T, Tsujioka H, Akasaka T.

(15) http://journals.lww.com/jhypertension/Abstract/2005/09000/Estrogen_reduces_endothelial_progenitor_cell.14.aspx Journal of Hypertension:September 2005—Volume 23—Issue 9—p 1699-1706 Estrogen reduces endothelial progenitor cell senescence through augmentation of telomerase activity Imanishi, Toshio; Hano, Takuzo; Nishio, Ichiro

(16) http://www.ncbi.nlm.nih.gov/pmc/articles/PMC1774098/?tool=pubmed Gut. 2004 July; 53(7): 1001-1009. Prevention of critical telomere shortening by oestradiol in human normal hepatic cultured cells and carbon tetrachloride induced rat liver fibrosis. R Sato et al. Department of Pathology, Iwate Medical University School of Medicine, Morioka, Japan

(17) http://circ.ahajournals.org/cgi/content/abstract/113/12/1605 Circulation. 2006;113:1605-1614.) Molecular Cardiology—Estradiol Enhances Recovery After Myocardial Infarction by Augmenting Incorporation of Bone Marrow—Derived Endothelial Progenitor Cells Into Sites of Ischemia-Induced Neovascularization via Endothelial Nitric Oxide Synthase—Mediated Activation of Matrix Metalloproteinase-9 Atsushi Iwakura, MD, PhD et al.

(18) http://projects.propublica.org/docdollars/states/massachusetts Dollars for Docs, What Drug Companies are Paying Your Doctor

(19) http://onlinelibrary.wiley.com/doi/10.1038/bjp.2008.272/abstract Resveratrol reduces endothelial progenitor cells senescence through augmentation of telomerase activity by Akt-dependent mechanisms L Xia, X X Wang, X S Hu, X G Guo, Y P Shang, H J Chen, C L Zeng, F R Zhang, J Z ChenArticle first published online: 29 JAN 2009 British Journal of Pharmacology Volume 155, Issue 3, pages 387-394, October 2008.

(20) http://www.ncbi.nlm.nih.gov/pubmed/20838231 J Cardiovasc Pharmacol. 2010 Aug 31. [Epub ahead of print] Silymarin Inhibits Endothelial Progenitor Cells Senescence and Protects Against the Antiproliferative Activity of Rapamycin. Preliminary Study.

Parzonko A, Naruszewicz M.Department of Pharmacognosy and Molecular Basis of Phytotherapy, Medical University of Warsaw, Poland.

(21) http://www.ncbi.nlm.nih.gov/pubmed/17312453 J Cardiovasc Pharmacol. 2007 Feb;49(2):111-5. Ginkgo biloba extract reduces endothelial progenitor-cell senescence through augmentation of telomerase activity. Dong XX, Hui ZJ, Xiang WX, Rong ZF, Jian S, Zhu CJ. Department of Cardiology, the First Affiliated Hospital, Medical School of Zhejiang University, Hangzhou, China.

(22) http://www.tasciences.com/pdf/Harley_CMM_final.pdf Current Molecular Medicine 2005, 5, 29-38 205 Telomerase Therapeutics for Degenerative Diseases. Calvin B. Harley* Geron Corporation, Menlo Park, CA, 94025, USA

(23) http://pharmalive.com/News/index.cfm?articleid=747325&categoryid=40 Sierra Sciences' Plan to Cure Aging is Validated by Newly Published Proof of Concept Experiment. "Telomerase activation technology promises to be the most significant advance in human health since germ theory."

CHAPTER 55

Low Dose Naltrexone LDN—The Latest Medical Scandal and Outrage

The Greatest Medical Discovery of the Century

No doubt, future medical history books will look back at the 20th century and conclude that the great medical discovery was the opiate receptor system in the brain, the brain's own production of these compounds called, endorphins, or endogenous opioids. The widespread medicinal use of the morphine class of opioid narcotics for pain relief is due to the fact that opioid receptors already exist in the brain and nervous system. The opioid drugs flood these receptors, blocking pain and sedating the nervous system.(1) Another key discovery was made quietly without fanfare by a humble New York internist, Bernard Bihari in the 1970's. (2-3) While working with drug addicts, he noted a beneficial effect from temporary blockade of opioid receptors, which produced a rebound increase in endogenous opioid production. The opioid blocking drug he used is called Naltrexone, an FDA approved drug developed by the government as part of its "War Against Drugs" campaign.(1-3)

This largely ignored and inexpensive off-patent drug called LDN has been used with great success over the past 20 years by various renegade physicians to cure or induce remissions in a host of seemingly unrelated diseases such as Multiple Sclerosis (4-6), Crohn's Disease (7), Systemic Lupus, Rheumatoid Arthritis, Pancreatic Cancer and Lymphoma. LDN has also been found useful in Autism, and halts progression to opportunistic infection in AIDS patients.(1)

Criticism from Mainstream Medicine

Paradoxically, LDN's ability to benefit so many seemingly unrelated medical conditions has been the greatest criticism from conventional mainstream medicine. If it sounds too good to be true, it probably is. However, since LDN is an FDA approved drug, off label use is allowed. LDN has virtually no adverse side effects, and based on my own short clinical experience prescribing LDN for Multiple Sclerosis (4-6), Crohn's Disease(7) and Ulcerative Colitis(38), I can report that although it does not work for all patients, it is amazingly effective in many. Even though it may sound too good to be true, in the case of LDN, I can assure you that, yes, it is all true.

Domination by Pharmaceutical Industry

The medical system's domination by the Pharmaceutical industry is clearly apparent by the scandalous and outrageous manner in which LDN has been ignored. Mainstream neurologists refuse to prescribe LDN for multiple sclerosis, instead using prednisone, and other useless medications. Mainstream gastroenterologists refuse to prescribe LDN for Crohn's and Ulcerative colitis, instead using prednisone, methotrexate and newer drugs like Remicade to inhibit the immune system, all with horrendous adverse side effects. Conventional oncologist refuse to prescribe LDN for cancer patients, preferring the more traditional chemotherapy, radiation and surgery, modalities which have changed very little over the past 60 years and although effective for a few selected cancers, largely ineffective for the vast majority of cancers and their relentless spread as metastatic disease.

A Mass Movement Driven by People, Not Pharmaceutical Corporations

An amazing thing is happening. In spite of lack of research funding by Big Pharma, a mass people power movement on the internet is creating a tidal wave of interest in LDN. A flood of anecdotal reports of LDN remission and cures have been posted in the internet, and in some cases published in the medical literature. (37) A series of LDN conferences have been organized, and have been highly successful. The 2008 LDN Conference speaker presentations may be viewed on You-Tube videos on the internet.(8-15) Jill Smith MD at Penn State University Hospital published a successful clinical trial of LDN for Crohn's disease in the American Journal of Gastroenterology.(7) This has blazed the trail for a whole series of new clinical trials. An army of dedicated volunteers are working selflessly to promote new clinical trials, to get the word out about LDN and to make a reality the eventual acceptance by mainstream medicine.

October 2008 Conference at USC Medical Center

LDN for Cancer—Dr Burton Berkson

At the October 2008 LDN conference at the USC Medical Center, Burton Berkson MD PhD presented his clinical experience with LDN which can be viewed on a You Tube video presentation.(8-15) Dr Berkson presents cases of successful remission from pancreatic cancer and B Cell lymphoma with LDN. Berkson also reported dramatic responses in cases of autoimmune diseases such as Rheumatoid Arthritis, Systemic Lupus and Dermatomyositis, as well as multiple sclerosis and inflammatory bowel disease. (8-15)

Lymphoma and LDN

One case report involves a lymphoma patient who experienced dramatic regression with LDN. This report by Berkson describes the treatment of a 61-year old man with biopsy-proven Lymphoma. His initial physical examination and PET/CT scan showed multiple large, metabolically active, pathologic lymph nodes that demonstrated complete resolution within 6 months of commencing therapy with Low Dose Naltrexone, taken as a capsule before sleep every night. The Pet Scans before and after LDN treatment showing regression of lymphoma can be viewed on a You Tube video.(11-15)

Pancreatic Cancer and LDN

Another case report involves pancreatic cancer which responded favorably to LDN. A 46-year-old man who was diagnosed with metastatic pancreatic cancer in October 2002. He was initially treated with a standard chemotherapy regimen by the local oncologist. However, after a single chemotherapy treatment, the patient experienced severe bone marrow suppression with low platelet and WBC counts, and could not tolerate any further chemotherapy. In addition, in spite of the chemotherapy, the cancer progressed. The patient then presented to Dr. Berkson, who promptly started treatment with intravenous Alpha Lipoic Acid (ALA), Low Dose Naltrexone (LDN), and a healthy lifestyle program. The Pancreatic cancer with metastases to the liver was followed with serial CAT and PET scans, and he has remained stable.(11-15) It is interesting to note that the cancer progressed rapidly when the ALA-LDN therapy was halted; however, the cancer stabilized quickly when treatment resumed. Serial Cat scans show no progression of hepatic metastatic lesions over three years.

How does LDN restrict pancreatic cancer?

A phase I clinical trial by Smith and Zagon using Opiate Growth Factor in advanced pancreatic cancer patients showed that OGF can be safely administered to patients with advanced pancreatic cancer. Basic science research by Dr. Zagon using molecular biology tools has answered this question.(16-34) Zagon found that Opioid Growth Factor and receptor inhibit growth of pancreatic cancer cells by influencing cellular replication during the G0/G1 phase of mitosis. Zagon found that this inhibition of cell replication in human pancreatic cancer involves a well known pathway in molecular biology, the p21-CKI pathway. This inhibition of cell replication can be obtained with Opioid Growth Factor itself, or with LDN. (16-34)

The Definitive Book on LDN

I recommend for you a book on LDN, "The Promise of Low Dose Naltrexone Therapy: Potential Benefits in Cancer, Autoimmune, Neurological and Infectious Disorders, by Elaine Moore and SammyJo Wilkinson. (1) The drug, Naltrexone, was developed in the 1960's as part of the government's War on Drugs, as a narcotics blocker intended as a treatment for narcotics addiction. However, narcotics addicts avoided it because of the narcotics withdrawal induced by the drug. However, over the years, Naltrexone found a niche for treatment and prevention of alcoholism. The usual tablet dosage is 50 mg, although some practitioners use a monthly injection for alcoholics. The book covers the use in LDN in the following disease categories (1):

Low Dose Naltrexone Use in Disease Categories(1)
Autoimmune Diseases
Multiple Sclerosis
Neurodegenerative Disorders
Cancer
Autism Spectrum Disorders
LDN in Wound Healing and Infections
The Immune System and LDN in HIV/AIDS

As of this date, this is the first and only book of its kind on LDN, and as such represents a milestone in the effort to bring LDN into mainstream use. Written by Elaine Moore, a high level science writer with a portfolio of previous accomplishments, her LDN book is perhaps somewhat technical and may be difficult for the untrained non-professional to follow. It delves into the sophisticated jargon of the medical research world. However, in addition to the esoteric technical sections of the book, there are also chapters devoted to the lay reader interested in learning how LDN can help them on a practical level. A listing of dispensing practitioners was included. The book is highly recommended for other health care practitioners who wish to get quickly up to speed in this new area of medicine which is destined to become the medical paradigm of the 21st century, casting a giant shadow over the rest of mainstream medicine.

LDN requires a prescription and is available at a few specialty compounding pharmacies.(35-36) For references and links, see my web site: www.bioidenticalhormones101.com

References for Chapter 55. Low Dose Naltrexone

(1) The Promise Of Low Dose Naltrexone Therapy: Potential Benefits in Cancer, Autoimmune, Neurological and Infectious Disorders by Elaine A. Moore, McFarland (December 1, 2008)

(2) http://www.ldninfo.org/bbihari_cv.htm Curriculum Vitae, BERNARD BIHARI, M.D. 29 West 15th Street New York, N.Y. 10011, (212) 929-4196 retired as of March 2007. Sadly, Dr. Bihari passed away on May 16, 2010.

(3) http://www.honestmedicine.com/2011/05/transcript-bihari-video.html Video of Dr. Bihari Released on the First Anniversary of His Death (May 16, 2011) Transcript of Dr. Bihari Video. Also see: http://www.megavideo.com/?v=S6HPUJZO

(4) http://www.ncbi.nlm.nih.gov/pubmed/20695007 Ann Neurol. 2010 Aug;68(2):145-50.Pilot trial of low-dose naltrexone and quality of life in multiple sclerosis.Cree BA, Kornyeyeva E, Goodin DS.

(5) http://www.ncbi.nlm.nih.gov/pubmed/18728058 Mult Scler. 2008 Sep;14(8):1076-83. A pilot trial of low-dose naltrexone in primary progressive multiple sclerosis. Gironi M et al.

(6) http://www.ldnresearchtrustfiles.co.uk/docs/BJNN.pdf Low-dose naltrexone as a treatment for multiple sclerosis by Tom Gilhooly, British Journal of Neuroscience Nursing, Vol. 5, Iss. 11, 13 Nov 2009, pp 494

(7) http://www.ncbi.nlm.nih.gov/pubmed/17222320 Low-dose naltrexone therapy improves active Crohn's disease.Smith JP, Stock H, Bingaman S, Mauger D, Rogosnitzky M, Zagon IS. Am J Gastroenterol. 2007 Apr;102(4):820-8. Department of Medicine, Pennsylvania State University College of Medicine, Hershey, Pennsylvania 17033, USA.

(8) 4th Annual LDN Conference 2008 You Tube Videos of Presentations http://www.youtube.com/watch?v=UNX3eeg4c_I&feature=player_embedded

(9) 4th Annual LDN COnference. LDN 2008 Sunny Sedlock O'Malley Interview corrdinator of 2008 meeting discusses how her fathers Multiple Myeloma went into remission with LDN

(10) http://www.youtube.com/watch?v=DAZ1fQKdOC8&feature=player_embedded 3rd LDN Conference Doctor Interviews 2007. Dr David Gluck gives overview of conference. 2007 3rd.

(11) http://www.youtube.com/watch?v=WqRwXEnPYKk October 11 2008 USC Medical Center. LDN 2008 Dr Burt Berkson Best of part 1.

Here are three videos of the meeting presentation by Dr Burt Berkson, a clinician using LDN, at the Oct 2008 LDN conference at USC Medical Center, in which he presents cases of successful remission from pancreatic cancer and B Cell lymphoma with LDN. He also notes most dramatic responses in cases of autoimmune diseases such as Rheumatoid Arthrisis, Systemic Lupus and Dermatomyosis, as well as multiple sclerosis and inflammatory bowel disease.

(12) http://www.youtube.com/watch?v=4bpRai9S03A&feature=related LDN 08 Dr Burt Berkson Part 2

(13) http://www.youtube.com/watch?v=BLoS_U85g0Y&feature=related LDN 2008 Dr Burt Berkson Part 3. Burt Berkson's publications of case reports of success with LDN for pancreatic cancer and B cell lymphoma:

(14) http://www.ldn4cancer.com/files/berkson-b-cell-lymphoma-paper.pdf Reversal of Signs and Symptoms of a B-Cell Lymphoma in a Patient Using Only Low-Dose Naltrexone. Integr Cancer Ther 2007; 6; 293. Burton M. Berkson, MD, Daniel M. Rubin, ND, FABNO, and Arthur J. Berkson, MD.

(15) http://www.ldn4cancer.com/files/Berkson_Pancreatic_paper.pdf The Long-term Survival of a Patient With Pancreatic Cancer With Metastases to the Liver After Treatment With the Intravenous Alpha-Lipoic Acid/Low-Dose Naltrexone Protocol by Burton M. Berkson, Daniel M. Rubin, and Arthur J. Berkson. INTEGRATIVE CANCER THERAPIES 5(1); 2006 pp. 83-89

(16) http://www.ncbi.nlm.nih.gov/pubmed/6640516 Cancer Lett. 1983 Nov;21(1):89-94. Opioid antagonists inhibit the growth of metastatic murine neuroblastoma.Zagon IS, McLaughlin PJ.

(17) http://www.ncbi.nlm.nih.gov/pubmed/6316064 Life Sci. 1983 Dec 12;33(24):2449-54. Naltrexone modulates growth in infant rats.Zagon IS, McLaughlin PJ.

(18) http://www.ncbi.nlm.nih.gov/pubmed/10592296 Brain Res. 1999 Dec 4;849(1-2):147-54. Cloning, sequencing, expression and function of a cDNA encoding a receptor for the opioid growth factor, [Met(5)] enkephalin. Zagon IS et al.

(19) http://www.ncbi.nlm.nih.gov/pubmed/11029512 Opioid growth factor regulates the cell cycle of human neoplasias.Zagon IS, Roesener CD, Verderame MF, Ohlsson-Wilhelm BM, Levin RJ, McLaughlin PJ.

(20) http://www.ncbi.nlm.nih.gov/pubmed/8620464 Cancer Lett. 1996 Mar 29;101(2):159-64. Inhibition of human colon cancer by intermittent opioid receptor blockade with naltrexone.Hytrek SD, McLaughlin PJ, Lang CM, Zagon IS.

(21) http://www.ncbi.nlm.nih.gov/pubmed/9066724 Cancer Lett. 1997 Jan 30;112(2):167-75. Opioid growth factor (OGF) inhibits human pancreatic cancer transplanted into nude mice.Zagon IS, Hytrek SD, Smith JP, McLaughlin PJ.

(22) http://www.ncbi.nlm.nih.gov/pubmed/6867737
Science. 1983 Aug 12;221(4611):671-3. Naltrexone modulates tumor response in mice with neuroblastoma.Zagon IS, McLaughlin PJ.

(23) http://www.ncbi.nlm.nih.gov/pubmed/6300232
Matthew, PM, Froelich CJ, Sibbitt WL, Jr., Bankhurst AD, Enhancement of natural cytotoxicity by beta-endorphin, J Immunol 130, pp.1658-1662, Apr 1983.

(24) http://www.ncbi.nlm.nih.gov/pubmed/6867737
Zagon IS, McLaughlin PJ, Naltrexone modulates tumor response in mice with neuroblastoma, Science 221, pp.671-3, Aug 12, 1983.

(25) http://www.ncbi.nlm.nih.gov/pubmed/6867737 Hytrek SD, McLaughlin PJ, Lang CM, Zagon IS, Inhibition of human colon cancer by intermittent opioid receptor blockade with naltrexone, Cancer Lett 101(2), pp. 159-64, Mar 29, 1996.

(26) http://www.ncbi.nlm.nih.gov/pubmed/8853403
Zagon IS, Hytrek SD, Lang CM, Smith JP, McGarrity TJ, Wu Y, McLaughlin PJ, Opioid growth factor ([Met5]enkephalin) prevents the incidence and retards the growth of human colon cancer, Am J Physiol 271(3 Pt 2), pp.R780-R786, Sep 1996

(27) http://www.ncbi.nlm.nih.gov/pubmed/6087062
Zagon IS, McLaughlin PJ, Duration of opiate receptor blockade determines tumorigenic response in mice with neuroblastoma: a role for endogenous opioid systems in cancer, Life Sci 35, pp. 409-416, 1984.

(28) http://www.ncbi.nlm.nih.gov/pubmed/6087062
Zagon IS, McLaughlin PJ, Opioid antagonist modulation of murine neuroblastoma: A profile of cell proliferation and opioid peptides and receptors, Brain Res 480, pp. 16-28, 1989.

(29) http://www.molecular-cancer.com/content/7/1/5
The OGF-OGFr axis utilizes the p21 pathway to restrict progression of human pancreatic cancer. Fan Cheng1, Patricia J McLaughlin1, Michael F Verderame2 and Ian S Zagon. Molecular Cancer 2008, 7:5

(30) http://www.pubmedcentral.nih.gov/articlerender.fcgi?artid=2613082&tool=pmcentrez Mol Biol Cell. 2009 January 1; 20(1): 319-327. The OGF-OGFr Axis Utilizes the p16INK4a and p21WAF1/CIP1 Pathways to Restrict Normal Cell Proliferation. Fan Cheng,* Patricia J. McLaughlin,* Michael F. Verderame,† and Ian S. Zagon

(31) http://www.ncbi.nlm.nih.gov/pubmed/18813788 Int J Oncol. 2008 Oct;33(4):751-7. Prevention and delay in progression of human squamous cell carcinoma of the head and neck in nude mice by stable overexpression of the opioid growth factor receptor. McLaughlin PJ, Kreiner S, Morgan CR, Zagon IS.

(32) http://www.ncbi.nlm.nih.gov/pubmed/18636152 Int J Oncol. 2008 Aug;33(2):317-23. Prevention and delay in progression of human pancreatic cancer by stable overexpression of the opioid growth factor receptor. Zagon IS et al.

(33) http://www.ncbi.nlm.nih.gov/pubmed/15014352 Anticancer Drugs. 2004 Mar;15(3):203-9. Treatment of advanced pancreatic cancer with opioid growth factor: phase I. Smith JP, Zagon IS et al.

(34) http://www.ncbi.nlm.nih.gov/pubmed/8853403 Am J Physiol. 1996 Sep;271(3 Pt 2):R780-6. Opioid growth factor ([Met5]enkephalin) prevents the incidence and retards the growth of human colon cancer. Zagon IS, Smith JP wt al. Sources for LDN

(35) http://www.thecompounder.com/index.php The Compounder Pharmacy 340 Marshall Ave Unit 100 - Aurora, IL 60506-2956 Phone: 630-859-0333 Fax: 630-859-0114

(36) http://www.skipspharmacy.com/sppress/?cat=8
Skip's Pharmacy LDN PAGE 21000 Boca Rio Rd Suite A-29 Boca Raton, Florida 33433 561-218-0111 800-553-7429 Fax: 561-218-8873

(37) http://www.ldninfo.org/index.htm LDNINFO Web site for low dose naltrexone information.

(38) http://www.drhoffman.com/page.cfm/795 One patient's UC Ulcerative Colitis success story, Nick's success story by Ronald Hoffman MD

CHAPTER 56

Predicting the Future of Medicine

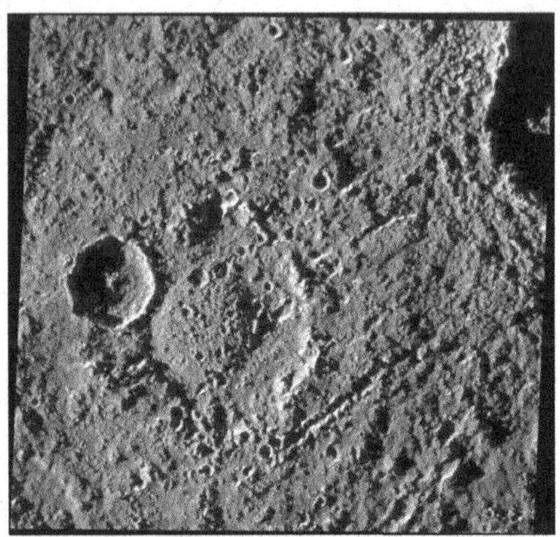

Surfaceofmoon, Callisto, photographed from the Gallileo spacecraft on its ninth orbit around Jupiter. Courtesy of NASA Jet Propulsion laboratory.

Predicting the future of medicine can be done using the same tools we use to predict the weather or anything else. In order to predict the future, we must first glean a few clues from the history books, and examine the major forces driving historical change over thousands of years.

The History of Western Civilization-A Few Milestones

Anthropologists argue over exactly what was the first major milestone in the development and success of humans as the dominant species on the planet. I think it was the appearance of language, the ability to verbalize and communicate complex thought. The exact moment in history when mankind first used language is unknown, but it must have been thousands of years ago.

The Invention of the Phonetic Alphabet

This event, as great it was, was followed many years later, by an even greater event, the invention of written language about 5,500 years ago. Literacy, and the use of the phonetic alphabet, provided the earliest technology to record and play back human thought. The human brain can be regarded as a recording device for sensory input, and has the capability to remember (or play back) images, sounds, smells, etc. However, our mental ability to remember and recall, to record and playback, is limited. Some form of amplification or enhancement would be useful, and this can be accomplished with an external recording device. The first external recording device was writing on clay tablets, and later on paper. In today's modern times, electronic audio and video recording has replaced the need to actually write the spoken words. However, we still rely on written transcripts as a remnant of the past.

Transition from Slavery to Freedom

Amazingly, the transition to literacy also marks transition from slavery to freedom. Throughout history, illiteracy has always been associated with slavery, and literacy with freedom, nobility and privilege. One of the earliest historical examples of this transition appears in the bible story describing the transformation of an illiterate group of slaves into a literate group of free men at Mount Sinai in the desert after they escaped from Egypt. Although written language makes possible enrichment of all forms of human thought, both in the realm of spiritual life and in the realm of natural science, we will restrict the following discussion to science, and focus on medical science.

College Graduation as Medieval Ritual

As I attended my son's college graduation a few years back, I was struck by the obvious symbolism denoting the dual transitions of the college student, from a state of illiteracy to literacy (with a degree in Arts and Letters), and the transition from a symbolic state of serfdom (poor college student burdened with college loans) to the freedom of a symbolic "Medieval Nobleman". The symbolism is completed by the medieval clothing of cap and gown. We will discuss individual freedom and government later on.

The Dark Ages—Knowledge Restricted

During early civilization, written documents were rare because paper was scarce and the method of reproducing written documents by hand was tedious and time consuming. Writing remained in the hands of a privileged few during a period called the Medieval Dark Ages. During this time, written language was the protected "intellectual property" of clergy and nobility who used written language for government, commerce and the expansion of scientific knowledge, as well as other purposes such as feudal warfare.

The Gutenberg Galaxy—Movable Type and the Renaissance

The prevailing state of affairs changed dramatically with the invention of movable type and the printing press by Johan Gutenberg in 1439, making written documents widely available. The printing press was a direct precursor to the Renaissance as explained by Marshall McLuhan in his book, "The Gutenberg Galaxy".(1-2) In every historical period, new technologies are at first afforded intellectual property rights and restricted to a privileged few. This technological innovation drives change. For example, the invention of movable type produced political and cultural upheaval. One might speculate that the fall of feudal monarchies and the rise of the democratic state were made possible by mass production of the written media leading to the Renaissance followed by the Enlightenment.

The Industrial Revolution—Increasing Life Expectancy

The Renaissance and Enlightenment culminated in the Industrial Revolution with new technological advances such as the steam engine, electricity, magnetism, electronics, radio, television, and finally, the computer chip and internet. The Industrial Revolution stood on the shoulders of the previous three centuries of scientific achievement. Mass production of goods and services lead to improved living standards, and increased life expectancy. From 1820 to present day, a life expectancy chart shows a linear increase in life span. (32) Before the Industrial Revolution, average life expectancy was only 35 years, going all the way back to the Roman Empire. After the Industrial Revolution, however, there was a sudden increase in life span, which was only 38 years in 1850, and increased to 70 in the year 2004.(27-28)(32) Today, we have a large population of citizens older than 50 years of age, a new phenomenon in the history of Western Civilization. These are the aging baby boomers. This linear increase in life expectancy and increasing older population is expected to continue, and serves as an important trend that is useful for predicting the future. According to Aldous Huxley, this overpopulation trend produces pressures toward global totalitarian government and loss of individual freedoms.

A Post-Industrial Second Medieval Dark Age

In spite of many impressive scientific and industrial manufacturing advances, the historical era of the post-Industrial Revolution shares many of the same features of the Medieval Dark Ages, such as restricted technical knowledge and increased levels of warfare. One of these shared features was the restriction of technical knowledge to the elite few, i.e. governments (military uses), multinational corporations, universities and professional groups such as physicians. Another shared feature was increased levels of warfare. The Dark Ages had their feudal warfare, and the post-Industrial Revolution had its series of wars as well. Thus, the era from the Post-Industrial Revolution to the end of the Cold War (the fall of the Berlin Wall) can be considered a second Medieval Dark Age. Perhaps the Internet Age will represent a Second Renaissance.

Global Warfare Following the Industrial Revolution

The first in a series of Post-Industrial Revolution Wars was the American Civil War in 1861-1864. Of course as we all know, the two opposing sides were the South, an agrarian society, economically dependent on the ancient concept of human slavery, and the Industrial North which depended on a more modern version of the master-slave relationship called hourly wage employment. Following the American Civil War, the series of post-Industrial wars continued globally with World Wars I and II.

Disruptive Science of Kuhn Leads to Atomic Bomb

In 1905, Classical Newtonian Physics gave way to the Einstein's Physics of Relativity, a scientific revolution described by Thomas Kuhn as "Disruptive Science" (29). This scientific revolution was required and needed to invent the Atomic Bomb. The decision by US president Harry Truman to use the new Atomic weapon on Hiroshima and Nagasaki, August 1945, marked the end of world wars and the beginning of the Atomic Age in which everyone globally lived in a state of anxiety that nuclear annihilation could be triggered at any time. In this new age, unrestricted global warfare threatened to destroy the entire planet, hence the creation of "Cold War" limited to the use of conventional weapons.

Centralized Information of the Mass Media

Media information during the 19th and 20th centuries originated centrally, was disseminated outward to the masses, and was non-interactive using the new radio and television. This created an opportunity for political or corporate gain through manipulation of the media. Government and corporate control of the media created a social and political climate aptly described by George Orwell's novel, "1984" in which perpetual global warfare was the norm. (3)(4) During the early 20th century, media content was copyrighted and protected by intellectual property law. Media ownership was limited to large corporations, excluding individuals from participating in this arena. This was reminiscent of the situation with medieval documents which were hand written, and restricted to a few noblemen and clergy who could read and write and could afford to maintain libraries. Ownership and control of modern media was in the hands of governments and large corporations. In the post Industrial Age, the Second Dark Age, individuals were passive recipients of information rather than interactive creators of information. This has been dramatically changed by the Internet Age in which any individual can publish a web site, blog or You Tube video.

Advances in Science and Medicine

The industrial revolution brought invention of instruments to extend human senses such as the light and electron microscope. This allows us to see the very tiny world of microbes, leading to microbiology and antibiotics. Although telescopes were invented centuries before, further refinement in satellites and radio telescopes gave us even more ability to see planets and stars on a very large scale. Further refinements in instrumentation allow visibility of the entire electromagnetic spectrum, allowing the human eye to see otherwise invisible aspects of the natural world. Turning these new instruments inward, for the first time, medical science can make images of the human body in the live state. X-rays, CAT scans, Ultrasound, Radionuclide and PET scanning all represent imaging with instruments which extend the senses to allow anatomic visualization inside the human body. (42)

Just as the world's great telescopes are restricted to a few privileged astronomers, medical instrumentation was restricted to a privileged few medical professionals who maintain the age old model of protecting and restricting technical knowledge. This created a social and political climate in the practice of medicine aptly described by Ivan Illich in his essay, Medical Nemesis in 1976. (5-12)

Although the history of medicine chronicles great achievements such as the conquest of infectious disease with invention of antibiotics and, advances in surgery with introduction of anesthesia and sterile technique, etc., critics of the medical system such as Ivan Illich and Robert Mendelssohn point out the disconnect between the promise of medicine and the reality. (42) This disconnect was perhaps best described by pediatrician Robert Mendelsohn MD in his 1979 book, Confessions of a Medical Heretic.(13-16) By the way, Mendelsohn was my medical school adviser in 1976. These two books by Mendelsohn and Illich perhaps best exemplify the Medieval Dark Age of Medicine, in which medical information is restricted to medical professionals and not to be shared with the layman.

The Revolutionary Impact of the Internet

In another form of Kuhn's "Disruptive Science", the Internet Age has turned everything upside down, and has brought the end of the Second Dark Age and created a Renaissance, representing a new openness of information. This is especially true in medicine, with the advent of the empowered autonomous e-patient. Rather than being centrally controlled, the new Internet media is now controlled by individuals empowered to publish their own web pages, blog or message board with video and audio streams, directly competing with conventional media in the form of television, radio and print media.

Empowering the Individual

The individual is now empowered as an owner of a personal audio/ video broadcast station on the Internet. Creating new content is as easy as writing on a computer screen, or uploading a video. On the internet, the individual has complete access to previously protected knowledge. New medical knowledge is being created on internet message boards and social networks. This new knowledge flows freely and is unprotected by intellectual property law. In the future, this body of public medical knowledge created on the internet will grow to immense size, dwarfing the current knowledge database. In comparison, the body of protected medical knowledge used by today's doctors and medical system will seem quite small in comparison to this new public internet based knowledge base. Here are a few examples:

Example 1: Although seemingly protected by copyright law, the music and movie industries experience huge losses from pirated music and DVDs available online.

Example 2: Secret corporate documents released during legal proceedings are deemed privileged by the court, yet are posted publicly on the internet (Zyprexa Documents) at huge personal cost to an individual. This information contradicts the corporate message of the drug companies and creates public outrage.

Example 3: Publication of the Rodney King video showing unjustified and cruel beating at the hands of the LA police contradicted the customary "resisting arrest" defense, and created public outrage.

Example 4: "Disease Mongering" Media Advertising by drug companies is exposed and unmasked by information on the internet. Disease Mongering is eventually abandoned by the pharmaceutical industry as self-defeating and embarrassing to corporate goals. Television drug advertising, and specifically disease mongering will be banned in the future by the government in response to public outrage.

> Example 5: An obscure doctor in Hong Kong publishes an article stating that acne resolves after taking vitamin B5. (37) The vitamin is safe, with no adverse side effects, and is widely available without a prescription. Thousands of acne sufferers try the vitamin B5 treatment and report their progress on hundred of acne message boards across the internet along with before and after digital photos. The net result is the creation of new knowledge on the efficacy of Vitamin B5 for acne. This knowledge is in the public domain and cannot be copyrighted or protected by intellectual property law. This is especially useful for vitamins, supplements and other natural substances which are generally regarded as safe, and yet will never generate enough money to pay for the expensive drug trials required for FDA approval.

Intellectual Property Laws?

Public display of pirated information on the internet represents a general assault on intellectual property law, which will be either revised or abandoned. These laws are ineffective at preventing the widespread dissemination of protected information. Although intellectual property laws are in effect and mostly respected and followed here in the US, the reality is that any kid with a video camera can copy a first run movie and post it on the internet. Anyone can buy a video recorder, record an event, and then publish the video on a blog or You-Tube, along with written narrative. Drug patents are now being violated internationally. For example, Ciprofloxin™ is sold off patent in India. Patrick Dixon says "*Trying to protect or copyright your own management ideas is last-century nonsense: absurd and illogical.*" (36)

New medical knowledge is created and shared interactively without concern for intellectual property laws. The internet gives us the "online community" in which individuals share written, audio and video information. This was previously the domain of specialized libraries restricted to privileged groups. Certain forms of knowledge have always been free of protection by intellectual property laws. For example, it is not possible to patent the alphabet, the English language, or the chemical structure of a natural substance.

The Doctor-Patient Relationship of the Future

Tom Ferguson MD describes the advent of a new type of doctor-patient relationship quite different from the old paternalistic one, in which the doctor is educator and participant, and recognizes an opportunity to learn from the expert e-patient, who engages in internet searches for medical information and may actually have more specialized knowledge than the doctor. The new doctor openly shares information with patients, and serves as educator.(21-22)

The Structure of DNA

Discovery of the structure of DNA was credited to Watson and Crick in 1953. However, the real work was done by Rosalind Franklin, an expert in x-ray crystallography who revealed the double helix structure of DNA. Unfortunately Rosalind died of breast cancer and never received proper credit. X-ray crystallography uses electromagnetic light not visible to the human eye to image molecular structures. (24) The discovery of the structure of DNA heralded a new age of molecular biology, and the Human Genome Project was started in 1990, and finished in 2000. This massive project sequenced the entire human genome.(25) Shortly thereafter, using sequencing technology, private companies began offering online genetic testing for individuals (without a doctor's prescription) who wish to know their genetic information. The first human genome sequence cost 300 million dollars. This will soon be offered online for under a thousand dollars.

What is DNA, and Why is it Important? (Deoxyribo-Nucleic Acid)

DNA controls the growth, metabolism and reproduction of the organism from embryo to adult. In essence DNA is the master controller, like the source code in your computer. Cell protein synthesis is controlled by DNA code and is the basis for all life. A new science called "Genome Sequencing" reveals the actual DNA code words controlling protein production in the cell. Defective, malfunctioning proteins are the result of damage and errors in the genetic code called "mutations". These mutations in DNA cause genetic diseases, or predispose to disease from environmental triggers. By understanding this process of genetic code and protein synthesis, medical science has tools to combat disease and improve health.

Hormonal Decline and Degenerative Disease

Bio-Identical human hormones are messengers which attach directly on the DNA strands, and "turn on" DNA protein synthesis. In the aging population (older than age 50), this lack of the hormone messaging from hormone deficiency results in "sleeping" DNA unable to do its job of instructing the cell to synthesize proteins. This, in turn, heralds the onset of degenerative disease from lack of reparative proteins. Replenishment of bio-identical hormone levels restores DNA protein synthesis, thereby delaying or reversing the onset of degenerative disease. This prevention, delay and reversal of degenerative disease with bio-identical hormone therapy has been described as "Anti-Aging Therapy". In reality, it is Anti-Degenerative Disease Therapy.

Chemically Altered Drug Paradigm is Rendered Obsolete by Advances in Bio-Technology

1) In the future, most patented drugs, which are chemically altered forms of naturally occurring molecules, will be rendered obsolete, or considered less desirable than natural counterparts. Many drugs available today will be replaced by more effective natural substances that have fewer adverse effects.

2) In the future, it will be universally recognized that chemically altered human hormones should never have been created, nor marketed to the population. In the future, chemically altered, synthetic hormones will be banned. These were found to cause cancer and heart disease in the 2002 Women's Health Initiative Study.

3) In the future, drug patents take on a new form. There will be a movement away from patents for an altered chemical structure. Instead we will see more patents for the manufacturing techniques

for non-patentable protein structures, vitamins and other natural substances such as human insulin and growth hormone (HGH).

4) In the future, medical interventions will focus on molecular biology, DNA genomics, protein synthesis and natural biochemical processes, making chemically altered hormones and drugs obsolete. Certain chemically altered drugs will always remain useful. However, these will be overshadowed by "functional medicine" which its focus on restoring normal cell physiology with natural substances found in the human biochemical pathways.

5) Randomized Controlled Trials: The drug company funded RCT (randomized controlled trial) is done for FDA approval of a new patented drug. After years of manipulation and falsification of data, the RCT will lose its luster as the Gold Standard and will be supplanted by other forms of medical knowledge such as cohort studies, epidemiology studies, basic science and animal studies, etc. Collections of large numbers of anecdotal reports on the internet will play an increasing role in highlighting adverse effects of drugs, and elevating natural substances to a more important role. Traditional medical knowledge in medical journals will be rivaled and displaced by collaborative knowledge created by e-patients on the internet.

The Rise of OrthoMolecular Medicine

In the future, Orthomolecular Medicine will enter the mainstream. This is a form of natural medicine, and a term coined by Linus Pauling in 1968, and championed by Abram Hoffer MD. By replenishing the body with higher concentrations of vitamin or mineral enzyme co-factors, enzyme efficiency increases, and thus correction of SNP (single nucleotide polymorphism) genetic variants and associated enzyme abnormalities can be accomplished with safe nutritional supplements.(19) In the future, medical treatment will be based on optimizing the functioning of human physiology and biochemistry, rather than limiting treatment to the use of drugs to block a specific enzyme or receptor. This is called Functional Medicine and natural substances will be preferred over drugs.

The Autonomous e-Patient and Reconfiguration of Medical Knowledge

The rise of the autonomous e-Patient is a new phenomenon, empowered by medical knowledge obtained on the internet, the e-patient knows more than the doctor, and may actually be helpful to the doctor, providing him with new knowledge. Social Networking of e-patients enhances knowledge and creates new medical knowledge which competes with and surpasses individual physicians. The exception, of course, being the physician technician such as the cardiac surgeon, or the invasive radiologist who maintains professional standing based on technical expertise. A special form of expert e-patient serves to guide others on the internet in social networks and message boards.(21)(22)

Online Genetic Testing

The use of confidential online genetic testing is available online without a doctor's prescription. Genetic testing will become mainstream, cheaper, and easier, and will provide more useful information as medical science uncovers more links between genetic variants and disease states. It will play a dominant role in the medicine of the future. When used by the individual, genetic testing predicts disease risk, and is helpful to avoid genetic diseases in potential offspring.

Personalized Medicine

Personalized Medicine is the combination of these two new powerful forces, Orthomolecular Medicine and Genetic Testing.(30) In the future, Personalized Medicine will expand and ultimately play a dominant role in medicine.(41) Example: Warfarin Genetic Testing allows improved calibration of Coumadin dosage to avoid bleeding complications. Drug metabolism testing allows for personal modification of drug dosage.

Health Care and Health Insurance—Transformation into a Public Utility

The health insurance industry makes its profit by denying health care to sick people, a criminal enterprise by any definition. Simply watch the Michael Moore Movie, "Sicko", for a preview of our dysfunctional health insurance industry. The movie convincingly suggests the entire system is broken and in need of major change. The only question is what will health insurance look like in 10-20 years? Will the industry survive? In the future, the health insurance industry will be regulated as a public utility, similar to the way the states regulate electric power utility companies. We all need electricity delivered to our homes, and we cannot function without it. Medical care is similar. If we need medical care, whether it is a blood transfusion, IV fluids, an operation for bowel obstruction or a simple antibiotic, we need it same as we need electricity for our homes and factories. We need it **NOW** and can't function without it. The health insurance industry will be recognized as a criminal enterprise which profits by denying health care to sick people. The corporate profit motive is a major problem. Currently, the health insurance industry can increase profit merely by adjusting the parameters on its "Denial Engine Software" to increase denial of medical claims. The solution is to remove the corporate profit motive and transform Health Care into a public utility, regulated by state insurance agencies. For more on health insurance see my previous article on this topic.(26)

The Future of the FDA

The FDA will either be eliminated as a government agency or changed into a new entity which will look entirely different from its current form. After all, if the FDA had done its job properly, synthetic hormones would have been banned from their inception as dangerous illogical replacements for human hormones. This practice of "selling" synthetic hormones to the American public is morally and ethically wrong.

The Future of the Economy, Energy and Government

Fifty years ago, Aldous Huxley predicted democracy and individual freedom would soon be replaced by an authoritarian, totalitarian government. (40-41) Huxley regarded overpopulation as the driving force behind this.

The Industrial Revolution and Cheap Energy

The abundance of cheap energy in the form of fossil fuels, together with the science and technology to harness this energy, in the form of machines such as the steam engine and the gasoline engine, essentially created the Industrial Revolution. Improvements in the standard of living since the Industrial Revolution of 1820 are largely responsible for increasing population growth, and increased longevity of the population. Global population doubling time is now only 50 years. Our victory over the forces of nature, paradoxically, has created the "Population Bomb". According to Aldous Huxley, this will lead to global totalitarianism, with the new technology in media, television, radio and Madison Avenue advertising, allowing the few to control the minds of the many.(40-41)(44-45) Perhaps he is right. However, Huxley lived before the Internet Revolution, and perhaps the openness and decentralization of the Internet Revolution will tip the balance in favor of individual freedom. The jury is still out on this one.

The End of Abundant Cheap Energy—Peak Oil

Much like any other natural resource on the planet, there is a limit to the amount of cheap oil available for exploitation. Exhaustion of cheap oil and declining reserves is called "Peak Oil", and the down slope of the oil reserve curve is where the pain of economic contraction begins. Many experts think the planet has already past this "Peak Oil" part of the curve, and we have entered the phase of economic contraction.

The Collapse Scenario

With our rear view mirror vantage point and knowledge of history, we are able to witness the ebb and flow of previous civilizations, and the "rise and fall" of ancient empires. We are not immune from the ups and downs of recurring economic cycles. The "Collapse Scenario" described in Dmitry Orlov's book, Reinventing Collapse, lists the stages of collapse. (50-52) The first stage is financial collapse, in which the volume of debt becomes too great for the economy to continue functioning with widespread default by both governments and private entities. Governments are then forced to pursue a hyperinflationary monetary policy to avoid default on massive debt, forcing debasement of their currency. This ends which an essentially worthless paper currency. This is followed by the stages of commercial, political, social and cultural collapse. (50-52)

Cold Fusion and More Cheap Energy

On the horizon, science and technology is racing to our rescue with a new energy technology, called "cold fusion" which holds the promise to restore "cheap energy" to the planet and rescue us from our collapse scenario. (53) Will "cold fusion" arrive in time to save the planet from global collapse? Stay tuned to find out.

Genetic Manipulation is Inherently Unsafe and Dangerous

In the future, (GMO) Genetically Modified Food will be recognized as unsafe, unsustainable, and immoral. In the future, GM seeds and crops will be abandoned. Attempts to genetically engineer plant or animal life will be outlawed. Genetic manipulation is inherently unsafe and dangerous, sort of like giving a loaded gun to a child. It may take one or two more centuries before our understanding of molecular biology and genetic engineering gives us the tools to actually do anything safely with it.

The Fluid Genome—The Human Genome Project

One of the unpredicted results of the Human Genome Project is the "Fluid Genome" of Dr. Mae-Wan Ho.(49) This Fluid Genome paradigm means that the genome is inherently unstable, and it is sheer folly to attempt to modify the genome of plants or animals with our current crude methods of genetic engineering. Likewise, the failure of gene therapy is due to the fact that our current methods are too crude to account for the fluid nature of the genome.

The Great Experiment of the 21st Century: Genetically Modified Food

A new human disease was identified in 1989 called EMS, Eosinophilia Myalgia Syndrome which killed 37 people and affected thousands. (45-46) This disease was eventually traced back to a Japanese company (Showa Denko) that had used genetically engineered bacteria to manufacture tryptophan, a naturally occurring amino acid food supplement. This is the first example of genetic modification transforming a normally safe and natural food into a Franken-Food causing a disease. There will be many others.

Nightmare Scenario for Medicine?

Here in the US, we now have widespread use of genetically modified food which is unlabeled and untested. Some of these genetically modified foods include Round-Up Ready corn, soy and canola and Bt corn which produces the Bt toxin. It is likely that these new genetically modified foods are causing allergic reactions, diseases, and infertility in the population. Therefore, you might think it would be prudent to label these GMO foods so that any new disease could be traced back to the cause. However, because of corporate control of the FDA regulatory process, the FDA has ruled GMO food to be "substantially equivalent" and no labeling or even safety testing required. We can be fairly sure that in the near future, medicine will be faced with a nightmare scenario of unexpected diseases caused by GMO food consumption. We can expect to see increases in food allergies, gastrointestinal disorders, inflammatory bowel disease, infertility and sterility, and other completely unexpected and unpredicted effects of GMO food consumption. Other nightmare scenarios caused by genetic manipulation include new epidemics caused by super bugs with antibiotic resistance, lethal super viruses, and bizarre forms of leukemia and other cancers caused by genetic manipulation in the laboratory accidentally or intentionally released into the environment.

The Future of Cancer

In the future, science will establish a greater understanding of the molecular biology and mechanism of cancer. In the future, aggressive cancer unresponsive to treatment will be cured with newer and more innovative cancer treatments which are based on the molecular biology of cancer. In the future, we will have an effective cure for aggressive cancer. For more on this, see my article on the Trophoblastic Theory of Cancer.

Conclusion

Since medicine follows the values of society in which it is practiced, the future of medicine depends on what kind of values our society will have in the future. If we value corporate profit, authoritarian government and devalue human life, then the future most likely holds in store for us the "nightmare scenario" aptly described in the novels, Brave New World by Aldous Huxley, and George Orwell's 1984. The 1971 George Lucas science fiction movie, THX 1138, is also to be included here under the nightmare scenario. On the other hand, if we retain our traditional values of human rights, preserving liberty, freedom, representational government, and value human life, then the future will be bright, with a "rosy scenario" and a true renaissance in the medicine of the future. In the final analysis, the future is up to all of us.

For references and links, see my web site: www.bioidenticalhormones101.com

References for Chapter 56. Predicting the Future of Medicine

(1) http://inventors.about.com/od/gstartinventors/a/Gutenberg.htm
Johannes Gutenberg and the Printing Press, About.com

(2) http://www.mcluhan.utoronto.ca/mcluhanprojekt/gutenberg2.htm
Gutenberg Galaxy by Marshall McLuhan divides history in four epochs: the oral tribe culture, the manuscript culture, the Gutenberg galaxy and the electronic age.

(3) http://www.mondopolitico.com/library/1984/1984.htm Online version of George Orwell's novel, 1984

(4) http://www.online-literature.com/orwell/1984/
Searchable Online version of George Orwell's 1984

(5) http://www.carj.ca/issues/2005-Feb/13/pg13.pdf
Lessons from Ivan Illich Editorial in Canadian Journal of Radiology CARJ

(6) http://www.mindfully.org/Health/Medical-Nemesis-Illich1976.htm Medical Nemesis:The Expropriation of Health. [Includes acknowledgements, introduction and Part1—Clinical Iatrogenesis] by IVAN ILLICH, Random House 1976.

(7) http://members.aol.com/pbchowka/medicalnemesis2006.html Medical Nemesis 2006 By Peter Barry Chowka.

(8) http://www.planetpapers.com/Assets/3621.php The quotation "the medical establishment is a major threat to health" was one devised by Illich in Medical Nemesis (1976 p11) where he attempted to explain the detrimental effects medical professionals and their procedures can have on the health of individuals.

(9) http://www.lewrockwell.com/wall/wall28.html A Turbulent Priest in the Global Village Ivan Illich, 1926-2002 by Richard Wall.

(10) http://brandon.multics.org/library/Ivan%20Illich/against_life.html BRAVE NEW BIOCRACY: HEALTH CARE FROM WOMB TO TOMB, By: Illich, Ivan, NPQ: New Perspectives Quarterly, Winter94, Vol. 11, Issue 1

(11) http://bmj.bmjjournals.com/cgi/content/full/311/7021/1652 BMJ 1995;311:1652-1653 (23 December) British Medical Journal. Death undefeated by Ivan Illich

(12) http://www.davidtinapple.com/illich/1990_health_responsibility.PDF Ivan Illich, HEALTH AS ONE'S OWN RESPONSIBILITY—NO, THANK YOU!

(13) http://www.whale.to/v/mendelsohn.html Dr Robert Mendelsohn biography.

(14) http://www.metzelf.info/Book%20Reviews/confessions.html Confessions of a Medical Heretic by Robert S. Mendelsohn, MD 1979 Reviewed by Mira de Vries

(15) http://www.cam.org/~rsilver/sickmed.htm Sickening Medicine A Book Review by Bob Silverman,

(16) http://www.furiousseasons.com/zyprexadocs.html Zyprexa Documents—Furious Seasons Blog.

(17) http://www.e-patients.net/e-Patients_White_Paper.pdf Tom Ferguson md and E-Patients

(18) http://www.orthomolecular.org/ Orthomolecular Medicine Web Site

(19) http://orthomolecular.org/library/articles/orthotheory.shtml Orthomolecular Theory by Linus Pauling, Ph.D. Journal Of Orthomolecular Medicine Vol. 7, No. 1, 1995

(20) http://www.acor.org/e-patients_wiki/index.php/Main_Page Wiki version of Tom Ferguson's White paper on e-patients

(21) http://www.e-patients.net/e-Patients_White_Paper.pdf PDF version of white paper e-patients by Tom Fergeson

(22) http://www.ba-education.demon.co.uk/for/science/dnamain.html Discovery of Double Helix of DNA by Watson and Crick

(23) http://www.genome.gov/ The Human Genome Project

(24) http://jeffreydach.com/2008/02/24/ fighting-the-abusive-practices-of-health-insurance-companies-by-jeffrey-dach-md.aspx Fighting the Abusive Health Insurance Companies by Jeffrey Dach MD

(25) http://www.infoplease.com/ipa/A0005140.html
Life Expectancy by Age, 1850-2004

(26) http://www.des.emory.edu/mfp/Kuhnsnap.html The Structure of Scientific Revolutions—Thomas S. Kuhn; University of Chicago Press in 1962.

(27) http://www.ageofpersonalizedmedicine.org/
The Age of Personalized Medicine

(28) http://www.globalchange.com/medicine.htm
Patrick Dixon 2002 Video, Future of HealthCare

(29) http://www.soc.upenn.edu/courses/2004/fall/soc007_hpkohler/readings/oepp02b.pdf Broken Limits to Life Expectancy Jim Oeppen and James W.Vaupe Science VOL 296 10 MAY 2002.

(30) http://www.youtube.com/watch?v=fXCT5DWPKOQ Patrick Dixon Future of Health Care—part 1 of 3. You tube videoparts 1-3

(31) http://www.ncbi.nlm.nih.gov/pubmed/7476595
Med Hypotheses. 1995 Jun;44(6):490-2. Pantothenic acid deficiency as the pathogenesis of acne vulgaris. Leung LH. Department of General Surgery, Hong Kong Central Hospital, Hong Kong.

(32) http://www.youtube.com/watch?v=X9M40dCHvLY
The Genomic Revolution and the Future of Medicine and Health. Dr. Richard Klausner discusses the topic of the Genomic Revolution and the Future of Medicine and Health. Recorded in Wolstein Audiorium on November 1, 2007.

(33) http://www.youtube.com/watch?v=c1KEFgD6Dtg
Karsten Staack made this video for some events in the Detailed Roadmap of the 21st Century

(34) http://www.cc.gatech.edu/~pesti/roadmap/ The 21st Century: What will it look like? This is a very entertaining look at the Future, with excellent music and interesting images, inspirational.

(35) http://www.youtube.com/watch?v=i0LvtQAQ6sc
Interview with Naomi Wolf, her book "The End of America" on the New York Times bestseller list.

(36) http://www.genome.gov/Pages/News/webcasts/Personalized_Medicine_files/0Media.asx Video on Personalized Medicine: How the Human Genome Era Will Usher in a Health Care Revolution Francis S. Collins, M.D., Ph.D. Personalized Medicine Coalition February 10, 2005

(37) http://books.google.com/books?id=_oDQ6yDO7kC&dq History of Medicine: A Scandalously Short Introduction By Jacalyn Duffin. University of Toronto Press 1999.

(38) http://www.hrc.utexas.edu/multimedia/video/2008/wallace/huxley_aldous_t.html Video 1958 Mike Wallace interview with Aldous Huxley author of Brave New World.

(39) http://www.hrc.utexas.edu/multimedia/video/2008/wallace/huxley_aldous.html Transcript 1958 Mike Wallace interview with Aldous Huxley author of brave new world.

(40) http://www.marshallmcluhan.com/
Marshall McLuhan Main Site

(41) http://faculty.law.pitt.edu/hibbitts/mcl.htm The life and work of Marshall McLuhan.

(42) http://www.youtube.com/watch?v=aqZNGYit3kY
Media professor/expert Paul Levinson on Marshall McLuhan. You Tube.

(43) http://scienceroll.com/2008/04/25/personalized-medicine-real-clinical-examples/ Personalized Medicine

(44) http://www.acceleratingfuture.com/michael/blog/ Transhumanism, AI, nanotechnology, and existential risk.

(45) http://unboundedmedicine.com/ Future of Surgery

(46) http://futurehealthtrends.blogspot.com/ Future Health Trends Blog

(47) http://www.i-sis.org.uk/fluidGenome.php Living with the Fluid Genome By Mae-Wan Ho Publisher: Third World Network 2003

(48) http://www.newsociety.com/Books/R/Reinventing-Collapse Reinventing Collapse, The Soviet Experience and American Prospects—Revised & Updated by Dmitry Orlov, New Society Publishers, 06-01-2011

(49) http://cluborlov.blogspot.com/2010/11/peak-oil-is-history.html Peak Oil is History, Nov1, 2010

(50) http://cluborlov.blogspot.com/2011/05/us-and-five-stages-of-collapse.html May 31, 2011 The US and the Five Stages of Collapse

(51) http://peakoil.com/alternative-energy/cold-fusion-validated-by-swedish-skeptics-society/ Cold Fusion Validated by Swedish Skeptic's

Appendix A.
Illustrations for Bioidentical Hormones 101 by Jeffrey Dach MD:

All illustrations can be found in the public domain on Wikimedia Commons.

(1) http://commons.wikimedia.org/wiki/File:Thyroide.jpg

Thyroid_gland_1.jpg This work is in the public domain in the United States because it is a work of the United States Federal Government under the terms of Title 17, Chapter 1, Section 105 of the US Code. See Copyright.

(2) Levothyroxine_2.jpg Levothyroxine Pills

http://commons.wikimedia.org/wiki/File:007815180lg_Generic_Levothyroxine.jpg

This image is a work of the National Institutes of Health, part of the United States Department of Health and Human Services. As a work of the U.S. federal government, the image is in the public domain. Generic Levothyroxine, Levothyroxine sodium 25 MCG Oral Tablet Imprint: 25;GG;331 Author: MOVA PHARMACEUTICAL CORPORATION http://upload.wikimedia.org/wikipedia/commons/thumb/a/a0/Thyroxine.svg/2000px-Thyroxine.svg.png

(3) Thyroxine_3.jpg

http://commons.wikimedia.org/wiki/File:Thyroxine.svg

Thyroxine Chemical Structure, 2D structure of thyroid hormone thyroxine, I, the copyright holder of this work, release this work into the public domain. This applies worldwide.

(4) Thyroid_Surgery_4.jpeg. Thyroid surgery, U.S. Navy photo by Journalist Seaman Joseph Caballero

http://commons.wikimedia.org/wiki/File:US_Navy_060527-N-3532C-092_USNS_Mercy_-_Deployment_2006.jpg

Republic of the Philippines (May 27, 2006)—A Navy doctor, an Aloha Medical Mission doctor, an Air Force dentist, Filipino nurse, and an Indian surgical technician work together aboard U.S. Naval hospital ship USNS Mercy (T-AH 19) to remove a thyroid goiter from a local resident during MercyUs humanitarian deployment to South and Southeast Asia, and the Pacific Islands. This file is a work of a sailor or employee of the U.S. Navy, taken or made during the course of the person's official duties. As a work of the U.S. federal government, the image is in the public domain.

(5) Adrenal_gland_5.jpeg

http://commons.wikimedia.org/wiki/File:Adrenal_gland_(PSF).jpg

Adrenal Glands . . . line art drawing of Adrenal gland, Source Pearson Scott Foresman, donated to the Wikimedia Foundation. This file has been (or is hereby) donated to the Wikimedia Foundation and released into the public domain by Pearson Scott Foresman. This applies worldwide.

(6) Sinking_Ship_6.jpg

http://commons.wikimedia.org/wiki/File:Pendleton_Sinking_Ship.jpg

Sinking Ship: Bow section of tanker SS Pendleton grounded near Pollock Rib lightship six miles off Chatham, Mass on the morning of Feb. 19, 1952." Date 19 February 1952. This image or file is a work of a United States Coast Guard service personnel or employee, taken or made during the course of that person's official duties. As a work of the U.S. federal government, the image or file is in the public domain.

(7) Ghost_7.jpg

http://commons.wikimedia.org/wiki/File:William_Hope_001.png

English: Man with the spirit of his second wife. National Media Museum Author William Hope (1863-1933). This image (or other media file) is in the public domain because its copyright has expired.

http://commons.wikimedia.org/wiki/File:Time_to_let_(her)_go!.jpg

Ghost of Mona by Author Fish Gravy Courtesy of Wikimedia Commons

(8) Ovary_8.jpg

http://commons.wikimedia.org/wiki/File:Illu_ovary.jpg anatomic drawing of uterus, right ovary and fallopian tube. This work is in the public domain in the United States because it is a work of the United States Federal Government under the terms of Title 17, Chapter 1, Section 105 of the US Code. See Copyright.

(9) RBC_9.jpg

http://commons.wikimedia.org/wiki/File:SEM_blood_cells.jpg

SEM Red Blood Cells image 35, caption: Left image: Scanning electron microscope image from normal circulating human blood. February 1982, Courtesy of Bruce Wetzel and Harry Schaefer of the National Cancer Institute.

(10)Frankenstein_10.jpg

http://commons.wikimedia.org/wiki/File:Frankenstein%27s_monster_(Boris_Karloff).jpg

Promotional photo of Boris Karloff from The Bride of Frankenstein as Frankenstein's monster. Date 1931(1931) Source Frankenstein promotional photo Author Universal Studios

(11)Mammogram_11.jpg

http://upload.wikimedia.org/wikipedia/commons/d/d0/Mammogram_showing_breast_cancer.jpg

Mammogram. The arrow on this mammogram points to a small cancerous lesion. A lesion is an area of abnormal tissue change. Date 23 October 2003(2003-10-23) Source NIH Senior Health

(12)breast_biopsy_12.jpg

http://commons.wikimedia.org/wiki/File:Surgical_breast_biopsy.jpg

Surgeons Performing a Breast Biopsy. Description: White woman patient is being operated on. Her nipple is being incised by the surgeon. The surgeon and an operating room attendant are visible (there may actually be two surgeons). A surgical biopsy is being performed to determine exact nature of solid tumor. National Cancer Institute Author: Linda Bartlett (photographer) AV Number: AV-8000-0512 Date Created: 1980 Reuse Restrictions: None—This image is in the public domain and can be freely reused. Source http://visualsonline.cancer.gov/details.cfm?imageid=2079 Author Linda Bartlett (photographer) This image is a work of the National Institutes of Health, part of the United States Department of Health and Human Services. As a work of the U.S. federal government, the image is in the public domain.

(13)testosterone_13.jpg

http://commons.wikimedia.org/wiki/File:Testosterone.svg

2D structure of testosterone 2009 Author: Harbin. I, the copyright holder of this work, release this work into the public domain. This applies worldwide. I grant anyone the right to use this work for any purpose, without any conditions, unless such conditions are required by law.

(14)Morphine_14.jpg

http://commons.wikimedia.org/wiki/File:MorphineAdvertisement1900.JPG

Advertisement for curing morphine addictions from Overland Monthly, January 1900 Date March 2008(2008-03) Source Extracted from PDF version of above on the Internet Archive Author Mike Cline. This media file is in the public domain in the United States. This applies to U.S. works where the copyright has expired, often because its first publication occurred prior to January 1, 1923. See this page for further explanation.

(15)prostate_15.jpg

http://commons.wikimedia.org/wiki/File:Gray1160.png

This faithful reproduction of a lithograph plate from Gray's Anatomy, a two-dimensional work of art, is not copyrightable in the U.S. as per Bridgeman Art Library v. Corel Corp.; the same is also true in many other countries, including Germany. Unless stated otherwise, it is from the 20th U.S. edition of Gray's Anatomy of the Human Body, originally published in 1918 and therefore lapsed into the public domain. Other copies of Gray's Anatomy can be found on Bartleby and also on Yahoo!. Caption: Prostate with seminal vesicles and seminal ducts, viewed from in front and above. (Spalteholz.) This image is in the public domain because its copyright has expired. This applies worldwide.

(16)Heretics_16.jpg People Burned at the Stake as Heretics, Medieval Period.

http://commons.wikimedia.org/wiki/File:People_burned_as_heretics.jpg

Group of chained me executed by burning while a crowd looks on. The artwork (as evidenced by the polearms and costume) seems to date from late 14th to mid-15th C, it could be a depiction of the burning of Cathar heretics by the Papal Inquisition in the Languedoc in late 12th to early 13th C, or could as easily depict the later execution of lapsed conversos by the later Spanish Inquisition. This image (or other media file) is in the public domain because its copyright has expired. This applies to Australia, the European Union and those countries with a copyright term of life of the author plus 70 years.

(17)selenium_17.jpg http://tin.er.usgs.gov/geochem/doc/averages/se/usa.html

Selenium Content in the soil USA http://tin.er.usgs.gov/geochem/doc/averages/se/usa.html

Selenium in Counties of the Conterminous States, U.S. Geological Survey, government agency public domain image.

(18)Brazilnut_18.jpg

Scientific American Supplement, No. 598, June 18, 1887 http://commons.wikimedia.org/wiki/File:Brazilnut1.jpg

Brazilnut1.jpg (378 × 400 pixels, file size: 26 KB, MIME type: image/jpeg) Brazil Nut—Project Gutenberg eBook 11662 Castanha do Pará. This image (or other media file) is in the public domain because its copyright has expired.

(19)Exhaust_19.jpg

http://commons.wikimedia.org/wiki/File:Exhaust.jpg

Exhaust from the tailpipe of a car. In this case, it is probably mostly water vapour that is seen. I, the copyright holder of this work, release this work into the public domain. This applies worldwide.

(20)Hashimoto_20.jpg

http://en.wikipedia.org/wiki/File:Hashimoto_Hakaru.JPG

1912 Photograph of Dr. Hakaru Hashimoto first to describe Hashimoto's Thyroiditis. Source: reprinted in: Hashimoto K. My father and his teachers. Endocr J. 49, 4, 389-91. 2002. Author Unknown. Public domain photo Courtesy of Wikimedia commons.

(21)lautrec_21.jpg

http://commons.wikimedia.org/wiki/File:Photolautrec.jpg

Photograph of Henri de Toulouse-Lautrec, one of the greatest painters of the Post-Impressionist period. B.1864—D.1901. Toulous Lautrec. This image (or other media file) is in the public domain because its copyright has expired.

(22)No_flame_22.jpg

http://commons.wikimedia.org/wiki/File:No_flames.png

No flame pictogram. Date 22 October 2006(2006-10-22) Source Composed using clip art elements. Author Michelet B Permission (Reusing this file) See below. I, the copyright holder of this work, release this work into the public domain. This applies worldwide.

(23)Depression_23.jpg

http://commons.wikimedia.org/wiki/File:Face-sad.svg Face-sad.svg Tango! Desktop Project. This work has been released into the public domain by its author, The Tango! Desktop Project (Contributors; FAQ). This applies worldwide.

(24)MonaLisa_24.jpg http://commons.wikimedia.org/wiki/File:Mona_Lisa.jpg The Mona Lisa 1503—1505 by Leonardo da Vinci (1452-1519), Medium Oil on poplar. Louvre Museum Paris. This work is in the public domain in the United States, and those countries with a copyright term of life of the author plus 100 years or fewer.

(25)Snake_River_25.jpg

Snake River by Ansel Adams. Ansel Adams The Tetons and the Snake River (1942) Grand Teton National Park, Wyoming. National Archives and Records Administration, Records of the National Park Service. (79-AAG-1) http://commons.wikimedia.org/wiki/File:Adams_The_Tetons_and_the_Snake_River.jpg

(26)Mine_Field_26.jpg US_Navy_Mine_Field. http://commons.wikimedia.org/wiki/File:US_Navy_explosive_ordnance_disposal_(EOD)_divers.jpg

A U.S. Navy explosive ordnance disposal (EOD) diver attaches an inert "Satchel Charge" to a training mine, during exercises in waters off Naval Base Guantanamo Bay, Cuba.

(27)http://commons.wikimedia.org/wiki/File:Pirate_Flag_of_Rack_Rackham.svg PirateFlag_27.jpg. The pirate flag of Jack Rackham (1682—1720) This file is from the Open Clip Art Library, which released it explicitly into the public domain, using the Creative Commons Public Domain Dedication.

(28)Harvesting_wheat_28.jpg caption: Harvesting in a wheat field, ca. 1900 Australia

http://commons.wikimedia.org/wiki/File:Harvesting_in_a_wheat_field_from_The_Powerhouse_Museum_Collection.jpg Photo is in public domain because copyright expired.

(29)DNA double helix #29 http://commons.wikimedia.org/wiki/File:DNA_simple2.svg I, the copyright holder of this work, release this work into the public domain. This applies worldwide.

(30) IV Bag_30.jpg http://commons.wikimedia.org/wiki/File:Infuuszakjes.jpg

I, the copyright holder of this work, release this work into the public domain. This applies worldwide.

(30)Marijuana_31.jpg marijuana plant,

http://commons.wikimedia.org/wiki/File:Marijuana.jpg

English: A photograph of hemp (Cannabis sativa L.) in Sherburne National Wildlife Refuge. A photograph of a cannabis plant credited to the United States Fish and Wildlife Service.

(31)Pseudomonas_31.jpg

http://commons.wikimedia.org/wiki/File:Pseudomonas_aeruginosa_SEM.jpg

Scanning Electron Micrograph of Pseudomonas aeruginosa. From the Centers for Disease Control and Prevention's Public Health Image Library (PHIL), with identification number #232. Content Providers(s): CDC/ Janice Haney Carr (Reusing this file) PD-USGov-HHS-CDC. This image is in the public domain and thus free of any copyright restrictions. As a matter of courtesy we request that the content provider be credited and notified in any public or private usage of this image.

(32)Callisto_32.jpg http://solarsystem.nasa.gov/multimedia/display.cfm?IM_ID=835 Callisto's Har Crater, NASA Solarsystem Collection http://www.nasaimages.org/luna/servlet/detail/nasaNAS~20~20~120965~227668:Callisto-s-Har-Crater http://en.wikipedia.org/wiki/File:Callisto_Har_PIA01054.jpg

Hár crater on Callisto, photographed by Galileo. Date 26 March 1998(1998-03-26)

Source http://photojournal.jpl.nasa.gov/catalog/PIA01054 Author NASA/JPL-Caltech

This image or video was catalogued by Jet Propulsion Lab of the United States National Aeronautics and Space Administration (NASA) under Photo ID: PIA01054. This file is in the public domain because it was created by NASA. NASA copyright policy states that "NASA material is not protected by copyright unless noted. Date: 4 Nov 1997. This image shows a heavily cratered region near Callisto's equator. It was taken by the Galileo spacecraft's Solid-State Imaging System on its ninth orbit around Jupiter. North is to the top of the image. The 105-km double ring crater in the center of the image is named Har. Har displays an unusual rounded mound on its floor. The origin of the mound is unclear, but probably involves uplift of ice-rich materials from below, either as a "rebound" immediately following the impact that formed the crater or as a later process. Har is older than the prominent 41-km crater superposed on its western rim. The large crater partially visible in the northeast corner of the image is called Tindr. Chains of secondary craters (craters formed from the impact of materials thrown out of the main crater during an impact) originating from Tindr crosscut the eastern rim of Har. The image, centered at 3.30S latitude and 357.90W longitude, covers an area of 245 km by 230 km. The Sun illuminates the scene from the west (left). The smallest distinguishable features in the image are about 294 m across. This image was obtained on 25 June 1997, when Galileo was 14,080 km from Callisto. Image Credit: Arizona State University Credit: Lunar and Planetary Institute

(33)old hospital_33.jpg http://commons.wikimedia.org/wiki/File:Erlangen_-_Frauenklinik.jpg

Postcard 1914 of old hospital in Germany "Erlangen—Frauenklinik." Courtesy of Wolfgang Sauber (Xenophon). This work is in the public domain in the United States because it was published (or registered with the U.S. Copyright Office) before January 1, 1923.

(34)placenta_34.jpg http://commons.wikimedia.org/wiki/File:Placental_cotyledon.png English: Structure of the placenta, with a placental cotyledon marked in rectangle. Date 23 November 2010(2010-11-23) Source File:Gray39.png Author Mikael Häggström. This faithful reproduction of a lithograph plate from Gray's Anatomy, a two-dimensional work of art, is not copyrightable in the U.S. as per Bridgeman Art Library v. Corel Corp.; the same is also true in many other countries, including Germany. Unless stated otherwise, it is from the 20th U.S. edition of Gray's Anatomy of the Human Body, originally published in 1918 and therefore lapsed into the public domain.

(35)Juan Ponce De Leon, PONCE_DE_LEON_35.jpg Wood engraving from Denison, John Ledyard, ed. Die illustrirte neue welt (New-York, H. Bill, 1858) [E45.D43 General Collections] Reproduction Number: LC-USZ62-3106. Library of Congress. This image (or other media file) is in the public domain because its copyright has expired. http://commons.wikimedia.org/wiki/File:PONCE_DE_LEON,_JUAN.jpg